Alternative Coca Reduction Strategies in the Andean Region

Office of Technology Assessment
Congress of the United States

Recommended Citation:

U.S. Congress, Office of Technology Assessment, *Alternative Coca Reduction Strategies in the Andean Region,* OTA-F-556 (Washington, DC: U.S. Government Printing Office, July 1993).

For sale by the U.S. Government Printing Office
Superintendent of Documents, Mail Stop: SSOP, Washington, DC 20402-9328
ISBN 0-16-041827-5

Foreword

Cocaine trafficking and abuse are formidable problems that disrupt social, economic, and political systems. Stopping the flow of cocaine through international black markets has proven impossible despite national commitments and international treaties. Strong demand continues to promote coca production and cocaine processing in supplying nations. This Report identifies opportunities for and constraints to reducing Andean coca production through: 1) improving U.S. alternative development efforts and 2) applying biological control technology (biocontrol) to eradicate illegally produced coca.

Coca has been important in South America for nearly 4,000 years and remains a critical element in traditional Andean culture. Today, coca dominates Andean economies, in part due to long-term social inequities and political and economic unrest. The ecological and cultural complexity of the Andean region precludes simple alternative development or coca eradication approaches. In this unsettled milieu, development assistance activities have promoted alternative agricultural systems incorporating high-value or multipurpose crops. Other interests have proposed that coca eradication is a necessary precursor to successful development. Although biocontrol may yield an undefined level of coca reduction, the technology is unlikely to result in coca eradication.

Several study conclusions have clear policy implications. First, development-oriented strategies for supply reduction have promise, but are unlikely to solve the cocaine problem without concomitant demand reduction efforts. Second, the extent and importance of the coca economy mean that single-sector development alone is insufficient to unseat Andean economic dependence on coca. Finally, the impact of a single organization on coca reduction is likely to be small, thus, coordination of the numerous bilateral and multilateral groups is a critical need.

The following congressional committees requested the Office of Technology Assessment to undertake a study of the potential for improving U.S. efforts to reduce coca production through development activities and biological control methods: the Senate Committee on the Judiciary and the House Select Committee on Narcotics Abuse and Control; Senator Orrin G. Hatch requested OTA to examine coca eradication by biocontrol. In addition, the House Committee on Agriculture endorsed the study.

OTA greatly appreciates the contributions of the workshop participants and authors of commissioned papers. We are especially grateful for the time and effort donated by numerous contributors who served as reviewers and as liaisons with the many groups and organizations involved in this issue. The information and assistance provided by those individuals proved invaluable to the completion of the assessment. As with all OTA studies, the content of the Report is the sole responsibility of OTA.

Roger C. Herdman, Director

Project Staff

Walter E. Parham
Program Manager
Food and Renewable Resources
    Program

Patricia J. Durana
Project Director

Elizabeth Turner
Analyst[1]

Catherine M. Torres
Research Analyst[2]

Jessica Wolin
Research Assistant[3]

ADMINISTRATIVE STAFF

N. Ellis Lewis
Office Administrator

Nellie Hammond
Administrative Secretary

Carolyn Swann
PC Specialist

Thomas Adamczyk
Detailee[4]

Karen Marston
Intern[5]

Susan J. Wunder
Contract Editor

[1]From February 1991 through September 1991.
[2]From June 1991 to present.
[3]From June 1990 through August 1990 and from June 1991 through July 1992.
[4]From July 1991 to September 1991
[5]From January 1991 to May 1991.

iv

Contents

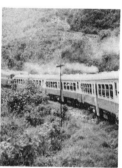

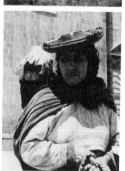

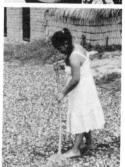

Summary, Issues, and Congressional Policy Options | 1

For at least 80 years, control and abuse of imported narcotic substances, in general, have been public policy concerns. International treaties have been largely ineffective in controlling production and trafficking of illegal drugs. The human "search for the high" fuels demand, and supply control has been nearly impossible. Cocaine abuse and its social and economic consequences have followed this legacy and reached disturbing proportions in the last decade.

INTRODUCTION

Narcotics control strategies commonly are divided into demand- and supply-reduction programs. Although controversy exists over which of the two is the most critical, a comprehensive narcotics control strategy includes education, treatment and rehabilitation, development assistance, interdiction, and enforcement components (figure 1-1). No single approach will solve the international narcotics problem, yet the proper mix of supply-and demand-control programs has yet to be identified.

Although most coca currently is produced in the Andean region of Peru and Bolivia (87 percent) and Colombia (13 percent) (59), it also has been produced in other South American countries (e.g., Ecuador, Brazil) and Central America. If coca production is reduced in the Andean region, new production areas would likely arise as long as cocaine and its derivatives remain attractive narcotics. Nonetheless, supply reduction could have a valuable role in an overall narcotics control strategy. The temporary disruption of supply could increase street prices and reduce accessibility. The time investment to re-establish a production and cartel system is likely to be large and could have a debilitating effect on the overall industry (10).

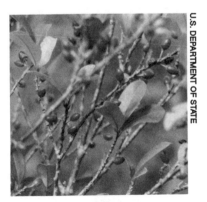

U.S. DEPARTMENT OF STATE

1

Figure 1-1—Components of a Comprehensive International Drug Control Strategy

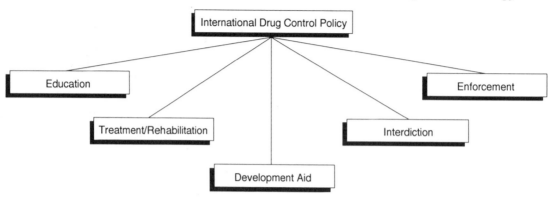

SOURCE: Office of Technology Assessment, 1993.

One potential strategy for reducing the flow of cocaine into the United States is to identify and support the development of alternative economic options for Andean producers of coca leaves and illegal coca-leaf products. This development-oriented strategy for supply reduction shows promise, but is unlikely to solve the cocaine problem without concomitant efforts in other areas such as drug law enforcement, interdiction, and education and rehabilitation of drug users.

Methods for coca eradication also are of interest in supply reduction strategies. Although eradication technologies focus on herbicide use, there is increasing interest in applying biological control methods to narcotic crop control. Some experts believe eradication must precede alternative development in the Andean nations. Others view coca eradication as futile and a threat to the culture and traditions of native Andean populations. Although key requirements, host country consent and cooperation currently are unlikely (57,58).

The economic, environmental, and sociocultural features of coca-producing countries profoundly influence supply reduction efforts. Developing suitable and effective approaches will require significant cooperative and coordinated effort among all concerned parties.

■ Cultural Context

Coca is a traditional Andean crop, with evidence of cultural significance dating from 2100 B.C. (11). Different coca-leaf varieties and associated chewing paraphernalia from succeeding centuries have been excavated in such varied areas as northern Chile and Costa Rica (40). Coca leaves are a critical element in the traditional Andean patterns of production and exchange between highlands and lowlands. Community and political solidarity were long maintained through these exchanges.

Chewing coca leaves has been practiced for thousands of years in the Andes and is still a pervasive cultural activity. Coca leaves are used to relieve fatigue, hunger, and a variety of human ailments (e.g., 87 percent of Bolivia's small town and rural population use coca leaf for health reasons (28)). Coca leaves figure symbolically in cultural and religious rituals and are an integral part of many daily social routines.

Today, transformation of this resource into a high-profit cash crop and its resulting steep price constitute a cultural threat and personal hardship for many indigenous Andeans. This situation may be exacerbated if coca eradication or substitution programs further restrict the availability of coca leaf for traditional use. Coca reduction efforts, thus, will involve providing for traditional needs, while precluding illegal use (43).

The Andean nations are increasingly concerned over the adverse impacts of cocaine on their societies. *Pasta básica*—an intermediate product of cocaine processing—generates effects similar to "crack" and consumption increases have been noted in some Andean countries. Further, *pasta básica* contains significant impurities (e.g., lead, sulfuric acid, kerosene) compounding adverse effects on users. In 1987, Colombia's Health Ministry estimated that 2 percent of the population were regular users and a United Nations report estimated Colombia may have one of the world's worst drug problems (14). Recent surveys indicate similar figures may apply to Bolivia. Within this heightened awareness of the adverse effects of illegal narcotics, alternative development may find greater acceptance.

■ Environmental Context

The Andean region is complex in terms of its geology, ecology, and cultural history. This complexity precludes simple or broadly applicable coca substitution or eradication approaches. The natural environmental diversity results largely from abrupt altitudinal changes common in the Andes. The region consists of a vertical succession of ecozones, ranging from rainforest and desert at the lowest levels to mountain tundra, snow, and ice at the highest. The Andes' enormous latitudinal and longitudinal range also makes for considerable variations in climate, soil, vegetation, and landuse (1).

The primary zones of illegal coca cultivation include the Chapare in Bolivia, the Alto Huallaga in Peru, and a variety of areas around the Cauca Valley in Colombia (figure 1-2). These areas are characterized by high rainfall, acidic soils, and altitudes ranging between 200 and 1,500 meters above sea level (masl). Many of these areas are inappropriate for agriculture, much less for characteristic coca cultivation (22). There are a number of environmental concerns arising from coca production: deforestation to establish coca fields, soil erosion and associated fertility losses,

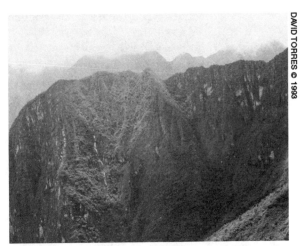

DAVID TORRES © 1993

Steep topography characteristic of the Andes gives rise to significant climatic variations over short distances.

heavy pesticide use, and subsequent movement of these chemicals to soil and surface and groundwater resources (3,22,29).

Chemical wastes from cocaine processing (e.g., kerosene, sulfuric acid, lime, calcium carbide, acetone, toluene, ethyl ether, and hydrochloric acid) also may impair terrestrial and riverine systems. These wastes can increase water pH, reduce oxygen availability, and lead to acute and chronic poisoning of fish (e.g., liver, heart, kidney, and brain lesions, and possible genetic mutations). An estimated 150 Peruvian streams and rivers have pollution levels exceeding the safety standards set by the World Health Organization (32).

Proposals for coca eradication using herbicides have been criticized for environmental reasons. Environmental reviews elaborating the potential environmental effects of chemicals have been prepared for specific herbicides identified as effective at eradicating coca species. However, the process has been less rigorous than that required for domestic activities under the National Environment Policy Act (NEPA). Substantial Peruvian opposition to the use of herbicides in the Amazon Basin resulted in cessation of U.S.-sponsored herbicide testing and data gathering in Peru (45). As a result, a complete analysis of the

Figure 1-2—Primary Coca-Producing Zones in Bolivia, Peru, and Colombia

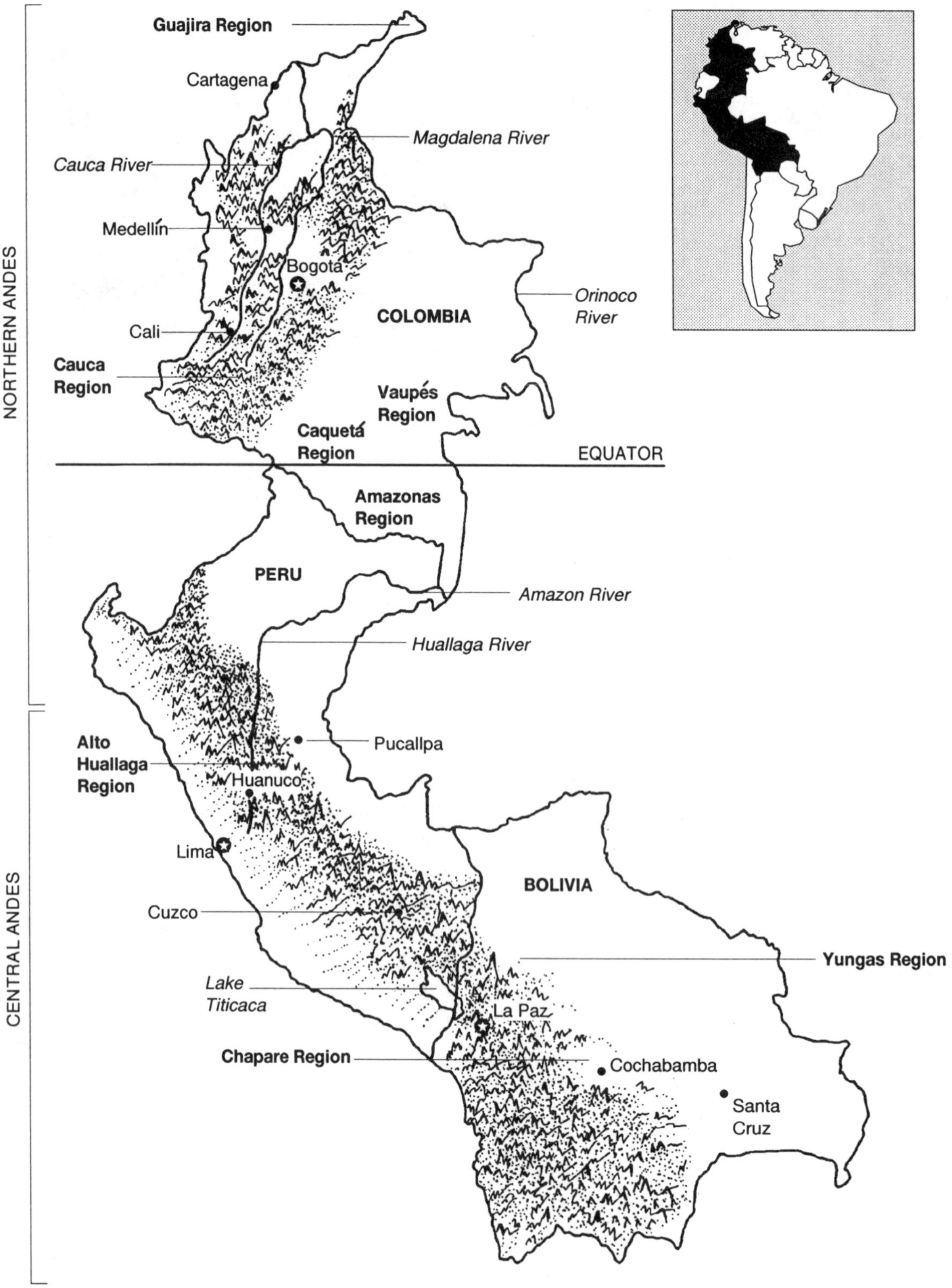

NORTHERN ANDES

CENTRAL ANDES

Guajira Region

Cartagena

Magdalena River

Cauca River

Medellín

Bogota

Cali

COLOMBIA

Orinoco River

Cauca Region

Vaupés Region

Caquetá Region

EQUATOR

Amazonas Region

PERU

Amazon River

Huallaga River

Alto Huallaga Region

Pucallpa

Huanuco

Lima

BOLIVIA

Cuzco

Yungas Region

Lake Titicaca

La Paz

Chapare Region

Cochabamba

Santa Cruz

SOURCE: Office of Technology Assessment, 1993.

potential impacts of herbicide use on future land and aquatic productivity is not available.

Biological control (biocontrol) has been identified as an alternative to chemical control of coca. The United Nations International Drug Control Programme identified biocontrol as a possible eradication method for narcotic crops nearly a decade ago, and interest continues in investigating the potential for this technology to control a variety of narcotic crops (54). Biocontrol relies on the use of biological agents to prey on an identified target and reduce its prevalence in the treatment area. However, some disagree about the potential for biocontrol techniques to achieve eradication. Biocontrol may provide an environmentally benign way to reduce coca cultivation, yet there are considerable social and political constraints to its implementation.

■ Social, Political, and Economic Context

Long-term social inequities and political and economic unrest contribute to coca's dominant role in the economies of Bolivia and Peru, the world's leading producers of coca leaf. Colombia, where a large cocaine trafficking industry has emerged, also exhibits extreme social and political instability. It is in this unsettled milieu that coca-dominated economies have flowered. However, each country has a unique set of contributing circumstances.

The cocaine economy—including production, processing, and transport—is extensive in Bolivia, Peru, and Colombia. The continuum from coca production to cocaine marketing involves different actors, with different values; their commonality is that each finds coca a ready cash source (35). Individuals deriving the greatest economic benefits from coca production (i.e., narcotics traffickers) have gained political power through a variety of mechanisms (e.g., bribery, land acquisition, farmer/cattlemen associations, assassinations) (14). The strong presence of numerous insurgency and terrorist groups compounds the difficulties Peruvian and Colombian national governments face in drug crop control efforts. As one analyst suggests:

> ...[the U.S. is] asking a country [Peru] that's fighting the Civil War and going through the Great Depression at the same time to suddenly take on Prohibition as well (4).

BOLIVIA

The progressive impoverishment of Bolivia's rural upland population, dating from the colonial period, was accelerated in the 1980s by severe drought and by agricultural and trade policies unfavorable to subsistence farmers. Many peasants were forced to migrate to other areas, including the Chapare—a center for coca cultivation. This influx of labor, and a general economic decline, affecting even middle-class Bolivians, helped spur a surge in coca-leaf production and processing as the only economic alternative for many financially-desperate Bolivians.

However, estimates of the population involved in the coca trade vary widely. For example, 20 percent of the Bolivian workforce was estimated to be involved in the coca economy in the late 1980s (24) whereas a 1990 report estimates only 7 percent (19). Nevertheless, the Bolivian coca economy annually generates as much foreign exchange (roughly U.S. $600 million) as all other exports combined (5).

Social and political inequities persist in Bolivia, such that peasant populations have meager educational and development opportunities, while an agrarian elite wields considerable political power and monopolizes the country's financial resources. This situation seriously constrains possibilities for the country's broad-based socio-economic development (27,30).

Although Bolivia operates under a democratically elected civilian rule, and is somewhat more stable politically than Peru or Colombia, the political situation is tenuous. Many national institutions, including judicial and law enforcement agencies, are weak, and the government has not been able to lift the majority of Bolivians out of poverty.

PERU

Recent peasant migrations from the Peruvian highlands to the coca-growing Alto Huallaga is the latest chapter in a long history of economically-induced migrations. Land shortages and/or lack of work in the highlands, as well as rapid population growth (beginning in the 1940s), have fueled the latest population movements into the eastern valley systems.

Coca cultivation has expanded in the Alto Huallaga, in part as a result of these migrations and in part due to the country's failing economy and severe international debt crisis. Coca production expanded considerably as economic conditions worsened in the late 1980s, softening the most profound economic and employment crisis in the republic's history. The coca economy continues to increase proportionally to the decline of the nation's legal economy (31).

Attempts at economic reform by the Fujimori Administration are undermined by pervasive political unrest, poverty, and an uncertain business environment. Alberto Fujimori ended 12 years of democratic rule in Peru when, supported by the army and police, he seized political power in a "pseudo-coup" (23). Peru's current state of extreme economic and political instability constitutes a domestic crisis that overshadows the importance of counternarcotic efforts in the minds of most Peruvians. Moreover, strong guerrilla movements in Peru's coca-producing areas make any counternarcotics initiatives extremely hazardous. In recent years, 10 workers for the U.S. Agency for International Development (AID) have been killed here (34).

COLOMBIA

Coca production has not been as widespread in Colombia as in Peru and Bolivia. Coca production, banned in 1947 after lengthy public debate, has re-emerged, however, paralleling the development of a large and lucrative criminal-run cocaine manufacturing industry, with exports netting close to U.S. $3 billion a year. The illegal drug industry has flourished in Colombia in part because State presence traditionally has been weak; guerrilla movements are strong, and political "clientelism" rampant, with increasing concentration of land, capital, and credit in the hands of an elite minority. As the gap between rich and poor has widened, so has that between written law and the economic behavior of the underground cocaine economy. Drug-related violence and corruption have undermined the country's courts, and police and customs service, as well as the military (8).

Colombia has enjoyed positive economic growth overall in the past four decades, but drug money now spreads corruption throughout the country's economy. Real estate and construction have been particularly heavily infiltrated by narcotics investors, who have had technologically modernizing but socially regressive impacts. For example, although they have introduced and financed new technologies for increasing economic productivity, they have also established paramilitary groups, discouraged peasant participation in the political process, concentrated land ownership, and laundered capital in investments with fast turnover rather than higher long-term yields (51).

Colombia's growth record was much better in the pre-cocaine era than it has been in the post-cocaine era. The trend today is toward declining economic productivity and reduced growth. Domestic drug violence and terrorism further undermine the country politically and economically. Today, Colombia is one of the most violent countries in the hemisphere. Strengthening and redefining the role of the State in Colombian society is central to the success of any drug-control policy.

■ Development Assistance and Coca Reduction

Development assistance seeks to create and extend alternative livelihoods, build local institutions, provide education and training, promote infrastructure improvements, and provide social services. The development goal in coca substitution programs is to assist countries dependent on a black-market economy to move toward legitimate markets. In the coca-producing countries, the focus largely has been on developing alternative agricultural systems incorporating high-value or multipurpose crops. However, existing national agricultural policies do not favor smallholders—those most commonly involved in coca production.[1] Fiscal realities result in focusing resources on areas of high population density. Conversely, coca-producing regions tend to be remote and sparsely populated and, within this environment, few opportunities exist for smallholders to be profitable in the legitimate agricultural market (2,27,34).

Early U.S. coca substitution efforts focused on producing regions in the Andean countries (i.e., Alto Huallaga in Peru, Chapare in Bolivia). Initial substitution efforts in Bolivia concentrated solely on farmers in the Chapare region through the Agricultural Development in the Coca Zones Project (ADCZP) and later under the Chapare Regional Development Project (CRDP). However, it became apparent the combination of an easily produced crop, stable market and marketing channels, and an abundant labor supply as a result of population migration were all fundamental to the increase of Chapare coca production. Thus, the CRDP was redesigned to include development in emigration zones through the Associated High Valleys component. This effort has been expanded further to encompass integrated regional development under the Cochabamba Regional Development Project (CORDEP) (figure 1-3). Similarly broad development efforts are likely to be needed in other coca-producing areas as well.

Numerous national and international organizations have been actively involved in coca substitution projects in South America. Their activities include basic and applied research on potential

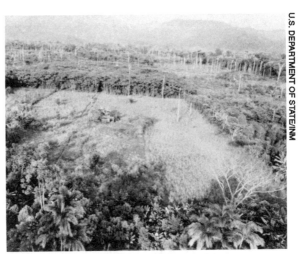

Small, remote landholdings characterize many coca-growing areas. Production units often are less than 2 hectares in size, such as this minifundia.

alternative crops, demonstration and extension of promising technologies to farmers, agroprocessing, and infrastructure development. Crop substitution approaches sponsored through the United Nations International Drug Control Programme are built on the concept of rural development that complements substitution efforts. While crop diversification alone may provide greater security for farmers compared with drug-crop monoculture, the transition to legal crops also requires concerted efforts in development of production practices, infrastructure, and markets (36).

The economics of coca is often seen as the primary constraint to widespread adoption of alternative crops. Coca profits are nearly twice that of identified high-value crops (e.g., peach palm) and at least four times greater than other traditional crops such as pineapple or citrus (61). However, declining prices at the producer level suggest coca may no longer be the most lucrative crop (18). Furthermore, such comparisons may be meaningless: the nature of coca production defies traditional methods of estimating profitability

---

[1] There are exceptions to this statement, most notably the long-range Colombian coffee policy designed to stabilize the national production system in light of the effects of the international market on prices and thus on producer earnings (18).

Figure 1-3—Evolution of the Cochabamba Regional Development Project (CORDEP)

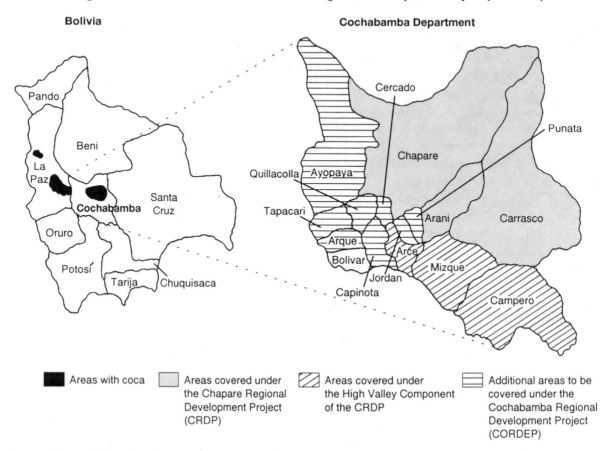

SOURCE: Office of Technology Assessment adapted from Development Alternatives, Inc., *Cochabamba Regional Development Project (CORDEP)—Bolivia,* technical proposal (Bethesda, MD: DAI, 1992).

because of its dependence on unpaid family labor (38).

A combination of legitimate crops suitable to the environmental and sociocultural features of the production region, market assurance, access to affordable credit, and a suite of social/human services (e.g., rural justice, school systems, health care) could be sufficient incentives for coca producers to adopt alternative systems (box 1-A). Removal of U.S. trade barriers for certain South American exports, for example, could promote crop substitution and development of value-added industry (9,3). To some extent, this has been accomplished under the recent Andean Trade Initiative (ATI). Revision of import quotas on certain commodities and tariff reductions on value-added products could complement the goal of the ATI.

In the past few years, crop substitution has become a subset of alternative development in the Andean countries as attention to industrial and marketing aspects has increased. Nevertheless, the focus remains on agriculture and related industries. The alternative development problem is complex, requiring attention to numerous variables, and not adequately addressed by any single approach. Long-term programs are needed that provide a range of options for potential participants.

Box 1-A—High-Value Legal Alternatives to Coca: Sericulture in Colombia

The economics of coca production has been perhaps the single most widely articulated obstacle to successful crop substitution efforts. However, some disagree over the need for a dollar-for-dollar equivalent to coca or if an integrated alternative development package based on legitimate crops, development of production and marketing infrastructure, and social service amenities is sufficient. However, combining a high-value, low-volume crop with clear market potential into an integrated development package may offer the greatest benefits.

Sericulture (silk production) in Colombia grew in 1970 as part of a diversification program sponsored by the Colombian Coffee Growers Federation (FEDERCAFE). By 1987, silk production was in progress in the Departments of Caldas, Risaralda, Valle, and Cauca, with a total production area of 124 hectares. A pilot plant was established in Timbio (Cauca) to process high-quality cocoons into export products, however, the plant subsequently closed due to technical difficulties (15).

The Colombian sericulture activities have been sponsored through a blend of national and international funding sources, primarily the Colombian Government and private sources and Korean investors. Currently, five silk-producing ventures exist in Colombia (i.e., COSEDA and COKOSILK, joint ventures between Colombia and Korea; COSILK, 100-percent Korean investment; and CAPULLOS and PROSEDA, 100-percent Colombian investment). The Colombian Government promotes sericulture by financing all technical assistance and providing credit opportunities at 28 percent interest. In addition, credit is available through FEDERCAFE and the Export Promotion Fund (PROEXPO) at 18 and 32 percent interest, respectively (15). The availability of sericulture technologies, technical assistance, credit, and markets suggests silk production could become an attractive alternative crop for some areas (15, 41).

A project currently underway in Colombia's Cauca Department is attempting to promote sericulture as an alternative to coca production for nearly 300 farm families in two small towns (Pan de Azucar and Santa Cruz). The project—Silk for Life—is sponsored by the Wisconsin Farmers Foundation, Inc. and works with local farmers and silk weaving groups and a weaving cooperative in Milwaukee, Wisconsin. The project site is characterized by small farms (about 8 hectares) and a lack of transportation and electrification systems. For at least a decade, coca has been incorporated in farmer's production schemes as a cash source. Nevertheless, today 40 pilot silk farms are operating under the Silk for Life project (16).

The project approach is based on basic rural economic development with goals of reducing coca production in the region and reviving the associated rural communities. The Silk for Life project offers a blend of technical assistance, credit, and marketing opportunities to support the producers:

- *Training*—Two model farms exist in the area, one in Timbio and one in Santa Cruz, to demonstrate sericulture techniques for potential adopters.
- *Technology*—Technical assistance is offered in basic sericulture techniques, energy systems, and organic farming.
- *Marketing*—Central marketing is organized for locally-produced cocoons.
- *Credit*—Materials for sericulture startup are available through the project on a 'barter' basis whereby the borrower repays the loan with cocoons after production has begun.

In addition to focusing on an economically attractive crop, this project has blended a variety of additional features into a single package to promote sericulture in Pan de Azucar and Santa Cruz, Cauca. The package includes generating support from local community leaders and incorporating community development features (e.g., electrification, transportation) that may have benefits beyond sericulture (16).

SOURCE: Office of Technology Assessment, 1993.

Opportunities exist to promote alternative development in the Andean region. Many of these are technically based, as in developing sustainable forestry practices suitable to current coca production regions. However, broad opportunities also exist for influencing the viability of coca reduction efforts more generally. These overarching issues include creating national incentives for participation in alternative development, gathering and making available information needed to support alternative development, coordinating donor activities, and pursuing integrated national development.

CREATING NATIONAL INCENTIVES FOR COCA REDUCTION

Technical feasibility alone will not guarantee success for coca reduction efforts. The political will of Andean nations is critical, as is the acceptance and support of Andean peoples. The Andean nations (Bolivia, Peru, and Colombia) operate with differing political agendas, and driving social, cultural, and economic forces. Also complicating substitution efforts is the fact that coca cultivation has enormous cultural and economic significance for Andeans. The chewing of coca leaves for social, medicinal, and religious/ spiritual purposes is an important and long-standing tradition that may inhibit acceptance of coca substitution programs.

Existing economic conditions in the Andean countries profoundly influence national ability to undertake coca reduction programs, including crop substitution and eradication components. Coca production contributes heavily to the national economies—in most cases comprising the greatest share of export income. Developing mechanisms to improve national economies could contribute to greater ability to enter into coca reduction programs. Such an effort is likely to require short-term economic relief and long-term economic development (58).

Another constraint to reduction efforts is the lack of governmental presence in rural areas,

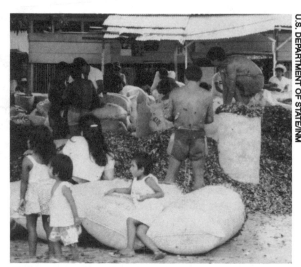

U.S. DEPARTMENT OF STATE/INM

Coca retains its cultural and social significance for many Andeans today. Here, coca leaf (hoja de coca) is being prepared for transport to legitimate markets to be sold for traditional use.

including provision of basic human services, rural justice, and other needed institutions. Local governments with leaders elected directly and held accountable by rural constituents could increase rural participation in the political process. Such efforts could reduce the environment where insurgency and lawlessness flourish.

Local grassroots organizations have played a large role in rural politics, particularly in Bolivia where local unions—*sindicatos*—have provided a means for rural inhabitants to voice their concerns and desires to a centralist national government. Nevertheless, assistance activities often do not make use of these local avenues of leadership and community cooperation. Acceptance of programs to reduce coca production could be enhanced through efforts to incorporate local groups in planning and implementation (27).

Support for U.S.-bilateral efforts in the Andean region is poor. Many Andeans perceive U.S. activities as heavy-handed attempts to solve our domestic narcotics problem on foreign soil. A key concern is that without commensurate demand reduction efforts, supply reduction merely increases costs to the Andean countries. Yet, U.S.

Table 1-1—Federal Drug Control Budget Authority
(billions of dollars)

	Supply	Demand	Percent demand of total
1981	$ 800	$ 350	30 %
1983	1,250	350	22.6
1985	1,700	400	19
1987	2,900	900	24
1989	4,000	1,600	29

SOURCE: M. Collett, "The Cocaine Connection: Drug Trafficking and Inter-American Relations," *Headline Series, Foreign Policy Association*, No. 290, Fall, 1989.

Federal expenditures focus on supply reduction (table 1-1). Analysts suggest that under these circumstances, multilateral activities are more likely to be publicly acceptable. In addition, public outreach and education efforts and greater coordination and cooperation with host countries could support these activities (57,58).

Issue: Lack of economic incentives at the national level hinders active participation in coca reduction programs.

The ability to carry out programs is inextricably linked to economic conditions. Some poorly paid public officials can be bribed to ignore illegal activities, poorly supported research and extension systems are unable to provide high-quality technical assistance to producers, and scarce alternative employment opportunities lead to participation in the coca trade. The level of bilateral debt owed by the Andean countries to the United States alone is significant and far outstrips their annual gross national products (GNPs) (table 1-2). Debt servicing hinders national government investment in needed development activities.

Generating political will to undertake coca reduction might be enhanced by providing general economic incentives to national governments. The current political and economic conditions of the Andean countries significantly reduce the ability of national governments to undertake coca reduction programs. Yet, without national commitment to improving opportunities for rural communities in general, and coca farmers specifi-

cally, potential for effective alternative development programs is greatly reduced (57,58).

Option: Congress could create "debt-for-drugs" swap opportunities for the Andean countries.

Providing bilateral debt relief in exchange for coca reduction achievements—"debt-for-drugs" swaps—has been suggested as an opportunity for improving supply reduction efforts, yet specific legislative action has not been taken. Examples of successful debt swaps suggest similar actions could be useful for coca reduction. The United States recently eliminated $371 million of Bolivian debt under the Enterprise for the Americas Initiative (EAI) (25). The EAI debt reduction component could serve as a model to develop "debt-for-drugs" swaps. National policy actions promoting preconditions for successful alternative development could serve as "collateral" for debt relief.

Conversely, if lessons from related activities involving national economic incentives are reviewed, possibilities for dramatic results from a "debt-for-drugs" program may seem less likely. For example, certification for U.S. development assistance funding has been used as a mechanism to motivate compliance with coca reduction goals and although it has elicited short-term reduction efforts, it has yielded little in overall supply reduction. Nevertheless, debt relief could provide a double service by increasing political will to undertake supply reduction and improving the fiscal ability of national governments to finance needed national projects.

Issue: Andean eligibility for U.S. development assistance is closely linked to coca reduction.

Eligibility for development aid is in part based on narcotics reduction achievements. Thus, at the national government level, the development goal may become secondary to a counternarcotics agenda—i.e., success may be measured by hectares of coca reduced rather than hectares of legitimate crops produced. Further complicating

Table 1-2—Andean Bilateral Debt With the United States
(In millions of dollars, as of 9/30/90)

	GNP	Debt:GNP ratio	AID	PL-480	CCC	EXIM	Total
Bolivia	$ 46.0	11:1	$ 331	$141	$ 0	$ 33	$ 505
Colombia	354.0	3:1	499	2	0	497	998
Peru	189.0	4:1	318	221	95	54	688
Totals			1,149	364	95	584	2,191

AID—U.S. Agency for International Development
PL-480—Agricultural Trade Development and Assistance Act of 1954 as Amended, "Food aid"
CCC—Commodity Credit Corporation
EXIM—Export-Import Bank

SOURCE: U.S. Department of the Treasury, "Enterprise for the Americas Fact Sheet," Washington, DC, September 30, 1990.

this situation is the reliance on narcotics data of questionable accuracy to support reduction claims.

Option: Congress could refocus certification requirements for development funding to include specific development objectives in addition to satisfying "coca clauses."

The basis of alternative development is to assist recipient nations to enter the international legitimate economy. Preconditions for achieving this goal have been identified and are part of many donor activities. However, some conditions can only partly be fulfilled by donors and require the firm commitment of host countries. For example, increasing local government presence, promoting rural justice, and providing social services for rural populations will depend largely on national government efforts, yet are critical for improving development opportunities. Refocusing assistance certification criteria on the achievement of these development goals could increase interest on the part of the host country.

However, placing additional burdens on national governments to achieve development goals to qualify for U.S. assistance might be unrealistic given economic and political conditions in the Andean region. Conversely, certification could highlight development objectives to the exclusion of coca reduction. Such an act is likely to require a significant increase in U.S. domestic enforcement, interdiction, and education to prevent increased narcotics abuse in the short term.

Issue: Lack of rural governmental presence hinders adoption of coca reduction programs.

Government presence generally is weak in rural Peru, Bolivia, and Colombia. National governments could choose to address this condition through policies that establish effective local governments and state control within the framework of the legitimate judicial system. An improved judicial system could facilitate development activities and offer increased human rights protection.

Rural government presence encompasses accountability to local political authorities by police and security forces, legitimizes support of the democratic process, and strengthens the judicial system. Administration of rural justice and control of national territory are critical for implementing development programs and development of popular support for substitution efforts. Common development assistance goals—institution building, providing social services, and improving standards of living—may contribute to increasing security in rural areas.

The U.S. Department of Justice and AID offer assistance to judicial institutions in the Andean countries through several programs intended to improve the administration, operation, and effectiveness of the country's judicial system. However, this assistance is a small part of the overall assistance budget.

Option: Congress could direct AID to increase its support to judicial institutions in the Andean nations through Justice Sector and Strengthening Democracy projects.

Greater presence of rural justice in current coca-producing areas could yield benefits in increasing stability by assuring those breaking laws would be properly adjudicated in an established legal system. AID justice-sector programs have been implemented since the mid- to late 1980s in Bolivia and Peru.

Achieving increased rural justice in the current social and political climates of the Andean region is likely to be difficult. A concerted effort is likely to require additional fiscal resources, and in areas where violence is significant, security needs would be paramount. Increasing military and police presence in some areas may not be perceived as a benefit at a time when militarization components of the ''drug war'' are unpopular.

Alternative Option: Congress could direct AID to increase the level of coordination/cooperation with local grassroots organizations.

Local community groups have and continue to play an important role in Andean rural politics. Grassroots organizations typically have strong support from local populations and understand local cultures, aspirations, and priorities. Groups such as the Bolivian *sindicatos* provide a mobilizing force for rural change and expression of concerns to the national governments.

Incorporating existing community groups and other grassroots organizations in planning and implementing alternative development programs could yield benefits in adoption rates. Bolivian crop substitution programs might work cooperatively with *sindicatos* to promote peaceful crop substitution and alternative development efforts. Such cooperative efforts would ensure local concerns were identified in project planning and encourage local understanding of the project process.

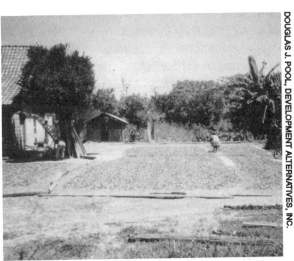

Coca farmers receive the lowest percentage of profit in the cocaine industry—perhaps as little as 1 percent. Here, a coca farmer in the Chapare is spreading the harvested leaves to dry them in preparation for sale.

However, diverse political parties may influence grassroot organization activities, and political conflicts between the state and these organizations may create difficulties for the organizations as development vectors. These features should be considered in project planning and approaches to deal with them identified to reduce any potential adverse impact on project effectiveness.

INFORMATION NEEDED TO SUPPORT ALTERNATIVE DEVELOPMENT PROJECTS

Setting realistic goals for coca reduction programs will depend, in part, on availability and accuracy of basic information on coca farmers and others linked to the cocaine economy. Identification of key targets for alternative development activities will be integral to increased effectiveness of U.S. development assistance. Several initial questions need to be addressed: What is the current and potential areal extent of coca production? Who and where are the populations economically linked to production? What are the appropriate levels of development (e.g., subsistence, semi-commercial, commercial) for these areas and populations? Additional decisions might further refine target groups (e.g., identifying what economic population should receive priority—poorest, borderline, or entrepreneurial). Information needed to support alternative development/coca reduction programs includes:

- Extent of the coca economy (including direct and indirect participants),
- Comparison of coca and alternatives, and
- Centralized and easily accessed source of information related to ongoing activities.

Issue: Inadequate information on the true extent of the coca economy hinders development of programs to reduce dependence.

Studies of the extent of the coca/cocaine economy are lacking and likely to be difficult to conduct. While estimates of the relative size and importance of coca to national economies exists, little information is available that identifies the subsectors dependent on coca/cocaine production, nor their level of dependence. Yet, such information could provide insights for development projects and improve opportunities for integrated development.

Collecting information that accurately identifies populations involved directly in coca production (through production, labor, transport), including the extent of dependence (i.e., part-time, seasonal, full-time), and survival strategies during low coca prices, is likely to be difficult. Existing information sources might provide an alternative to new information-gathering activities. Information on coca farmers in the Chapare exists through the Cooperative Agreement on Human Settlements and Natural Research System Analysis (SARSA). Although somewhat dated, similar information exists for farmers in the Alto Huallaga. This resource could be reviewed and evaluated within the context of improving identification of target populations for alternative development programs.

Option: Congress could direct the U.S. Department of State, Bureau of International Narcotics Matters, and AID, cooperatively, to develop comprehensive coca industry profiles that *identify populations and economic sectors directly and indirectly linked to coca production and their relative level of dependence and use this information to direct development projects to high priority targets.*

Profiles could be developed using existing information gathered through activities of both agencies. AID and its contractors have accumulated a wide array of information on coca producers and farm laborers. The U.S. Department of State has focused more on those involved in the additional aspects of transport, processing, providing precursor chemicals, etc. This information could be pulled together to create a comprehensive profile of the breadth of the coca economy and provide an outline of key populations/sectors that ultimately will be affected by coca reduction programs. Such an outline could provide an agenda for future international development planning as well as a resource for a national development strategy.

Additional funding could be made available to allow profile development without adding the burden on agency staff. In addition, some activities and populations may be more transient than can be incorporated readily into such analysis. The segments of the coca trade that are likely to be excluded or insufficiently described also could be identified in the overall effort. Mechanisms to assure the profile information is used in future project planning also would be needed.

Issue: Lack of accurate economic studies comparing coca with other potential alternatives hinder efforts to promote adoption of renewable resource-based alternatives to coca.

Coca is a traditional Andean crop, relatively easy to produce and sell, and provides a good return on investment. Although coca prices fluctuate, traditional economic analyses suggest they are high relative to legitimate agricultural commodities that are more visibly affected by global markets. These conditions make identifying and promoting alternative crops difficult.

Although alternative crops, products, and activities exist, information on the market potential of many of them is lacking. However, such information could facilitate identifying priorities for alternative development efforts. Additionally, economic analyses of other alternatives such as forest products, wildlife, and fisheries as compared with coca and alternative crops could be used to identify additional opportunities for specific regions.

Option: Congress could direct AID, cooperatively with the U.S. Department of Agriculture, Economic Research Service, to undertake economic studies of renewable resource-based alternatives environmentally suitable to coca-producing areas that have not been evaluated economically to date.

Alternatives to be evaluated economically (e.g., agroforestry, forestry, extractive reserves, alternative crop plants, animals, etc.) could be identified by AID, along with regional characterizations describing existing production opportunities and constraints. For example, if tropical hardwood production provides an environmentally suitable and high-value opportunity in certain regions, but is constrained by lack of processing or harvest mechanisms, these features could then become development priorities.

Studies would be prepared and filed with AID's Office of Evaluation, Center for Development Information and Evaluation (CDIE) and available to prioritize activities in the Andean region. The information could be made freely available to international development assistance groups and used to promote adoption and assist in developing appropriate incentives for adopters.

However, the fluctuation of global markets may complicate such analyses. Thus, opportunities and analyses may only be accurate for short periods, making rapid turnaround a high priority. Additional pressures on staff time could result in reduced attention to ongoing priorities.

Issue: Lack of a centralized information source on alternative development activities

hinders improved project planning and implementation.

A lack of institutional memory within AID, and other bureaucratic constraints, work against incorporating lessons learned from past activities into new project plans. The AID project approach incorporates numerous technical and contract groups and information gathered by these groups may or may not reach CDIE files. Thus, potential lessons learned from early activities may not be used to improve current projects or the design of future projects. Stringent requirements for filing project studies and reviews along with improved training of AID personnel, emphasizing area history, could promote use of "lessons learned" materials. Additional requirements for contractors to generate logs of activities and results from their efforts could be useful in future program planning. AID could strengthen its requirements for filing contractor reports and other project-related information with CDIE to assure that this resource is easily available for future project development.

Option: Congress could direct AID to establish and maintain an interpretive database on institutional experiences and development project evaluations in the Andean region.

A large body of information exists on development in the Andean region, but much of this information is "gray literature" and can be difficult to access. AID currently is developing a management information system (MIS) database on AID alternative development projects in the Andean region to improve its ability to measure the impact of these efforts. The system will be updated semi-annually and will include a variety of economic and project data. This effort could be expanded to incorporate the activities of other donor groups operating in the Andean region, thereby supporting improved donor coordination. Once established, project planning could require a database search to identify potential cooperative opportunities.

However, by incorporating the broad array of activities, database development and maintenance tasks would be increased dramatically. Additional financial resources might be needed and without additional appropriations could come at the expense of more applied activities. In addition, the ongoing United Nations effort to develop a Sustainable Development Network (SDN) could complement AID's MIS effort. The SDN effort is intended to assist less developed countries to develop and maintain data on domestic development activities with an ultimate goal of developing a global network.

DONOR COORDINATION

The narcotics problem is immense, and the impact of one donor is likely to be small. Many bilateral and multilateral groups are actively working toward a variety of development and coca control goals. Coordination of the numerous organizations involved in the Andean countries poses a difficult problem, yet it could yield large benefits in achieving comprehensive counternarcotic and development goals. The Organization of American States identified the need for a coordinating body for early development efforts in the Chapare to coordinate the activities of nearly 54 donor organizations. The need for such coordination throughout the Andean region remains.

Issue: Lack of donor coordination has reduced the effectiveness of rural development and crop substitution efforts in Andean drug-producing nations.

Uncoordinated donor activities can result in duplicative or counterproductive efforts. Development funds may be spent on similar projects without incorporation of ''lessons learned.'' Similarly, lack of coordination can reduce opportunities for efforts aimed at solving mutually identified problems and preclude potential for expanded efforts or building on current activities. ''Reinventing the wheel'' may have high costs in overall terms of donor funding.

Option: Congress could direct the U.S. Department of State to establish a coordinating committee comprised of U.S. development agencies, those receiving U.S. funds for development activities, and national government counterparts to improve coordination of development programs.

A variety of U.S. agencies and international institutions, and multilateral banks receive U.S. funding for development activities in the Andean region (e.g., AID, InterAmerican Foundation, World Bank, InterAmerican Development Bank, United Nations). A committee composed of representatives of these organizations could be created to develop a unified alternative development approach for the United States and ensure that activities complement one another or at least do not work against each other. Such a committee could be responsible for setting a development agenda, prioritizing needs, and linking similar activities among cooperating groups.

However, coordination by committee can be time-consuming. Scheduling meetings and preparing committee reports would add to staff duties. Further, authority would be needed to ensure committee findings and recommendations were adequately considered by individual implementing agencies. Such additional bureaucratic processes are unlikely to be popular among implementing agencies.

Issue: Coordination between enforcement and development activities is inadequate.

Diverse or conflicting goals and operations of the numerous agencies (e.g., U.S. Department of State, Drug Enforcement Administration) active in the Andean nations have adversely affected local response to development activities. For example, non-development operations have led to some distrust of development personnel in certain locales. Thus, coordination of all agency activities may be required to improve acceptance of U.S. development groups. Enforcement typically is dependent on maintaining a certain level of secrecy and, possibly, coordination with development activities would be seen as potential "leaks." Nevertheless, these two activities necessarily complement one another and, without coordination, have the potential to detract from each other's effectiveness. Coordination of enforcement and development activities should occur at high levels, with clear separation at the field application level.

Option: Congress could create an interagency coordinating body composed of representatives of the agencies involved in development and enforcement in the Andean countries (e.g., AID, InterAmerican Foundation, U.S. Department of State, Drug Enforcement Administration).

A coordinating group with representatives from the agencies involved in development and supply control activities in the Andean region could promote unified direction for U.S. efforts. Congress could choose to create a separate task force or place the responsibility under an existing agency. The Office of National Drug Control Policy currently coordinates agency activities related to international and domestic demand control, interdiction, and financial systems, and thus may be an appropriate entity to coordinate the broader picture of narcotics-related activities. However, as an executive branch office, congressional investigation and oversight of committee activities could be curtailed.

INTEGRATED NATIONAL DEVELOPMENT

The extent and importance of the coca economy in the Andean nations strongly influences the ability of narrowly focused, short-term efforts to achieve promising results in coca substitution. Development groups have identified a variety of goals ranging from the highly specific (e.g., building agroprocessing plants) to more general (e.g., increasing rural incomes), but all are based on general rural development. Achieving this goal, however, requires development activities to

fulfill a broad number of needs concomitantly. For example, whereas the crop substitution efforts in the Chapare region concentrated on identifying high-value crops, little effort was invested in developing processing, transport, and marketing mechanisms. This has changed under the current project (i.e., CORDEP), however, and a regional development approach has been embraced.

Alternative development programs could be enhanced further through integrated development strategies that expand options for those involved in the coca economy. Development, agricultural or otherwise, in the Andean countries might best be approached in terms of economic diversification. Diversification of local and regional economies could include agricultural options, light industry, and service operations.

Should efforts continue to focus on narrowly circumscribed regions and solely agricultural opportunities, the chances for coca reduction success will be similarly narrow and circumscribed. Rural development alone may be insufficient to extricate these countries from their economic dependence on coca production. Increasingly, urban poor have become involved in the coca economy as farmworkers, processors, and transporters.

Issue: Short-term project cycles reduce the potential for effective, integrated alternative development efforts.

Alternative development is not a short-term problem nor likely to be solved with short-term solutions. The transition time from coca to alternative production systems is likely to be lengthy and programs or projects must consider this investment time. Moreover, incremental substitution programs are likely to be more attractive to potential participants. Efforts likely will need to be long-term irrespective of the approach taken to promote alternative crops or livelihoods. Nevertheless, short-term project cycles are standard in U.S. development activities, in part, driven by financial management requirements.

Option: Congress could expressly identify "no year" funding status for AID crop substitution projects to remove the current constraints associated with fiscal year spending and short-term project deadlines.

Long-term project cycles could contribute to a sense of continuity for program participants and recipient countries. Such stability could contribute to reducing the perceived risks associated with adoption of alternative systems. Long-term project cycles could also assure efforts are not redirected based on political changes.

However, cross-year funding could complicate bureaucratic requirements and increase budgeting difficulties. Such a change would also require concomitant changes in project reporting, evaluation, and review to ensure that despite longer timeframes, project difficulties are noted and resolved expeditiously.

Issue: Development activities designed to reduce coca production have been created with insufficient understanding of the existing sociopolitical, economic, and environmental conditions of recipient countries.

Alternative development programs largely have been developed by U.S. agency personnel. Yet, the existing sociopolitical, economic, and environmental conditions of the Andean countries significantly influence whether or not these programs will succeed. Program components may be based on counternarcotics goals, rather than the underlying development needs to shift black-market economies to legitimate markets. In large part, this might be addressed by increasing the level of host nation participation in program development.

Option: Congress could create an International Andean Commission responsible for developing an integrated strategy to reduce economic dependence on coca.

This commission would be interdisciplinary, composed of technical experts from the United States, Andean, and other concerned foreign nations. The group would serve as a long-term inclusive coordinating organization unencumbered by U.S. programs, but including NGOs, private-sector, and grassroots and stakeholder organizations to oversee long-term development programs. The commission could address practical technical needs for successful development and be responsible for oversight of impacts of development activities.

Congress could create a similar commission composed of domestic agencies and U.S. representatives of the Multilateral Development Banks (i.e., InterAmerican Development Bank, World Bank, etc.). However, such a commission may appear strictly bilateral, which is already unpopular in host countries. Further, it may be no more able to solve development problems without a significant Andean presence.

IMPROVING CROP SUBSTITUTION EFFORTS

The importance of coca in the national economies of the Andean countries suggests development efforts narrowly focused on improving agricultural opportunities alone are unlikely to achieve broad coca reduction goals. The Cochabamba Regional Development Project (CORDEP) has expanded crop substitution efforts in the Chapare region to diversified agricultural development throughout the Cochabamba Department. However, the current effort does not adequately address alternative development for participants in the coca trade in nearby departments also involved through cocaine elaboration and as migrant workers.

Existing information on the extent of the economy, populations, and sectors dependent on coca indicate it is broadly distributed. Over the long term, single-sector development is unlikely to create stable national development of the kind needed to shift economies to legitimate enterprises nor fulfill the economic diversification goal of alternative development. Thus, alternative

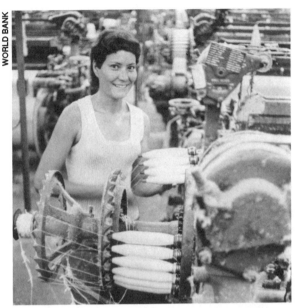

Developing value-added industries, such as this textile factory in Medellín, is one mechanism to diversify economies and increase the value of locally produced raw materials.

development efforts for Andean countries need to incorporate options for nonagriculturists as well.

This thinking has already been articulated in AID documents (55), although not yet demonstrated through implementation. Opportunities may exist in developing mineral resources, light industry, etc. to diversify economies, particularly for the urban populations currently involved in the coca chain. This issue is beyond the scope of the present study, yet is likely to be critical for achieving coca reduction goals. This might be addressed in part by expanding the range of resource-based alternatives and undertaking actions to ease the transition from coca-based to legal livelihoods.

■ Expanding the Range of Alternatives

The Andean countries have a wide range of renewable resources that could be developed to increase economic opportunities for producers. Indeed, many coca-growing areas are more suitable to some of these options than traditional agriculture. For example, in the Alto Huallaga, most coca is produced on steep slopes where agriculture is environmentally, if not economically, unsuitable. In the Chapare region of Bolivia, logging was the primary economic activity until the mid-1970s when coca expansion eclipsed the industry (39). However, the existing development thrust is largely agricultural. Projects that focus on forest, wildlife, and aquatic resources, integrated resource use, and related industries are likely to require an expertise-building period prior to implementation.

Issue: Agricultural alternatives have focused on export markets to the exclusion of domestic market opportunities.

The value of smallholder agricultural production in the Andean countries is low relative to other sectors. To some degree this is the result of national food policies that maintain low-cost food for urban areas (6). In addition, some analysts suggest competition with P.L. 480 (The Agricultural Trade and Assistance Act of 1954, as amended) food imports may also contribute to this condition (26,58). Increasing the value of domestic agriculture through domestic policy adjustment could have larger beneficial effects on national agriculture generally and rural economies and crop substitution specifically.

Import substitution may offer an opportunity to diversify markets for some producers involved in substitution programs and contribute to increasing national food supply. This approach has generated some success in a cooperative project among the Food and Agriculture Organization, the United Nations International Drug Control Programme, and the Pakistani Government in developing alternative employment for opium cultivators. Similar activities could be undertaken in the Andean region with long-term goals of increasing the value of agriculture domestically as well as internationally.

Option: Congress could direct AID to increase attention to import substitution opportunities

in crop substitution to meet local and national market needs.

Although cropping systems incorporating staple crops exist, most effort seems to be placed on developing export agriculture. International agricultural research centers (IARCs) in the Andean region *(Centro Internacional de la Papa, Centro de Investigación y Mejoramiento de Maíz y Trigo, Centro de Investigación de Agricultura Tropical)* have developed improved cultivars and production practices for several staple crops (e.g., potato, corn, rice) and could provide a valuable technical resource for development activities.

However, increased attention to local and national markets could come at the expense of attention to possibly higher-priced export markets, if an appropriate balance is not defined. Further, without concomitant agricultural policy reforms that increase the value of domestic agriculture, available national markets may be inadequate incentive for producers to shift to legitimate crops.

Issue: Greater investment in Andean agricultural research and extension is needed.

Enhancing agricultural profitability in the Andean nations will require a continuing and significant investment in research and extension to develop alternatives and demonstrate techniques and technologies to potential adopters (12). Research and extension activities were large components of early crop substitution efforts in Bolivia and led to numerous alternatives for coca farmers. However, this effort has declined and continued devotion of funding to long-term research and extension activities is hampered by pressure to produce immediate results. Small-scale farms are largely the rule in coca-producing zones and opportunities to intensify their production are needed.

Although several IARCs conduct research on crop improvements directly applicable to the Andean region, there are no similar institutions focusing on integrated farming systems such as polyculture and tree crop research (agroforestry)

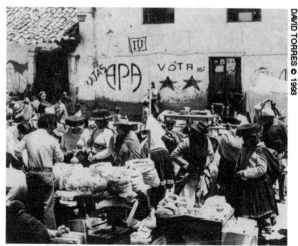

Access to external markets is highly dependent on adequate transport infrastructure. Largely, agricultural commodities produced in coca-growing regions are sold at the farm gate or in local markets such as this one in Peru.

(33). One Consultative Group on International Agricultural Research institute focuses primarily on agroforestry—the International Council for Research on Agroforestry (ICRAF), however, it is located in Kenya, hundreds of kilometers distant from tropical wet forests ecologically similar to those of the eastern Andean foothills. Agroforestry research previously carried out in Peru by North Carolina State University largely was an offshoot of traditional agricultural research, yet highlighted the importance of perennial tree crops in tropical agriculture. These efforts have ceased, however; largely due to violence in the area.

Option: Congress could authorize funding through AID for development of an integrated farming system research center (IFSRC) in the Andean region.

An IFSRC could support efforts to develop improved traditional agriculture systems. Several IARCs in Latin America could provide a valuable resource in development of an IFSRC in the Andean region. IFSRC research could focus on highly productive crop combinations, improved water and nutrient management, cultivar improvements, and agronomic research to identify appropriate production practices to assure quality products to meet market requirements.

Research and extension activities could emphasize the local and national research centers to promote institution building and skill development, thereby improving the potential for activities to continue after direct assistance is withdrawn. Agronomic management research could be oriented to on-farm, farmer-participation production trials, involving the local farm population in direct participatory research. Extension activities could emphasize on-farm demonstration and farming systems to maximize the diffusion of new technologies and practices to rural adopting populations.

Development of a full-scale research center is likely to be costly. Yet opportunities to pool resources of many donors could alleviate the financial burden and contribute to a larger effort and wider use and acceptance of the institution. Alternatively, financial investment in the *Instituto Boliviano de Tecnología Agropecuario-Chapare* (IBTA-Chapare) could be increased. This institution has undertaken alternative crop research for nearly a decade and already contains substantial expertise. However, since IBTA-Chapare is a Bolivian institution, it may be difficult for practioners in other areas to access.

Issue: Insufficient attention has been placed on developing forest resource exploitation options.

The importance of sustaining tropical forest resources has been highlighted in the last two decades and recently was underscored by the United Nations Conference on Environment and Development. Bolivia, Colombia, and Peru have substantial areas of remaining natural forests with potential for biodiversity conservation and forest management (33). For example, the value of forest products (e.g., nuts, fruits, latex) harvested from an extractive reserve can be longer-term and significantly higher than that offered by one-time logging operations or conversion to agricultural production (48). Opportunities also exist for "chemical prospecting" in tropical forests to identify compounds with commercial potential. Sustainable timber exploitation technologies also exist and have been demonstrated in the Palcazu Valley in Peru. Such innovative operations could be tested and adapted to other forest areas. Despite these potential opportunities, efforts will be needed to increase the understanding of tropical forest management, specifically in the Andean region (33).

Forestry opportunities have now taken a more prominent position in U.S. alternative development efforts in Bolivia (21) and would be appropriate for other coca-producing areas as well. Full-scale research centers in relevant Andean forests are needed, however, to promote forestry activities. Initial activities could focus on existing forest management technologies that seem successful, such as those at the experimental level in the Palcazu Valley, Peru (52). Such an effort, however, would require significant financial investment over a 10-to 20-year period.

Option: Congress could authorize funding through AID to establish a full-scale, state-of-the-art, tropical forest research experiment station in the Andean countries.

While a number of tropical forest research stations exist worldwide, none are in the humid tropical Andean region. Given increasing concern over conservation of the Amazonian rainforest, this would seem to be an appropriate site. A major tropical forest research center could be located in a humid tropical Andean region and several sub-centers could be located in other places to conduct site specific activities and adaptation of identified technologies. These experiment stations could concentrate on conservation and forest management technologies that use forests and species native to the coca-producing regions. The U.S. Forest Service, Institute for Tropical Forestry in Puerto Rico could provide a valuable resource for research station development.

Concomitant with on-site research efforts, education and training opportunities could be made available for conservation, forest, and protected area scientists from tropical countries. Professionals trained at those stations could fulfill necessary roles in development and extension of forest management systems to local populations.

Issue: Insufficient attention has been placed on examining potential wildlife and wildland resource use options.

Wildlife-centered economic development has become more acceptable and research efforts are being undertaken to determine sustainable yields and appropriate husbandry practices. Techniques for raising/producing certain wildlife species have been developed and are easily incorporated in rural communities with little capital investment. For example, experimental programs for ranching of green iguanas have now spread from Panama to other neotropical countries (7,62). Licensing and protection mechanisms that make farming and ranching of wildlife more profitable than taking from the wild are being implemented in the region (46). The International Union for the Conservation of Nature and Natural Resources and other international resource organizations are working to create viable legal markets for wildlife and wildlife products in conjunction with protecting habitats and wild populations.

Wildlife-based tourism has grown at least 20 percent annually since 1980 (58,99), and has been described as a reasonable approach for sustainable wildland development. Tourism offers an opportunity to earn foreign exchange and provide employment for local communities. Where tourism is developed properly, it may have a greater potential for generating local income than most traditional farming or ranching activities.

Option: Congress could direct AID to provide assistance for wildlife industry development in the Andean countries.

Efforts could include extension of production techniques, development of educational materials, and programs on potential benefits from farming or ranching and the needs for resource

conservation to support such development. Market identification and logistical needs to meet markets will be critical for industry development. Existing programs have tended to be production-oriented, as were the initial crop substitution efforts.

Coordination with other donors in the Andean region could contribute to developing an adequate support structure to handle transport and marketing opportunities for producers. Further, areas suitable for wildlife production may lie outside the current region of AID focus, yet are of interest to other donors.

Option: Congress could direct the U.S. General Accounting Office to review current U.S. trade regulations affecting wildlife and wildlife product imports in light of changing production methods.

Current regulations on wildlife imports have been based primarily on wild-gathering as opposed to established ranching and farming systems. Size and quantity restrictions suitable under these conditions may not be appropriate when trade is not affecting wild populations. A review of existing trade regulations on wildlife and wildlife products could evaluate potential adverse effects of existing regulations on developing wildlife industries.

Option: Congress could direct the U.S. Park Service, U.S. Forest Service, and U.S. Fish and Wildlife Service to give priority to Andean participants in their respective international nature tourism training programs.

Training programs offered by the U.S. Park Service and the U.S. Forest Service to foreign government officials currently focus on cultural and nature-based tourism and buffer zone management. Programs might be expanded to include training opportunities for professional guides, operators, and protected area staff to promote sustainable development of wildlands. Training should include land-use planning, environmental impact analysis, and tourism monitoring system development to improve the abilities of national governments to determine optimum tourism growth and sustainable tourism industries. Without these capabilities, the tourism industry is likely to be short-lived or encounter significant problems (7).

Issue: Aquatic resource development has received little attention in development efforts.

Potential exists to expand fishery production in the Andean region to offer an alternative to coca production and provide additional protein sources for national populations. The numerous lake and river systems contain a variety of harvestable organisms and, with application of appropriate technology, their productivity could be enhanced (47). Past fishery development projects have focused on high-value species and have for the most part been unsuccessful (37). Efforts to promote subsistence aquaculture in Bolivia were similarly unsuccessful. Nevertheless, international efforts could focus on artisanal fishermen to maximize occupational opportunities. Although fisheries may not be significant in some coca production regions, they could increase in importance within the context of national development.

Constraints to developing Andean fisheries are largely due to a lack of information on the extent and quality of the various resource systems, level of resource extraction, and fishermen themselves. Significant postharvest losses characterize existing artisanal fisheries due to shortfalls in handling, processing, and storage technologies and transport infrastructure (47).

Option: Congress could direct AID to conduct an aquatic resource inventory for the Andean countries to complement ongoing alternative development programs.

An aquatic resource inventory was contracted by AID in 1983. Although the survey focused on the Chapare region, it could be updated within the context of alternative development opportunities in general and similar efforts could be undertaken

for other coca-producing zones. A cooperative effort involving AID, the U.S. National Oceanic and Atmospheric Administration, International Sea-Grant Program, and the Andean countries could inventory existing aquatic resources and identify potential for improving production and harvest opportunities.

Alternatively, the Andean countries could take advantage of existing international expertise in aquatic resource management and development. International research organizations, such as the International Center for Living Aquatic Resource Management (ICLARM) that conducts research on tropical fishery management and production, could be tapped to assist in fishery development. Congress could promote such support through funding to ICLARM and increased collaboration with U.S. and Andean universities to conduct applied research on aquaculture development appropriate to the Andean countries.

■ Easing Transition to Alternative Livelihoods

Strategies to enhance coca-substitution efforts must address a wide variety of constraints from production to marketing. Producers are unlikely to cease coca production in favor of alternative crops or activities if they cannot be assured that a market exists and that the mechanisms for production, harvest, processing, and transport are in place. Nevertheless, the current support structure to sustain alternative livelihoods is lacking or inadequate in several areas: insufficient technology and technology transfer, lack of markets and marketing assistance, unavailable or unaffordable credit, and inadequate agroprocessing facilities and transportation systems (20,49).

A guaranteed sufficient quantity and quality of product must be available to interest international markets. This has been a difficulty to date, although efforts to expand production areas and increase use of modern production technology are underway. Promoting producer organizations offers an opportunity for smallholders to combine products to reach the necessary threshold level and, thereby, enter a market. Contract farming may provide a long-range prospect for assuring sufficient product quantity. While this approach can be very successful, it requires firm commitment on the part of agroprocessors and advanced agronomic understanding of crop requirements to achieve standard product quality.

Revision of credit programs could improve the opportunities for smallholders to obtain financing for entering legitimate production systems. Credit revisions could mimic current U.S. subsidy programs, providing loans to farmers at lower rates than those currently available in the Andean countries. Such an effort, with planned obsolescence as a goal, could be relatively short term, provide appropriate grace periods prior to repayment (i.e., allow for real production to occur), and perhaps augment or replace current coca eradication payments as a method of inducing change.

Issue: Existing terms for agricultural credit reduce its availability and discourage farmer investment in improved legitimate systems.

There are a number of disincentives to investment in agricultural production improvements in the Andean region; these stem largely from national economic and political conditions (e.g., rural poverty, risks to personal security). Yet, one mechanism open to U.S. and multilateral organizations to improve investment opportunities is to increase the availability and affordability of agricultural credit. Coca farmers tend to be smallholders, often without land title, few personal capital resources and, thus, little access to normal routes of credit. Recent actions by national governments have improved the outlook for gaining land title, but, bureaucratic constraints make the process slow.

Within the context of coca-substitution programs, opportunities for credit exist; however, evidence suggests insufficient attention has been paid to developing appropriate credit packages for coca farmers. Loan rates are high, in some cases collateral terms are difficult to meet, and

repayment schedules seem unrealistic for resource-poor farmers. Credit availability and affordability could be further attenuated under alternative development programs that expand the range of resources exploited, processed, and marketed.

Option: Congress could direct AID to amend the current credit Grant Agreement process to require the private voluntary organization (PVO) selected to include host country participation in developing credit terms.

Credit components of development projects are intended to improve opportunities for the target population to participate in the planned intervention. However, in some cases, credit terms restrict the ability of individuals to participate. For example, existing credit under CORDEP is made available through a grant agreement between AID and a private voluntary organization. However, the terms of credit are so high that credit is essentially unavailable for most smallholders (49). The existing Grant Agreement process used by AID could be amended to ensure host countries are adequately involved in development of credit eligibility requirements, loan rates, and repayment schedules.

Credit could be made available on a "suspensory loan" basis. This would allow a proportion of the capital sum normally repayable to be written off over 5 years, or some other term depending on the activity. The scheme could replace the current "payment" for coca eradication in the production phase and might also promote full private-sector involvement in the region's development. The cost to AID or national governments would be unchanged, but funds would be guaranteed to go into productive development, which is not assured under the present system (49).

Issue: Additional effort is needed to promote private investment in value-added processing.

Increased agricultural productivity is likely to do little for producers' economic well-being if they cannot effectively and efficiently apply postharvest technologies. Such applications will be necessary for alternative crops to become significant in terms of total agricultural exports. Success, in part, depends on establishing cost-effective postharvest processing, enhancing producer efficiency through reduced production costs and increased yields, and improving access to markets. The United States has provided support for processing facilities with respect to crop substitution efforts (table 1-3). Creating incentives for marketing these products could complement this investment. Loans to the private sector at realistic interest rates could promote entrepreneurial activity, and ultimately replace the need for AID and other contributing institutions to maintain the present high level of investment in infrastructure and agroindustry.

Option: Congress could direct the Overseas Private Investment Corporation (OPIC) to make the Andean region a priority.

OPIC promotes U.S. investment in developing countries by providing insurance against numerous risks, financing investment projects, and providing investment counseling. OPIC could develop a portfolio of opportunities in the Andean region to make available during counseling to encourage investment in the Andean region.

Increased investment could expand the array of employment opportunities in the Andean countries. However, if approached without sufficient planning, it could lead to haphazard growth and potentially complicate national economic development. Mechanisms for coordinating investment and development efforts could address this potential problem. For example, investments for agroprocessing of alternative crops could be coordinated with AID and national governments to ensure the production, processing, and transportation components are synchronized.

Option: Congress could reduce tariffs on value-added products from the Andean countries for 10 years to promote development of the processing industry.

Raw materials tend to be less valuable than processed materials, and processing activities can increase national employment opportunities. Typically, tariffs increase as products move through the processing chain (i.e., raw materials generally are subject to lower tariffs whereas processed items have higher tariffs). This aspect of U.S. trade policy has been suggested to reduce incentive for development of value-added industry in exporting nations. An examination of tariff policies on value-added products that might be exported by the Andean Nations is needed to determine if this policy adversely affects development of processing industries.

Value-added processing provides a multiplier opportunity for economic improvement. The United States could foster development of such industries by providing preferential treatment for value-added products associated with alternative development programs under the authority of the Andean Trade Preference Act. Such an action could be given a specified lifetime, long enough to allow industrial development and stabilization. As capability increases with experience, opportunities for Andean extension into other national and international markets could improve. Other countries that currently participate in alternative development might be induced to provide similar preferential opportunities.

Issue: Lack of infrastructure hinders success of alternative development efforts.

Inadequate infrastructure exists to support alternative development (e.g., paved roads, postharvest handling, storage facilities, agroprocessing plants). Yet, infrastructure development tends to be approached slowly because of the potential benefits that might accrue to coca transporters (i.e., roads are seen as potential landing strips for narcotics traffickers). Despite the fact that infrastructure development might initially contribute to the coca economy, alternative development and production cannot occur without the availability of adequate transportation and marketing routes.

Table 1-3—Value-Added Processing Investment in the Chapare Region

Industry	Source of finance	Dollar value capital	Comment
Coffee pre-processing	AID Project 412	$ 73,835	Started in 1980; Project 412 in 1990.
Latex pre-processing	INC - AID	32,900	Started in 1970; Project 412 in 1990.
Tea processing	China - 1984	108,000	In production.
	AID Project 412	166,728	
Glucose plant	Universidad Mayor de San Simon/UNDCP	307,174	Installation now underway.
Vinegar plant	Universidad Mayor de San Simon/UNDCP	175,298	Installation now underway.
Yuca and banana drying	AID Project 412	73,897	Not yet in operation.
Banana and kudzu drying	Universidad Mayor de San Simon	105,572	Starting production.
Mint oil extraction	AID Project 412		Starting production.
Lemon balm plant	AID Project 412	103,200	Working; low oil return per hectare.
Milk plant	Public Law 480 UNDCP	3,200,000	Project incorporates health aspects.

SOURCE: B. McD. Stevenson, "Post-Harvest Technologies to Improve Agricultural Profitability," contractor report prepared for the Office of Technology Assessment, May 1992.

However, significant fault has been linked to the methods and approaches used by U.S. and multinational development groups to develop land transportation routes in the tropics. Adverse environmental impacts associated with road-building in South America are highly visible (e.g., increased erosion, forest loss, poaching). Increased attention to developing mechanisms to mitigate such impacts should be included in project design and planning.

Option: Congress could direct AID to increase support for improving rural-urban trade networks, including roads, trucking, communications, and postharvest handling facilities.

Primary constraints to marketing alternative crops and products largely are linked to inadequacy or lack of infrastructure. Increasing capability to handle, process, and transport products to domestic and international markets could improve the ability of alternative resource exploitation activities to compete with coca. Increased attention would be needed to address the potential environmental impacts of infrastructure development, particularly road systems.

This is likely to be a long-term and costly endeavor, requiring a substantial increase in financial resources for assistance projects. Additional burdens on staff time could reduce efforts on production-related activities. Nevertheless, without ability to move products effectively and economically, alternative products are likely to remain at a disadvantage relative to coca.

Issue: Meeting food quality and safety requirements for agricultural exports can pose difficulties for some alternative crop producers.

Increased share in the international market can contribute to improving the economies of the Andean countries. Although crop substitution components of alternative development programs have focused on export markets, additional effort is needed to assist producers and processers to meet the quality and safety criteria required in the international marketplace (53).

The United States maintains a broad range of trade policies, ranging from import quotas and tariffs to complex food safety, sanitary, and phytosanitary requirements. Meeting these requirements is often difficult for developing nations. Assistance in developing capacity for meeting these standards could contribute to increased competiveness of Andean products. Assisting the Andean countries in improving their competitiveness in international markets could yield additional benefits by increasing their range of trading partners, encouraging foreign investment, and improving national food systems.

Option: Congress could direct the U.S. Department of Agriculture, Animal and Plant Health Inspection Service (APHIS) and Food Safety Inspection Service (FSIS) and the U.S. Department of Health and Human Services, Food and Drug Administration (FDA) to assist the Andean countries to improve the quality and safety of agricultural export products.

Authority for entering into international cooperative work exists primarily for APHIS, although FDA and FSIS possess limited authority for providing assistance. Current APHIS cooperative efforts are designed to assist developing countries meet U.S. inspection standards and quality requirements and thereby facilitate imports to the United States. Similar activities among FDA, FSIS, and the Andean countries could address other processing and marketing areas.

However, increasing agency responsibility without a commensurate increase in fiscal resources could come at the expense of the primary mission. Funding and responsibilities could be increased for a specified period to provide training and development of expertise in the Andean countries with periodic reports to Congress that evaluate the program's progress.

Issue: Lack of product quantity hinders smallholders from entering large, high-value agricultural markets.

Despite the existence of alternative crops, production remains at low levels that inhibits entrance into lucrative markets. Opportunities are needed to expand the production base to increase product availability or aggregate the production

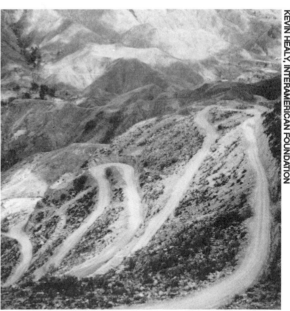

KEVIN HEALY, INTERAMERICAN FOUNDATION

Steep topography and difficult road conditions in many rural areas may hinder expanded production of renewable resource products by limiting easy access to inputs and markets.

of numerous smallholders. Strong producer organizations could overcome the problem small individual producers have in negotiating just prices for their product.

Option: Congress could direct AID to increase efforts to encourage producer organizations in the Andean region in order to reach product quantity thresholds for international marketing.

Lack of sufficient product quantity has constrained international marketing of some products of ongoing substitution programs. Producer organizations can provide an opportunity for groups of smallholders to consolidate production quantity to meet the needs of larger markets. For example, cocoa cooperatively produced and processed in the Alto Beni, Bolivia has been successful in competing in the international cocoa market. Ongoing alternative development efforts could be required to increase the focus on supporting producer groups for other alternative crops as well. However, increasing product quantity must be accompanied by ability to move these products quickly and efficiently to markets to realize benefits from such an effort.

Alternative Option: Congress could increase funding for the InterAmerican Foundation to expand efforts in grassroots development in the Andean region.

The InterAmerican Foundation (IAF) has extensive experience in grassroots development in South America and many of its projects have demonstrated success (e.g., El Ceibo, see chapter 4). IAF has provided assistance for a broad range of cooperative activities including agricultural, textile, and handicrafts and such economic diversification could generate benefits beyond increasing product quantity for outside markets.

BIOLOGICAL CONTROL OF COCA

Coca eradication is seen by some as a necessary precursor to successful alternative development (57), whereas others view it as a futile attempt to curtail cultivation of illegal narcotic crops. Regardless, quantitative goals of a coca eradication strategy in the Andean region do not exist. It has not been determined what level of coca removal is required to achieve domestic supply-reduction goals.

Interest in the potential benefits of a biological control (biocontrol) approach to coca reduction is evident. Biocontrol may offer the least environmentally damaging and longest-term means of reduction, although the current state of the technology suggests likely levels of reduction will be difficult to determine. Predation levels evident in laboratory experiments do not necessarily translate into similar effects in the field. Thus, biocontrol cannot guarantee specific results (47, 57). Further, as long as coca remains an attractive crop, it is likely farmers would take measures to protect their investment.

U.S. activities abroad that involve a regulated substance, such as herbicides or biocontrol agents, require an environmental analysis under Executive Order 12114—either an Environmental Impact Statement (EIS) or a less rigorous Concise Environmental Review (CER). However, the choice of document is at the agency's discretion. Experience with herbicide testing in Peru suggests significant sociopolitical constraints will be difficult to overcome without increased attention to rigorous testing and safety features for candidate coca control agents (13).

Several key technology factors hinder development of biocontrol agents: lack of inventories of potential agents, incomplete understanding of the efficacy of biocontrol (i.e., what level of reduction might be achieved through deployment of an agent), lack of understanding of what level of control is required to achieve "success," and lack of containment mechanisms. These needs could be addressed through a highly focused research and development effort, but, such an effort would be conditional on host country cooperation.

∎ Coordination and Cooperation

Coordination and cooperation among donor and host countries will be critical elements for effective research and development of a coca biocontrol program. Traditional biocontrol development methodology includes search and identification of existing predators, screening for host-specificity, and testing. The search activities could be undertaken in the target range and other locations; however, efficacy testing needs to be conducted in the implementation site or sites with similar environmental characteristics.

Issue: Insufficient coordination and cooperation with potential host countries in planning and design of eradication programs reduces support for implementation.

Experience with herbicide testing in Peru suggests significant government and public participation will be necessary for a successful coca eradication effort (56). Incorporating public review and comment periods, broad dissemination of environmental impact reviews and methodologies, and coordination and cooperative efforts with national groups will be key.

The United Nations International Drug Control Programme (UNDCP) investigations into potential narcotic crop control opportunities highlight host country involvement and agreement. Currently, UNDCP is evaluating biocontrol potential through expert group meetings. Any activities that might result from these investigations will be conditional on host country agreement and cooperation in all phases (50). The U.S. Department of State notes similar agreements would be sought for U.S. bilateral eradication activities in the Andean region but currently little likelihood exists for obtaining them (57).

Option: Congress could create a multinational commission, with representatives from donor and host countries, that would manage the research and development of a biocontrol agent for coca and the implementation of any coca reduction program.

Creation of a multinational commission could provide for substantial host country involvement in developing a biocontrol program and perhaps overcome public resistance that was evident in the earlier chemical control research. Such a commission could be composed of U.S., Andean, and other interested country scientists and narcotics control policymakers. The commission could be responsible for overseeing the development and implementation of a coca biocontrol program, including determining acceptable levels of risk, desirable levels of control, and necessary testing and screening precautions. Such an international commission would serve to improve the coordination and cooperation of the various donor and host countries.

However, developing a commission could be a lengthy process. Competing agendas among participants could make agreement and direction difficult. Setting a lead country or chairman could alleviate some difficulties, yet, it could also give the commission an appearance of being dominated by single-member concerns or motivations. Nonetheless, without such cooperation and coordination, research and testing of potential agents

is also likely to be slow. Further, without host country agreement for implementation, any research runs the risk of being moot even before it is completed.

■ Information Needs for Decisionmaking

Information to support wise decisionmaking is fundamental to undertake a biocontrol program. Basic informational needs include identification of:

- The level of reduction necessary to fulfill supply reduction goals,
- The role of coca in the Andean ecosystem, and
- Potential environmental impacts of a biocontrol program.

Issue: Lack of understanding of the level of reduction necessary to achieve supply reduction goals hinders establishment of clear target levels for eradication efforts.

The extent of coca reduction necessary to achieve supply reduction goals in the United States has not been identified and, given the questionable accuracy of historical data on coca production, it is likely to be difficult to derive. Nonetheless, setting goals and identifying mechanisms for reduction programs may require this type of information. For example, biological control of coca, while suggested as an environmentally benign alternative to chemicals, may only achieve low coca reduction in the short term. Information on how this level of reduction would affect overall cocaine availability could be used to determine feasibility of such an approach.

Option: Congress could direct the U.S. Department of Energy, through its National Laboratory System, to conduct a supply/demand analysis to identify the relative level of coca reduction required to achieve domestic supply reduction goals.

The National Laboratory System has substantial resources for computer modeling and could be directed to create an integrated computer model to simulate the effects of several reduction scenarios on U.S. cocaine supply. Although numerous variables confound precision of such a model, resulting information could identify high-low scenarios to provide bounds for coca reduction objectives.

However, such a model would likely be based on existing narcotics data, the accuracy of which is questionable. Data on coca and cocaine are notoriously suspect, leading to widely varying estimates of the area under production, area eradicated and newly planted, potential leaf yields, and conversion rates from leaf to paste and cocaine hydrochloride. Thus, existing data used in such an analysis could lead to a ''garbage in-garbage out'' product yielding little new insight. Improved data collection could address this problem, although it would likely be a lengthy process. Alternatively, in the near term results could be given a ''percent confidence'' rating while new data-gathering activities were undertaken.

Issue: Little is known of the role of coca in the Andean ecology. Thus, determining potential adverse impacts of coca eradication is difficult.

Generating support for biocontrol efforts will require placing adequate attention on addressing the concerns of the potential host countries. Environmental concerns have been highlighted in previous activities and are likely to continue to play an important role. Information on the role of coca in the complex Andean environment would be important in determining the feasibility and appropriateness of a biocontrol program. This information could provide needed background information to help national government decisionmaking on the biocontrol of coca.

Option: Congress could direct the U.S. Department of Interior, Fish and Wildlife Service to conduct ecological studies of coca's role in the Andean environment cooperatively with host country counterparts.

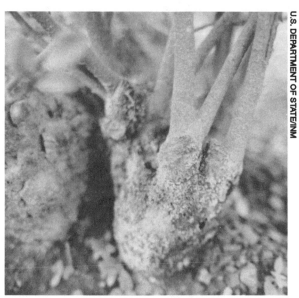

Some fungi and lichens are natural coca pests that may significantly reduce the plants' productive life. Here, lichen covers the stem of a coca shrub.

Financial and technical support could be provided for a comprehensive study of coca in the Andean environment. Cooperative efforts among U.S. and Andean scientists could identify the range of coca species of interest and the role wild counterpart plays in local ecology. This information would be a logical counterpart to potential host screening studies on candidate agents and could further be used to determine potential areas of concern with biocontrol activities. However, such a study would require site visits in hazardous areas (e.g., Alto Huallaga) for observing and characterizing coca ecology. Substantial efforts would be required, in some cases, to assure participant safety in such a study.

Issue: The current environmental assessment process applied to U.S. activities in foreign countries is inadequate to identify the broad range of potential environmental impacts that might be associated with biocontrol efforts.

Despite government agreements during the 1987 herbicide testing in Peru, local populations and environmental groups felt inadequate opportunity existed for their input and discussion (56). The resulting public outcry over the potential adverse environmental effects of the tested herbicides was significant. Similar situations are likely to occur with a biocontrol program if inadequate attention is given to local participation in the environmental impact review process.

Determining potential environmental impacts of a biocontrol program will require a rigorous assessment effort. The instrument under which these environmental reviews currently are required (Executive Order 12114) allows agency discretion to undertake a Concise Environmental Review rather than a more comprehensive Environmental Impact Statement is as required under National Environment Policy Act (NEPA) for domestic actions (13).

The legal status of NEPA with respect to the extraterritorial environmental impacts of Federal programs remains in doubt. However, it is clear Federal agencies involved in the proposed coca eradication program will be required to prepare some kind of environmental evaluation, either under NEPA or Executive Order 12114. Experience demonstrates the value of this environmental analysis can be enhanced if the relatively rigorous procedural requirements of NEPA are followed. In particular, the agency should ensure full public participation throughout the assessment process, environmental assessment early in the decision-making process, full discussion of alternatives and mitigation techniques, consultation with experts within and outside of government, and that the results of the assessment are meaningfully considered by involved decisionmakers.

Option: Congress could choose to expand the authority of the National Environment Policy Act to include U.S. coca control activities in foreign countries.

A rigorous environmental review process could alleviate some of the public resistance to coca control efforts. The Environmental Impact Statement (EIS) process required domestically could be an appropriate process for examining the full array of potential impacts of a coca eradication method. However, expanding the U.S. Environmental Protection Agency's responsibility to include international EISs, would increase agency workloads substantially and would likely require a concomitant increase in staff and financial resources. Further, technical expertise for outlining requirements and reviewing EIS's would be needed and could create a lengthier process. Changes in the process may be necessary to account for environmental differences between U.S. and Andean environments.

■ Technological Feasibility

Biocontrol methodologies exist, but there are considerable technological constraints to rapid implementation. Investigations into possible herbicides continue to be the primary focus at the Federal research and development level (45). Thus, if a biocontrol program is to be pursued, an extensive research and development period could be needed. Ongoing research is classified and conducted by the U.S. Department of Agriculture, Agricultural Research Service and cooperating agencies.

Option: Congress could direct the U.S. Department of Agriculture to balance funding resources for crop control research between herbicides and biocontrol.

Currently, biocontrol research is treated as part of an overall eradication method research program. Division of funds and activities are agency-discretionary and largely focused on chemical research. Nevertheless, balanced attention to both opportunities could be undertaken to assure neither development is disadvantaged if host country agreement is forthcoming.

Alternative Option: Congress could place responsibility for coordinating a broad-based national research and development program for biocontrol with the Office of National Drug Control Policy, Counterdrug Technology Assessment Center (ONDCP/CTAC).

There are numerous public and private research resources that could be appropriate to undertake or participate in biocontrol research. Currently, responsibility for development, oversight, and coordination lies with the U.S. Department of Agriculture. Responsibility for a broad-based research and development effort could be placed with ONDCP/CTAC, which holds responsibility for counternarcotic enforcement research of which eradication is one aspect. Coordination with the numerous Federal agencies appropriate to the preconditions for development (e.g., USDA, DOE, DOS) could be undertaken by ONDCP/CTAC to expedite efforts. However, recent Administration actions have downsized ONDCP significantly and without concomitant efforts to rebuild the Office, such a task might not be feasible.

Alternatively, Congress could choose to halt new programs for coca biocontrol research and continue existing programs under maintenance budgets conditional on the outcome of the UNDCP efforts in biocontrol. U.S. intellectual and financial resources could be directed to assist the United Nations effort if host country agreement were obtained. Such an approach would ensure the program was multilateral and assure the Andean countries of an international forum within which their concerns or grievances over biocontrol or coca eradication in general could be heard.

CHAPTER 1 REFERENCES

1. Alford, D., "The Geoecology and Agroecosystems of the Northern and Central Andes," contractor report prepared for the Office of Technology Assessment, March 1991.
2. Alvarez, E., "Opportunities and Constraints to Source Reduction of Coca: The Peruvian and Bolivian Macro-Economic Context," contractor report prepared for the Office of Technology Assessment, March 1992.
3. Alvarez, E.H., "Reasons for the Expansion of Coca Exports in Peru," paper presented at the Congressional Research Service Panel on Cocaine Production, Eradication, and The Environment: Policy, Impact, and Options," U.S. Congress, Library of Congress, Congressional Research Service, Washington, DC, Feb. 14, 1990.
4. Andreas, P. "Peru's Addiction to Coca Dollars," *The Nation* Ap. 16, 1990, p. 515, In: McClintock, 1992.
5. Andreas, P., Brown, E.C., Blachman, M.J., and Sharpe, K.E., "Dead-End Drug Wars," *Foreign Policy*, 1992, pp. 106-128.
6. Ardila, P., "Beyond Law Enforcement: Narcotics and Development," *The Panos Institute*, February 1990, pp.1-8.
7. Ashton, R.E., Jr., "Potential Use of Neotropical Wildlife in Sustainable Development," contractor paper prepared for the Office of Technology Assessment, December 1991.
8. Bagley, B.M., "Opportunities and Constraints to Source Reduction of Coca in Colombia: The Political Context," contractor paper prepared for the Office of Technology Assessment, April 1992.
9. Bagley, B.M., "Dateline Drug Wars: Colombia: The Wrong Strategy," *Foreign Policy*, No. 77, pp.154-171, winter 1989-1990.
10. Bagley, B.M., "Colombia and the War on Drugs," *Foreign Affairs*, fall 1988, pp. 70-92.
11. Bray, W., and Dollery, C., "Coca Chewing and High Altitude Stress: A Spurious Correlation," *Current Anthropology* 24(3):269-282, 1983, In: Reeve, 1991.
12. Chavez, A., "Andean Agricultural Research and Extension Systems and Technology Transfer Activities: Potential Mechanisms to Enhance Crop Substitution Efforts in Bolivia, Colombia, and Peru," contractor paper prepared for the Office of Technology Assessment, December 1991.
13. Christensen, E., "The Environmental Impact Process and Coca Eradication Programs," contractor paper prepared for the Office of Technology Assessment, August 1991.
14. Collett, M., The Cocaine Connection: Drug Trafficking and Inter-American Relations, *Headline Series* Foreign Policy Association, No. 290, fall, 1989.
15. *Colombia Exporta*, "Colombia and the World Silk Market," 1991, pp. 44-49.
16. Conway, P., "Silk for Life Project Proposal: Common Sense Crop Substitution in Colombia," Milwaukee, Wisconsin, January 1991.

17. Cuellar, F.H., private consultant, personal communication, Santafe de Bogotá, Colombia, September 1992.

18. Cuellar, F.H., "Incidencia del cultivo de coca en la economia Colombiana y comparación con los casos de Peru y Bolivia," Instituto Interamericano de Cooperación para la Agricultura, Santafe de Bogotá, Colombia, 1991.

19. DeFranco, M. and R. Godoy, "Economic Consequences of Cocaine Production in Bolivia: Historical, Local, and Macroeconomic Perspectives." (Boston, MA: Harvard University, 1990).

20. DeVincenti, J., "Infrastructural Needs to Support Agricultural Alternatives to Coca in Bolivia," contractor paper prepared for the Office of Technology Assessment, December 1991.

21. Development Alternatives, Inc., "Cochabamba Regional Development Project (CORDEP) Bolivia: Technical Proposal," Submitted to AID under RFP No. Bolivia 92-001, Bethesda, MD, January 21, 1992.

22. Dourojeanni, M.J., "The Environmental Impact of Coca Cultivation and Cocaine Production in the Peruvian Amazon Basin," paper presented at the Congressional Research Service Panel on Cocaine Production, Eradication, and The Environment: Policy, Impact, and Options," U.S. Congress, Library of Congress, Congressional Research Service, Washington, DC, Feb. 14, 1990.

23. The Economist, "Getting Away with It," 323(755):44, April 18, 1992.

24. The Economist, "The Cocaine Economies: Latin America's Killing Fields," October 8, 1988, pp. 21-24.

25. Hatfield, L.Z., "Bolivia's New Legislation Attracts Foreign Investment," Business America March 23, 1992, pp. 19-20.

26. Healy, K., InterAmerican Foundation, Rosslyn, VA, personal communication, September 1992.

27. Healy, K., "Opportunities and Constraints to Source Reduction of Coca in Bolivia: The Political Context," contractor paper prepared for the Office of Technology Assessment, March 1992.

28. Healy, K., "The Boom Within the Crisis: Some Effects of Foreign Cocaine Markets on Bolivian Rural Society and Economy," D. Pacini and C. Franquemont (eds.), Coca and Cocaine: Effects on People and Policy in Latin America, Cultural Survival Report 23 (Peterborough, NH: Transcript Printing Company, 1986) pp. 101-143.

29. Jacoby, T., Miller, M., and Sandza, R., "A Choice of Poisons," Newsweek, December 1988, p. 62.

30. Kraljevic, I., "Migration, Social Change, and the Coca/Cocaine Economy in Bolivia," contractor paper prepared for the Office of Technology Assessment, February 1992.

31. Larrain, F., and Sachs, J.D., "International Financial Relations," Paredes, C. and J. Sachs (eds.), Peru's Path to Recovery (Washington, DC: Brookings Institution, 1991) In: Alvarez, 1992.

32. Mardon, M., "The Big Push," Sierra, November/December 1988, pp. 66-75.

33. McCaffrey, D., "Biodiversity Conservation and Forest Management as Alternatives to Coca Production in Andean Countries," contractor paper prepared for the Office of Technology Assessment, August 1991.

34. McClintock, C., "Opportunities and Constraints to Source Reduction of Coca in Peru: The Political Context," contract paper prepared for the Office of Technology Assessment, September 1991.

35. Morales, E., "Coca and Cocaine Economy and Social Change in the Andes of Peru," Economic Development and Cultural Change 35(1):143-161, October 1986.

36. O'Carroll, P., "Crop Substitution," International Drug Report, United Nations, Geneva, February, 1978, p. 4.

37. Orlove, B., and LeVieil, D., "Some Doubts About Trout: Fisheries Development Projects in Lake Titicaca," In: B. Orlove, M. Foley, and T. Love (eds.), State, Capital, and Rural Society: Anthropological Perspectives on Political Economy in Mexico and the Andes (Boulder CO: Westview Press, 1989) In: Schroeder, 1991.

38. Painter, M., Institute for Development Anthropology, personal communication, August 1992.

39. Painter, M., and Bedoya-Garland, E., "Institutional Analysis of the Chapare Regional Development Project (CRDP) and the Upper Huallaga Special Project (PEAH)," contractor paper prepared for the Office of Technology Assessment, July 1991.

40. Plowman, T., "Coca Chewing and the Botanical Origins of Coca (Erythroxylum spp.) in South America," In: D. Pacini and C. Franquemont

(eds.), *Coca and Cocaine: Effects on People and Policy in Latin America*, Cultural Survival Report 23, (Peterborough, NH: Transcript Printing Co., 1986).

41. Rao, C.B.J., "Sericulture and Silk Production in Bolivia, Peru, Ecuador, and Colombia," paper submitted to Corporacion Andina de Fomento, Caracas, Venezuela, January 31, 1990.

42. Raymond, J.S., "A View from the Tropical Forest," R. Keatinge (ed.), *Peruvian Prehistory: An Overview of Pre-Inca and Inca Society*, (Cambridge, England: Cambridge University Press, 1988); in Reeve, 1991.

43. Reeve, M.E., "Traditional Roles and Uses of Coca Leaf in Andean Society," contractor paper prepared for the Office of Technology Assessment, July 1991.

44. Rosen, D., "Potential for Biological Control of Coca," contractor paper prepared for the Office of Technology Assessment, November 1991.

45. Rosenquist, E., U.S. Department of Agriculture, Agricultural Research Service, personal communication, August 1992.

46. Ross, P.R., Executive Officer, Crocodile Specialist Group, personal communication, 1991, In: Ashton, 1991.

47. Schroeder, R., "Fishery/Aquatic Resources in Bolivia, Colombia, and Peru: Production Systems and Potential as Alternative Livelihoods," contractor paper prepared for the Office of Technology Assessment, October 1991.

48. Smith, E., "Growth vs. Environment," *Business Week*, May 11, 1992, pp. 66-75.

49. Stevenson, B.McD., "Post-Harvest Technologies to Improve Agricultural Profitability," contractor paper prepared for the Office of Technology Assessment, May 1992.

50. Szendri, K., United Nations Drug Control Programme, Vienna, Austria, personal communication, August 1992.

51. Thoumi, F., "Opportunities and Constraints to Source Reduction of Coca: The Colombian Macro-Economic Context," contractor paper prepared for the Office of Technology Assessment, April 1992.

52. Tosi, J.A., Jr., "Integrated Sustained Yield Management of Primary Tropical Wet Forest: A Pilot Project in the Peruvian Amazon," Tropical Science Center, Costa Rica, 1991, In: McCaffrey, 1991.

53. Turner, E., "Primer on U.S. Agricultural and Trade Policies: Opportunities and Constraints to Crop Substitution in the Andean Nations," contractor paper prepared for the Office of Technology Assessment, February 1992.

54. United Nations Commission on Narcotic Drugs, Report of the Expert Group Meeting on Environmentally Safe Methods for the Eradication of Illicit Narcotic Plants, meeting held in Vienna December 4 - 8, 1989, E/CN.7/1990/CRP.7, Dec. 14, 1989.

55. U.S. Agency for International Development, "Lasting Solutions to the Transnational Drug Problem: The Role of Development in the Counter-Drug War," July 1991, p. 21

56. U.S. Congress, Library of Congress, Congressional Research Service, *Cocaine Production, Eradication, and The Environment: Policy, Impact, and Options*, seminar held on February 14, 1990, Washington, DC.

57. U.S. Congress, Office of Technology Assessment, Biological Control of Coca, Workshop held January 23, 1992, Washington, DC.

58. U.S. Congress, Office of Technology Assessment, Agricultural Alternatives to Coca, Workshop held September 30 - October 1, 1991, Washington, DC.

59. U.S. Department of State, Bureau of International Narcotics Matters (INM), *International Narcotics Control Strategy Report* (Washington, D.C.: U.S. Department of State, 1992).

60. U.S. Department of the Treasury, "Enterprise for the Americas Fact Sheet," Washington, DC, September 30, 1990.

61. Villachica, H., "Crop Diversification in Bolivia, Colombia, and Peru: Potential to Enhance Agricultural Production," contractor paper prepared for the Office of Technology Assessment, April 1992.

62. Werner, D.I., "The Rational Use of Green Iguanas," *Neotropical Wildlife Use and Conservation* (Chicago, IL: Chicago University Press, 1991) In: Ashton, 1991.

Factors Influencing Coca Reduction Initiatives | 2

T he Andean region is complex in its geology, ecology, and cultural history. This complexity precludes simple or broadly applicable coca substitution strategies. Successful, cooperative, counternarcotics efforts among the United States and Andean countries require careful consideration of all of these factors. This chapter examines the biophysical, cultural, socio-political, and economic conditions that may affect the success of efforts to reduce coca cultivation in Bolivia, Peru, and Colombia.

GEOECOLOGY OF THE NORTHERN AND CENTRAL ANDES

Clear understanding of the biological and physical environments in the Andean region is critical for appropriate design of projects to eradicate or offer alternatives to coca. The natural environmental diversity of Bolivia, Peru, and Colombia results largely from the abrupt altitude changes in the Andes mountain system (2). There is a vertical succession of ecozones, ranging from rainforest and desert at the lowest levels to mountain tundra, snow, and ice at the highest (104). The enormous latitudinal span (approximately from 10 degrees north to 40 degrees south along the western edge of South America) and longitudinal breadth (approximately between 80 degrees west and 60 degrees west) also make for considerable variations in climate, soil, vegetation, and land-use (104). Thus, the local and regional diversity of biophysical environments requires that any project be site-specific (2).

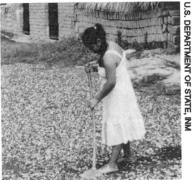

U.S. DEPARTMENT OF STATE, INM

■ Andean Geography and Geology

The Andean *cordillera* (mountain range) divides the South American continent into Atlantic and Pacific drainage systems and is part of a great band of active crustal uplift that circles the Pacific Ocean. The Andes are among the youngest mountains on Earth, and consequently, soils are generally shallow, stony, and undifferentiated (104). Extensive volcanic and earthquake activity has characterized the region's geologic history, and this activity continues today (84). Any technologies dependent on the land's surficial characteristics—e.g., road-building or soil identification and use—must deal with the geologic variability, as well as the instability of the area due to ongoing mountain-building (2).

The Andean *cordillera* is made up of many interwoven ranges, which include high intermontane plateaus, basins, and valleys. Colombia, Peru, and Bolivia are located within the Northern and Central Andean ranges (figure 2-1).

The Northern Andes extend from coastal Venezuela and Colombia to northern Peru and contain several broad ecosystems falling into four altitudinal belts, the highest and coldest of which rises to 4,500 meters above sea level (masl). The Northern Andes subregion is distinguished from the rest of the region by higher relative humidity and greater climatic symmetry between the eastern and western flanks of the range (2).

The three main warm ecosystems of the Northern subregion are the upper *montaña* (mountain) slopes, the intermediate-level coffee belt, and the foothills. The upper *montaña* slopes, with their vast, dense forests, have experienced little adverse human impact. However, in some areas, deforestation may have contributed to increased stream flow and erosion. Precipitation is heavy, averaging 4,000 mm per year, and physical and chemical weathering and erosion can be intense. The coffee belt, immediately below the upper *montaña*, has been profoundly modified by coffee plantation agriculture. The best coffee soils are developed on volcanic ash, which is sensitive to erosion. The low Andean foothills are relatively humid with annual rainfall of at least 2,000 mm and a mean annual temperature of at least 24 degrees C. Low-productivity, lateritic soil covers much of the area, particularly in cleared fields where maize, manioc (*yuca*), plantain, and cocoa are cultivated.

The Central Andes extend from northern Peru to the Antofagasta Province in Chile and Catamarca Province in Argentina. They are characterized by a succession of agricultural zones with varied climatic conditions along the mountains' flanks and by large, high-altitude plateaus above 3,500 masl, which do not occur in the Northern Andes. Variously called *puna* or *altiplano*, these plateaus, separated and surrounded by higher mountains, were the heartland of the pre-Columbian Andean empire (2).

The soil fertility of the northern *altiplano* generally is good (147). The western Central Andean ranges are relatively arid with desert-like soils, whereas the eastern ranges are more humid and have more diverse soils (26). The eastern slopes of the Central Andes in many ways are similar to the wet forests of the Northern Andes. Unlike the Northern Andes, however, these slopes have a dry season (2).

The *altiplano* and *páramo* (heathland) are broken by river valleys. Cutting deep into the lofty plateaus, these valleys descend 2,000 to 3,000 meters, often in a few tens of kilometers, and create areas of highly distinctive relief, climate, habitat, and agricultural uses. The upper ends of the valleys merge with the high plateaus. Their middle slopes and alluvial plains are temperate, referred to as *kichwa* by indigenous Andean peoples. Lower parts of the valleys, the

Figure 2-1—Generalized Geographic Map of Andean Coca-Producing Countries

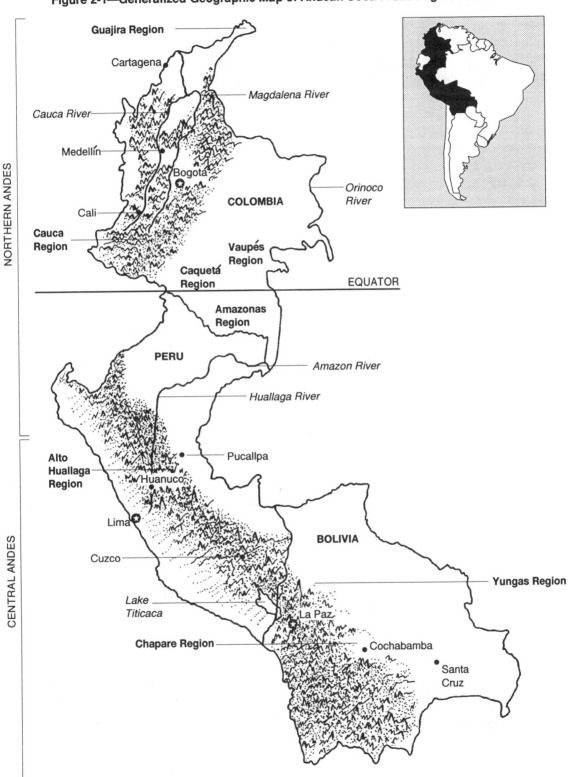

SOURCE: Office of Technology Assessment, 1993.

yungas, can be wet or hot and dry as a result of rain-shadow.[1]

Unlike regions of gentle topography (e.g., the central United States or Amazon basin), where regional climatic variation can be determined from a few widely spaced measurements, regions with extreme topographic and climatic features (e.g., the Andean *cordillera*) make regional projections difficult (2). For example, while air temperature generally decreases with increasing altitude, variability of mountain topography can produce much lower-than-expected air temperatures at any altitude.

Some general climatic patterns, however, are discernible in the Andes. For example, with increasing distance south of the equator the seasonality of precipitation increases, whereas the total annual amount generally decreases. Humidity commonly increases with increasing altitude, but only to some intermediate altitude (e.g., approximately 1,000 masl on the eastern slope of the Ecuadoran Andes at the equator) above which it declines (92). The variability of mountain terrain also affects precipitation, such that conditions of extreme wetness and aridity may exist in close proximity. Annual temperatures in upper reaches of many Andean valleys may average 8 degrees C with frequent nocturnal frosts, whereas lower levels may average as high as 24 degrees C, with no frost. Related to this temperature gradient is a pattern of greater rainfall at the valley heads, and less rain at lower altitudes, resulting in part from mountain rain-shadow effect (2).

The weather patterns of the Andean *cordillera* and Amazon basin in general reflect movements of high and low-pressure "cells" associated with the Intertropical Convergence Zone, a low-pressure trough that moves further north and south on a seasonal basis. Precipitation is high throughout the year in the highlands and on the coast in the Northern Andes. South of central Ecuador, at about the latitude of Guayaquil, coastal aridity increases, culminating in the Atacama desert of northern Chile. In the Central Andes, highland precipitation is seasonal, and amounts are approximately one-half those measured in the northern Andes. The aridity of the Central Andean coastal zone is the result of the drying effect of the cold Pacific Humboldt current, and the southern Pacific high-pressure cell (59). Much of the southern portion of the Central Andes in Bolivia is also arid. The dry season causes soil moisture deficits and diminished stream flow for a part of each year.

■ Andean Agroecosystems[2]

At the regional or macroscale level, vegetation patterns in the Northern and Central Andes tend to reflect climatic zones determined by latitude and altitude. At the local or mesoscale level, however, this correspondence becomes less precise, as local variations in soil type, slope, drainage, climate, and human intervention come into play.

Most of the Northern Andes can support lush vegetation because of the high humidity and relatively high temperatures. Tropical rainforests and other types of evergreen and deciduous forests dominate this subregion, with considerable symmetry of vegetation types on the eastern and western flanks of the mountains. The lowest slopes support agriculture year-round, producing, for example, bananas, *yuca,* and cocoa.

Aridity reduces vegetation growth and agricultural options in some areas of the Central Andes. The Atacama desert region of the coastal plain, for example, is one of the driest places on Earth. However, the lower valley floors of the Central Andean western ranges, and the lands at the foot

---

[1] Rain-shadow occurs when moist easterly winds lose their moisture as they pass over the high, cool peaks and plateaus. As the air descends from the *puna* or *páramo*, the temperature rises and its moisture-bearing capacity increases, resulting in a desert condition below 1,500 masl in most interior valleys of the Andes (2).

[2] *Agroecosystem* is a term used to describe natural ecosystems modified by human agricultural activities (2).

of the mountain slopes, along the coast, are densely populated and support intensive, high-yield cultivation of cash crops including maize, rice, cotton, tobacco, garden vegetables, peppers, sugar cane, and fruit trees. Irrigation water is provided by the numerous streams that drain the western slopes. The eastern slopes of the central Andes have vegetation types similar to that of the northern Andes (2).

A significant portion of the Andean population lives within the Central Andes' eastern valley systems and *altiplano*. Settlements and farming are concentrated toward the upper end of the inter-Andean valleys for several reasons: the primary subsistence crops are acclimatized to these altitudes; drought and frost are less common than in the lower and upper altitudinal extremes; and access to the grazing lands of the *puna* and *páramo* is relatively easy (31).

ANDEAN AGRICULTURAL PRODUCTION

Humans first altered the Andean landscape some 12,000 to 15,000 years ago as hunters and gatherers (146). By 3,000 to 4,000 years ago, the original nomadic, hunting and gathering way of life had been supplanted by a village-based agro-pastoral economy (95). Pre-Columbian agricultural productivity was achieved largely through specialized adaptation of food crops to the myriad of local microenvironments. Indigenous farmers planted numerous varieties of each crop in a single field, or in neighboring fields, so that if one variety performed poorly, several others might provide an adequate yield (42). Virtually all productive land was used for crop production. These two strategies led to a sufficiency of food supplies throughout the Andean highlands.

From the onset of human occupation, the varied Andean environments led to vertical arrangements of settlements, production regimes, migrations, and political organizations. Patterns of verticality derive from the classification of different agricultural zones, based on their climatic conditions (31,32,107,145). For example,

the inhabitants of the Uchucmarca valley in Northern Peru recognize seven agro-climatic units that are distinguished according to altitude, moisture, temperature, vegetation, land tenure, crop assemblages, and agricultural technologies (31,32).

The Spanish conquest of the Andean region produced severe dislocations in the indigenous pattern of resource exploitation. The arriving Spanish found a highland Andean agricultural complex that focused on the intensive hoe cultivation of maize, squash, beans, and hot peppers (chiles). Fiber was secured from the *cabuya,* cultivated on the drier leeward sides of the mountain valleys, and from American cotton, cultivated in the lowlands, along with coca and sweet manioc (21). The principal root crop was the small Andean potato.

The Spanish developed urban centers and introduced exotic plants and animals in the Northern and Central Andes. Forced clustering of the semi-dispersed indigenous settlement patterns, exploitation of the large resident labor force, and establishment of the Iberian grazing ethic also followed. Large landed estates (*haciendas*) were developed in the *altiplano* belt for animal husbandry. In the hot, humid *yungas*, land clearing was facilitated by the introduction of iron tools, and maize, sugar-cane, and pigs were raised for urban markets (2).

Displacement of indigenous people to marginal lands that began in the colonial period continued under subsequent regimes. Invariably, the best lands of the region (e.g., flat, fertile valley bottomlands) were claimed by the existent rulers, and often were designated pasture for livestock. Many indigenous people who had lived on these lands were forced to move to remote, inhospitable, forested slopes. Others were reduced to landless laborers, or *colonas*, on the *haciendas*. Thus, throughout the Northern Andes, the logical spatial relationships of agricultural production were reversed. The broad, level bottom lands so suitable to the cultivation of staple foodstuffs were given over to pasture and meat production, or commercial crops such as sugar cane destined for foreign markets. Highland plots, more suitable as pasture or forest, were cultivated, with consequential damage to the natural vegetation. Harvests were meager and had to be transported, on the back of either man or beast, to distant urban markets (43).

Competition for land between *haciendas* and peasant communities became a common and sometimes violent feature of rural society in the Central Andes. The concentration of land ownership, uneven population distribution and land-use, feudal subjugation of many peasants, and rise of a large pool of displaced, landless peasants created a legacy of inequality that still prevails in the region (19,61,141). The dichotomy between the urban dweller, or civil servant of Spanish descent, and the rural Indian peasant—between the lowland centers of power and the powerless inhabitants of the eastern Andean slopes—persists, with significant implications for any attempts to alter agricultural practices in coca-producing regions (2).

In more recent times, the so-called "green revolution" has had mixed blessings. For instance, production of some crops (e.g., banana, rice, and maize) and of poultry has increased dramatically in the Andean region (16,78,82). However, this increased agricultural production occurred among the large landowners of the region, with few benefits accruing to the impoverished subsistence sector (43).

A significant modern-era land-use change has been the opening of eastern lowland regions in the Northern Andes for agricultural use. For centuries, fear of disease and reluctance to leave the secure highland social structure deterred highlander settlement of lowlands. With their worsening economic plight in modern times, however, an ever-increasing number of highland Indians are moving eastward along every major river valley (46). In spite of endemic shortages of good roads, legally recognized land titles, credit, education, electricity, and modern health and sanitation services, highlander colonization of the Orinoco

and Amazon basins serves the interests of the individuals and nations involved and can be expected to continue (43).

Today, the basic pattern of Pre-Columbian land use and agricultural practices, as modified by the Spanish, remains more or less intact in the Central Andes. Commercial agriculture tends to be concentrated in flat, lowland areas, at least in part due to high transportation costs and difficulties applying mechanization to farming on valley and mountain slopes. This mitigates in favor of mountain crops that are hand-cultivated, easily harvested, and easily transported with low spoilage, one example being coca.

COCA-PRODUCING ECOSYSTEMS

Potentially, 10 to 20 percent of the Andes mountain range (7,250 kilometers in length) is suitable for coca production, and these areas are concentrated in an altitudinal belt from sea level to about 2,000 masl, extending from Colombia to Bolivia. Coca grows best at temperatures averaging above 15 degrees C, with high precipitation, but does not require evenly distributed rainfall. Coca can be grown in a wide variety of soils, but is sensitive to poor drainage and intolerant of frost or drought. In addition, a wide range of soil pH levels can be tolerated by coca (i.e., *E.coca* var. *coca*, the most important source of cocaine, will tolerate pH levels as low as 4.3 and as high as 8.0 (54)).

Coca cultivation is concentrated in and along deep valleys that cut into the eastern slopes of the Northern and Central Andes, and coca is the most important agricultural product of the hot, often dry lower reaches of the *yungas* (31). Other warm ecosystems with a potential for coca growth are found between sea level and 2,200 masl in the northern Andes, which are characterized by a sub-Andean or tropical *montaña* at higher limits and wet forest at lower levels. These regions are heavily populated, particularly in the "coffee belt" (2).

Coca bushes are stripped of their leaves up to six times a year, and the leaves are then dried and transported to the highlands by porters, pack animals, or trucks. Some highland communities control territory in the coca-producing valleys, and may establish satellite communities there. Several times each year, they journey to these fields to tend their coca, or to work as laborers in the fields of relatives and fellow villagers (107).

Much of the land involved in coca production is sloping, and its suitability for other agricultural uses will depend on factors such as slope steepness, soil type, and water availability. Water quality problems now exist in some Andean watersheds, largely as a result of discharges associated with mining and agricultural activities, and high rates of natural erosion from the region's geologic instability and climatic variability (102,114). The extent to which new agricultural practices may contribute to these water quality problems can only be determined by basin-specific monitoring programs in the affected watersheds (2).

■ Environmental Impacts of Coca Cultivation and Processing

The adverse environmental consequences of coca cultivation and processing often are cited as a problem in the Andean nations (14,53). Because most data are anecdotal, and on-site research is problematic, the degree of environmental damage that directly or indirectly can be attributed to coca cultivation and cocaine processing remains undetermined. However, the few available information sources point to significant differences between damage from coca cultivation and cocaine processing.

COCA CULTIVATION

Little is known about the role of coca in the ecology of the Andean rainforest, or about the environmental impacts of coca cultivation. Impacts are likely to differ from one growing area to another, given variations in ecology, culture, and cultivation practices. Today, no formal comparative study exists of even the most notable coca-growing regions (i.e., the Alto Huallaga of

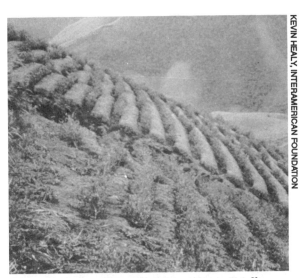

KEVIN HEALY, INTERAMERICAN FOUNDATION

Terracing is a traditional, more environmentally benign means of growing coca still practiced most notably in the Bolivian Yungas.

Peru and the Chapare of Bolivia). Despite this lack of information, three factors seem key to determining coca cultivation's environmental impact: geographic area, types of external inputs and frequency and intensity of their use, and cultivation practices.

Experts argue that deforestation is the most visible damage caused by coca cultivation. Some older coca production regions (e.g., the Yungas, Bolivia) continue to produce coca along well-constructed terraces that reduce soil erosion potential. However, these practices are not employed in the newer coca-growing regions. In many areas coca is grown on unterraced plots with no barrier to soil loss from heavy rains. Migrants to these regions may use slash-and-burn practices to clear forested areas. Between the early 1970s and the late 1980s, an estimated 700,000 hectares (about 2,700 square miles) of Amazon rainforest were deforested as a direct or indirect result of coca cultivation (53).

The potential consequences of deforestation associated with coca cultivation are numerous. Habitat loss and decreased species diversity are often a direct result of destruction of tropical forest. In addition, the rise in soil temperatures and decrease in organic matter and soil nutrients, resulting from slash-and-burn practices, can make the area hostile to revegetation. In the Alto Huallaga in Peru, tropical forest burning causes extensive air pollution, and smoke layers have been observed covering the valley in August and September (14).

The most devastating effect of deforestation in the Andean region may be extensive soil erosion. Clearing tropical forest areas for agricultural expansion without investing in soil conservation can severely disrupt biological productivity and start a self-reinforcing cycle of degradation. For example, soil erosion reduces soil fertility, which in turn can reduce growth of cover plants, leading to more soil erosion and to rapid depletion of diversity as the site becomes suitable for fewer species.

The cultivation practices, tillage and weed control, can increase the potential for soil erosion. Tillage loosens the soil and leads easily to erosion. Whether coca seeds or seedlings are planted, the soil remains largely unprotected from heavy rains. Furthermore, the soil around the coca plants is weeded regularly to reduce competition for the minimal nutrients available. These practices leave the soil in coca plots almost continually bare during the production years, and the results are increased soil temperatures, reduced development of soil microbial populations, and long-term exposure of the soil to wind and rain erosion. Finally, the leaves of the coca plant are stripped periodically (e.g., three to six times per year), thereby removing whatever protection the canopy might offer.

As a result of soil erosion, sediment-laden runoff may flood lowlands, overcome the nutrient trapping capability of wetlands, and damage associated aquatic systems by smothering bottom communities and decreasing oxygen availability to other organisms. Floods, avalanches, and landslides have been attributed to the increased soil erosion found in the coca-growing areas of the Andean foothills. Exceptionally heavy rain-

Table 2-1—Pesticides Commonly Used in Coca Production

Common name	Trade name	Percent used
Carbaryl	Sevin	70%
Metamidophos	Monitor	15
Decamitrina.........	Decis	10
Monocrotophos	Azodrin	5

SOURCE: J. Antognini, Research Leader, Tropical Science and Research Lab, U.S. Department of Agriculture, "Remarks," U.S. Library of Congress, Congressional Research Service, *Cocaine Production, Eradication and the Environment: Policy, Impact and Options Hearing,* February 14, 1990 (Washington, DC: U.S. Government Printing Office, 1990), p. 3.

Table 2-2—Dimensions of Pollution from Coca Processing in the Alto Huallaga Valley[a]

Material	Quantity (in millions)
Acetone	6.4 l
Carbide	3.2 kg
Kerosene	57 l
Quicklime	16 kg
Sulphuric Acid	32 l
Toilet paper	16 kg
Toluene	6.4 l

[a] Based on estimated quantities of these substances in Alto Huallaga Valley rivers and streams in 1986.

SOURCE: M. Buenaventura, "Victims of the Drug Trade," U.S. Library of Congress, Congressional Research Service (CRS), *Cocaine Production, Eradication, and the Environment: Policy, Impact, and Options,* February 14, 1990 (Washington, DC: U.S. Government Printing Office, 1990), pp. 143-148.

fall in November 1987 caused devastating landslides killing animals and people as well as ruining roads, villages, and productive land throughout coca-growing regions (14).

Pesticides and fertilizers used in coca cultivation may cause environmental and health problems as well. Synthetic pyrethroids, carbaryl, and paraquat are a few of the pesticides used to control insects and weeds in coca fields (135) (table 2-1). Some of these chemicals are known to be mobile in soils, thus increasing the potential for contamination of groundwater resources. Pesticides adsorbed on soil particles may be carried to nearby aquatic systems during heavy rains common in many production regions. Similarly, nitrate from fertilizers is highly mobile in the soil and that not

Table 2-3—Cocaine Processing Chemicals and Potential Environmental Effects

Chemicals	Characteristics
Carbide compounds	• Highly toxic to organic tissue, can raise water's pH to toxic levels.
Kerosene	• Oily liquid, pungent odor. • Only moderately toxic to living organisms, but if present in surface water for a long time can produce chronic adverse effects in amphibians and fish. • Problems may arise from inhalation or ingestion. • Reduces dissolved oxygen levels in the water.
Sulphuric acid (H_2SO_4)	• Highly corrosive, toxic, oily liquid. • Extremely harmful to organic tissue. • Dissolves easily in water. • Fish and plants may suffer from acute sulfuric acid poisoning.
Toluene (C_7H_8)	• Highly soluble in water and very toxic. • Harmful to fish and amphibians.

SOURCE: M. Buenaventura, "Victims of the Drug Trade," U.S. Library of Congress, Congressional Research Service, *Cocaine Production, Eradication, and the Environment: Policy, Impact, and Options Hearing,* Feb. 14, 1990 (Washington, DC: U.S. Government Printing Office, 1990), pp. 143-148.

taken up by vegetation may leach to groundwater or be transported to nearby surface waters much the same as pesticides. Agrichemical contamination of water resources can lead to adverse effects on human, plant, and animal health (136).

Evidence suggests that coca production can lead to serious erosion problems and reduce land productivity. However, data comparing the environmental impacts of coca production with those of other crops are lacking. The environments in which coca is produced may be just as easily damaged, or perhaps more so, from legitimate agricultural activities that are as likely to involve deforestation, heavy tillage, and extensive agrichemical inputs (135). Coca is a perennial shrub and once planted can provide some soil stabilization during its productive life (10 to 18 years), annual grains on the other hand would result in tillage and harvest once a year. In this comparison, coca may be more conserving of resources.

COCA PROCESSING

Although little concrete data exist illustrating the damage caused by coca processing, it is clear that the chemicals used to process coca leaves into coca paste and, later, cocaine can have considerable adverse impacts on the Andean environment. Data gathering alone poses some problem because some of the items used in processing also have legitimate uses (e.g., kerosene, toilet paper, lime) (table 2-2). Estimates may be based on overall consumption under the assumption that the items are purchased for illegal purposes although clearly for some items this may not be the case. In any case, coca and cocaine processing methods employ a variety of toxic chemicals (e.g., toluene, sulfuric acid) that, if released in sufficient quantities, could harm the immediate surroundings and ecosystems far removed from the processing site (table 2-3).

In the first phase of coca processing, the dried leaves are soaked in a solution of sulfuric acid and water. The resulting acid fluid, which now contains the alkaloids (one of which is cocaine) from the leaves, is decanted and mixed with a chemical base (e.g., lime or sodium carbonate) to neutralize the acid, and finally with an organic solvent (kerosene). The mixing is repeated, as needed, until the solutions have yielded an expected amount of coca paste. In the process, thousands of gallons of polluted water may be dumped onto the land or into nearby rivers and streams (105). Thus, primary processing chemicals may contaminate soil and ground- and surface water supplies (53). Such contamination also has taken place in the course of enforcement

**Table 2-4—Inputs Required to Prepare
a Kilogram of Coca Paste**

Material	Quantity		Price ($U.S.)
Coca leaves	150-170	kg	$100.00
Kerosene	26.5	l	7.00
Lime	8	kg	1.50
Sodium carbonate	1	kg	4.00
Sulfuric acid	5	kg	10.00
Water	1,300	l	—
Total cost			122.50

SOURCE: R. Henkel, "The Cocaine Problem," *Bolivia After Hyper Inflation: The Restructuring of the Bolivian Economy* (Tempe, AZ: Arizona State University, Center for Latin American Studies, 1990). *Author's note:* Data provided by informants familiar with the cocaine industry in the Chapare region, August 1989.

efforts, when coca processing chemicals sometimes have been dumped on the ground and into nearby waterways.

Although there is no accurate account of the amount of dumping, estimates have been made based on the amount of chemicals needed to process a kilogram of coca paste (table 2-4). Further estimates have been made for the amount of chemicals used throughout the processing chain to transform coca leaf into cocaine hydrochloride (table 2-5). While these figures are not likely to illustrate the degree of the problem adequately, they help to identify areas of concern.

CONCLUSION

Although little documentation of environmental degradation caused by coca cultivation and processing exists, it is clear that these activities have significant potential to damage the Andean environment. Deforestation and soil erosion are two of the most notable effects of coca cultivation, whereas chemical contamination of soils and surface and groundwater seem likely results of coca-processing. Human and wildlife populations in coca growing and processing areas may suffer the consequences of these environmental impacts.

Concrete data on the degree of contamination from processing activities is needed to determine the level of risk to human and wildlife populations. A comprehensive assessment of the environmental damage caused by coca cultivation and processing in the Andean countries could identify the relative environmental risks from both activities. Although recent efforts in Bolivia have sought to identify the impacts of processing activities on terrestrial resources (largely soils), additional effort is needed to quantify overall ecological impacts. National support for coca reduction might increase if coca cultivation and processing-related activities are shown to be adversely affecting the Andean resources and thus reducing alternative development options.

When compared with the destructive practices of some other agricultural and nonagricultural industries in the Andes, however, the potential quantity of land degradation and pollution attributable cocaine industry becomes somewhat less striking. The destructive land-use practices observed among coca growers could occur in the case of any other "booming" export crop, and likely stem more so from the social and economic marginalization of coca growers than the illegal status of their livelihood (108).

TRADITIONAL ROLES AND USES OF COCA LEAF

Ritual importance of coca leaf in traditional religious and social activities, and traditional and mainstream medical and therapeutic applications are concerns of some sectors of the Andean population. Chewing unprocessed coca leaves has long been a pervasive Andean cultural tradition. Generally, a dry leaf of cultivated coca contains less than one percent of the alkaloid cocaine.[3] Thus, although related, cocaine hydrochloride and raw coca leaf are unique substances whose pharmacological and cultural uses differ significantly.

---

[3] Amazonian coca contains less than 0.5 percent of the alkaloid cocaine; chemical analysis showed the cocaine content in "Huánaco" or "Bolivian" coca, the principle source of the world's cocaine, to vary from 0.23 to 0.93 percent (112).

Table 2-5—Estimated Quantity of Chemicals Used to Process Coca Leaf Into Cocaine Hydrochloride in 1990

Processing stage	Inputs (in millions)	Low/high			
		Regionwide	Bolivia	Colombia	Peru
Coca leaf to coca paste	Kerosene (l)	567/776	108/317	—/45.8	—/413
	Sodium bicarbonate (kg)	1.2/1.64	0.23/0.67	—/0.10	—/0.87
	Ammonia (l)	5.56/7.62	1.06/3.12	—/0.45	—/4.05
Coca paste to coca base	Sulfuric acid (l)	9.94/13.6	1.90/5.57	—/0.80	—/7.24
	Potassium permanganate (kg)	0.24/0.32	0.05/0/13	—/0.02	—/0.17
Coca base to cocaine HCl	Ethyl ether (l)	15.8/21.7	1.06/3.12	13.6/17.4	—/1.16
	Acetone (l)	7.89/10.8	0.53/1.56	6.78/8.69	—/0.01

SOURCE: U.S. Department of State, Bureau of International Narcotics Matters, *Narcotics: The Environmental Consequences* (Washington, DC: Department of State, 1991).

Many indigenous Andeans chew coca on a daily basis as a mild stimulant to allay fatigue and hunger, and coca leaves are used by indigenous and non-indigenous people for medicinal purposes. Coca leaves are also an important part of offerings made in cultural and religious rituals and are a critical element of traditional Andean patterns of production and exchange between highlands and lowlands. Community and political solidarity were long maintained through these exchanges.

The desire for products of the *montaña*, particularly coca, is a longstanding, basic part of Andean culture, and so the commercial ties survived the fall of empires (115).

■ History of Coca Leaf in Andean Society

The earliest archaeological evidence of coca use, found in southwestern Ecuador, dates from about 2100 BC (uncorrected radiocarbon dating) (112). Different coca leaf varieties and associated chewing paraphernalia from succeeding centuries have been excavated in such widely spread areas as Northern Chile and Costa Rica (112). Prior to European settlement, major areas in Peru, from the north coastal subtropical desert zone to the southern coca-producing areas of Sonqo, were coca production zones for the Inca state (30,107). In Inca times, coca was a sacred plant. The Inca symbolically associated coca with the color green, itself evocative of the rainy season, spirits of the dead, love amulets, and in general, with supernatural forces (151). This symbolic context of fertility, outside forces, and the divine realm continues to have significance in contemporary ritual coca use (116).

Although initially opposed by colonial clergy, coca chewing in the indigenous population spread even further during the first years of Spanish occupation (125,126). Wherever coca production brought significant revenue, as in Bolivia and Peru, attempts at suppression gradually were abandoned (22). Evidence suggests coca consumption was encouraged by mining interests to help miners withstand harsh working conditions in high-altitude silver and tin mines (101, 116). The transformation of coca into a commodity during the colonial period represented a clear break with the indigenous pattern, and has parallels with the current crisis (116).

■ Ritual and Medicinal Uses

Traditional coca chewing is not an isolated or relic phenomenon (table 2-6). Coca is the focal element in all traditional religious rituals surrounding interaction between humans and supernatural forces, such as supplication and divination. It is employed for religious purposes by the Quechua-speaking peoples of the Peruvian Andes and the Aymara of Bolivia, as well as the

Table 2-6—Traditional Coca Use in the Andean (A) and Tropical Forest (TF) Regions[a]

	Colombia				Peru					Bolivia					
Coca users →	Chibchan (Paéz)	Tukanoan	Tupian (Witoto)	Macro-Chibchan (Kogi)	Quechua	Aymara	Non-Indian Peruvians	Arawakan	Tupian (Witoto)	Quechua	Aymara	Miners (Indian and Non-Indian)	Non-Indian Bolivians	Tacanan (Araona)	Guaraní (Chiriguan)
Regions →	A	TF	TF	TF	A	A	A	TF	TF	A	A	A	A	TF	TF
Means of obtaining coca															
Cultivation															
Trade		X	X	X					X					X	X
Cultivation and trade	+				X	X	X	X		X	X	X	X		
Frequency of use															
Daily, by men and women	X				X	X				X	X				
Daily, by men only		X	X	X				X	X			X			
Form or method of use															
"Chewed"	X	X	X		X	X		X	X	X	X	X		X	X
Powdered		X	X												
Smoked with tobacco	X			X				X	X						
Purpose of use															
Social rituals	X	X		X	X	X				X	X	X			
Ritual healing	X				X	X				X	X				
Divination					X	X	+	X		X	X				
Medicinal					X	X	X	X		X	X	X	+		
Labor exchange or wages					X	X				X	X	X	X		

[a] This table is illustrative, not exhaustive.

KEY: X= present. += occasional or possible.

SOURCE: M.E. Reeve, "Traditional Roles and Uses of Coca Leaf in Andean Society," contractor report prepared for the Office of Technology Assessment, July 1991.

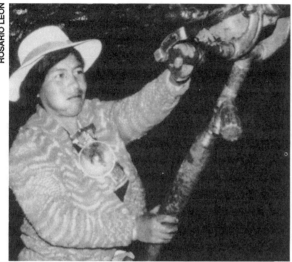

Traditional coca use by Andean miners has persisted since colonial times. Here, a Bolivian miner chews coca, indicated by the bulge in her cheek, while working.

Tukanoans of the Colombian Amazon, who inhabit the Vaupés, Caquetá, and Paraná river regions (116). Even those who do not chew coca on a daily basis use it periodically in rituals. For instance, most native Andeans believe that certain activities, such as sowing and harvesting, require ritual offerings of coca be made to those lending their labor (122).

Apart from its religious significance, coca is almost universally regarded by indigenous peoples as a food, and native explanations of the coca's value are grounded in physiological rather than cultural factors (97). The persistence of the coca habit can be understood if it has been critical for the adaptation and survival of native Andeans under high altitude conditions (29). When Western scientists began studying coca at the turn of the century, they focused on cocaine hydrochloride. The applicability of unprocessed coca leaf as a modern pharmaceutical product was not pursued and, following the abolition of cocaine, coca leaf was not available for scientific investigation

in the United States and Europe (112). Nevertheless, the utility of traditional coca consumption for Andean populations cannot be ignored. Three physiological benefits of coca use (for relief from altitude sickness, as a remedy to vitamin deficiencies, and in conserving body heat), are specifically appropriate to Andeans who must endure the stresses of high-altitude labor and a low-protein diet (29,64,101). Evidence does not support claims that long-term traditional use is harmful (86). Rather, the multiple advantages of coca use indicate that it has a strong positive role in Andean health (box 6-A) (112,116).

A much higher percentage of the Bolivian population regularly consumes the unprocessed coca leaf for daily sustenance than is involved in the illegal production, transport, marketing, processing, and trafficking of the coca leaf and its derivatives. Coca leaf is used by eighty-seven percent of the inhabitants in the small towns and rural communities of Bolivia for some 40 different health remedies (76). Between $1^1/_2$ and 2 million people chew coca in Bolivia alone (34,76). Similar, or greater figures also apply to Peru.[4]

■ Traditional Patterns of Coca Leaf Production and Distribution

In traditional Andean society, coca is critical to the smooth functioning of daily interaction and ritual affirmation of kin group exchanges. Most coca chewing takes place within the daily routine and is carried out according to a specific ritual pattern (3,125). A coca exchange will seal a social contract, whether it be an agreement to share labor (*anyi*), a marriage contract, or acceptance of a political office (3,22). Coca also is used as wages or payment for services outside of *anyi* in place of less stable Andean currencies (23,35).

Production of coca is intricately linked to the wider pattern of Andean agricultural subsistence that depends on interregional trade networks that

---

[4] There is comparatively less available information on the extent of contemporary use of coca leaf among Andean peoples of Colombia and the Amazonian regions (116).

Box 2-A—Traditional Use of Coca Leaf

Ritual Religious and Medicinal Importance

- *Divination:* As part of the complex of beliefs surrounding its power to see and communicate with the supernatural, and its association with the realms of ancestral and spiritual forces, coca is used by diviners to bring divine knowledge to the communities they serve. Throughout the Andes today, coca continues to be a major medium for divination, sought by indigens and non-indigens.
- *Supplication:* Coca is used as an offering to propitiate supernatural forces, and to ensure agricultural and animal fertility and personal well-being; it is also ritually offered during marriage negotiations, and to the dead at burial.
- *Traditional medicine:* Coca use is integral to practices of traditional healers and herbalists throughout the Andean and Amazonian regions. Though they practice nonconventional (non-Western) medicine, traditional healers and herbalists do not operate within the indigenous sphere alone.

Widespread Therapeutic Importance

- *Anesthetic/antiseptic:* Indigens and non-indigens apply coca topically as a local anesthetic; coca also has antiseptic qualities. The cocaine alkaloid has been shown to exert a powerful bactericidal action on gram-negative and coccus organisms.
- *Curative/preventative remedy:* Coca tea, consumed by indigenous and non-indigenous Andean people, alleviates the symptoms of altitude sickness; combats the effects of hypoglycemia; and helps prevent various lung ailments (an attribute of particular significance to the mining population). For example, chewing coca leaves is believed to limit inhalation of silicates that cause silicosis.
- *Dietary supplement:* Coca leaves contain vitamin A and significant amounts of B1, B2, and C; they also contain calcium, iron, and phosphorus, in either the leaves or the calcium carbonate customarily taken with the leaves. Leaf chewing helps alleviate nutritional deficiencies of a diet consisting principally of potatoes.
- *Stimulant:* Coca gives energy for work, reduces physical discomfort and fatigue, alleviates hunger, sharpens mental processes, and, at high altitudes, helps the chewer keep warm.

SOURCE: Adapted from M.E. Reeve, "Traditional Roles and Uses of Coca Leaf in Andean Society," contractor report prepared for the Office of Technology Assessment, July 1991.

move food and coca between distinct ecological zones. Exploitation of distinct zones, called "verticality," is a critical concept symbolically and in terms of subsistence strategies (107). From prehistoric times, coca has been the major crop grown by Andean peoples in the lowest of the principle ecological zones, and trade of coca for highland goods has bound communities and kin groups across the zones. Studies of modern Andean subsistence strategies demonstrate that this pattern has been preserved.

The exchange of coca and food is an ancient strategy and coca traders were a nexus of the regional integration promoted by this lowland/highland exchange (35,38). Even prior to the cocaine boom, coca was the largest trade item involved in most of the Peruvian market economy (125). Peoples participated in this market if for no other reason than for the coca needed to obtain agricultural labor. Additionally, outside of the markets, an active trade in coca has traditionally been part of the household activity of temporary migrants to the lowlands. Highland Quechua and Aymara households each year traveled to the lowlands with their products (meat, livestock, cereals, and produce) and traded them for coca and other tropical products. The informal market sector traditionally has been of significance in terms of promoting regional integration and in stimulating small-scale production of an agricultural surplus (72,99).

However, operation within this traditional pattern is now a risky business largely because of the emergence of a black market for coca leaves, with which traditional users must compete (3). In Peru, for instance, coca transported in greater quantity than is necessary for immediate personal use is subject to confiscation. As the number of traditional commercial traders has diminished, subsistence agriculturalists have increased their trips, perhaps to move smaller quantities of coca leaves at a time or to take advantage of the opportunities for wage labor (105). Other traditional users find they must make do with fewer supplies of coca leaf, and use substitutes, making proper performance of ritual obligations more difficult (116).

■ Cultural Ramifications of Illegal Coca Trade

The persistence of coca chewing in Andean Bolivia and Peru is linked most closely to cultural continuity, and follows the linguistic patterns of Quechua and Aymara (30). However, as economic pressures have provoked increased fragmentation of land holdings, temporary or permanent migration to coastal and tropical forest areas, and delocalization of food production and distribution, individuals are cut off from the traditional work and life patterns of their natal community (*ayllu*) and face a "crisis of the traditional ideology" (116). While poverty and migration likely will continue to disrupt rural, indigenous Andean communities, the international cocaine industry has been instrumental in corrupting the traditional role of coca.

In the cocaine trade, wage laborers are paid more often in *pasta básica* (coca paste) than money or unprocessed leaf. *Pasta básica* is an intermediate, unrefined coca derivative that is highly addictive. It contains numerous chemical impurities accumulated during cultivation and processing (e.g., pesticides, kerosene, sulphuric acid), and is presumed to have serious health effects (75). The practice of smoking *pitillos*,

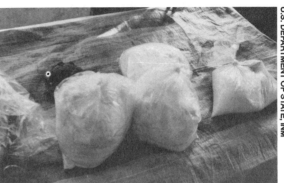

More than just impure cocaine, pasta básica de cocaína *is cheap, widely available, and highly addictive, attributes which underscore its potential to be a significant public health problem in coca-producing countries.*

coca paste mixed into tobacco cigarettes, has spread among urban and rural youth, and across economic boundaries (85,86,94). Another health risk of the cocaine trade, which has affected poor, teenage male peasants in particular, is caused by the process of making *pasta básica*. Thousands of unemployed youth seek work as *pisadores*, those who stomp the coca leaves in a chemical soup. Exposure to *pasta básica* processing chemicals over the numerous hours required for paste-making causes damage to *pisadores'* feet and may pose other, as yet unknown, health risks (75).

■ Cultural and Economic Implications for Coca Reduction

A recent study in Bolivia found that among traditional agriculturalists and miners, 13 percent said their productivity would decrease without coca, and 16 percent said they would fall ill (39). Laboratory testing of the effect of coca chewing on individuals indicate that there is no significant difference in actual work efficiency, but that it may slightly increase endurance in work performance, acting much like caffeine and amphetamines to produce central body stimulation (72). Still, further restrictions on the availability of coca leaf for traditional use could, at the very least, increase the difficulty of traditional Andean cultures to fulfill ritual religious and social activities. Furthermore, 40 percent of the Bolivians studied believed that ''people would rebel in some way or another'' (39).

Indeed, coca leaf has become an important focal symbol in the indigenous struggle for self-determination, a significant political movement already active in Bolivia. The ongoing effort for cultural equity by indigenous Bolivians often includes support for or approval of traditional use of coca leaf; concurrently, the Bolivian peasantry have used what political power and organization they have as a means of fighting coca eradication efforts and bans on coca cultivation (76).

In addition to cultural factors, economic and political factors need to be carefully considered in evaluation of any action which would alter the current situation. Unless illegal demand is removed, regulation of legal coca cultivation and trade likely will be too great a challenge for the Andean countries. Restrictions on all coca-related activity then will likely continue, to the detriment of traditional users (116).

SOCIAL, ECONOMIC, AND POLITICAL ASPECTS OF COCA CULTIVATION

Bolivia and Peru share the distinction of being the world's leading producers of coca leaf, a condition spurred in both countries by long-term social inequality, and political and economic unrest. Over time, the appeal of coca leaf cultivation was heightened by national agricultural policies that promoted agricultural production for often unstable international markets while discouraging production for domestic markets. Small farmers in Bolivia and Peru, who grow the bulk of nationally consumed food products, were particularly hurt by agricultural and rural development policies.

In contrast, Colombia's involvement in the cocaine industry mostly has been confined to cocaine processing and international trafficking. Numerous aspects of Colombia's history contrib-uted to creating an enormous advantage for enterprising Colombian criminals in these activities, and Colombia's narcotics traffickers remain the industry's chief beneficiaries.

How all these problems are linked might best be understood by briefly examining some of the social, political, and economic developments in Bolivia, Peru, and Colombia that have motivated involvement in the cocaine industry most directly. For Bolivia and Peru these developments will be discussed mainly in the context of settlement in the Chapare and the Alto Huallaga regions.

▌ Bolivia

The development of coca activity is very much within the framework of the political and economic history of Bolivia (5). Stagnation of Cochabamba's upland valley agricultural economy is a development problem and periodic source of crisis that dates from Bolivia's colonial period.

Within the colonial economy, agricultural areas supplied mining and administrative centers with food and fiber (109). Then, as now, smallholding farmers frequently undercut large estates, because they did not attach a value to their own labor, and could sell their produce at prices the large estates could not match profitably. In fact, large estates could only count on making money in drought years, when smallholders were obliged to consume most of what they grew. Because their landholdings were small and located in the least favorable areas for agriculture, many smallholders could not support themselves from farming, despite the fact that they dominated the markets for agricultural products in most years. As a result, smallholding farmers became heavily dependent on off-farm sources of income early in Bolivian history (91).

This social context effectively discouraged investment in agriculture and contributed to worsening imbalance between the agricultural and mining sectors of the economy.[5] For large landowners, their estates were essentially collateral for investment in other economic activities. For smallholders, revenues not immediately consumed were also invested in off-farm activities. Economic opportunities were not plentiful, however, and worried government officials constantly sought ways to bring new life to the agricultural economy through development schemes.

The imbalance between the agricultural and mining sectors was exacerbated by several events during the 20th century. With completion of the railroad linking Cochabamba with ports on the Pacific coast in 1917, centers of craft production could no longer compete with manufactured imports, and many had to seek employment in the mines. Large estates contracted labor on behalf of mines, frequently obliging part of their resident peasant population to work there. The relationship with the mines was strongly influenced by international ore prices. During periods of high ore prices, the agricultural areas of central Bolivia exported large numbers of people to the mining centers, and then reabsorbed many of them when ore prices declined (48,73).

NATIONAL AGRICULTURAL POLICY AFTER 1952

The problems faced by agricultural areas deepened in 1953 when the *Movimiento Nacionalista Revolucionario* government enacted agrarian reforms that substantially redistributed land in the upland areas and released peasants from the political domination of large estates. The reforms did not address productivity of peasant labor; in fact, although more rural people had land, the conditions for earning a living on that land were as unfavorable as before, owing to the absence of government policies to assist smallholders.

Conversely, land concentration reoccurred as a consequence of economic growth in the new export agricultural sector (140). Larger land holders in the eastern lowland areas of Bolivia, such as the Santa Cruz department, were encouraged and financed to expand and modernize a commercial and largely export agriculture industry. Bolivia was the world's largest recipient of U.S. foreign assistance under the Point Four program during the 1950s (77). Economic development policy focused on expanding the export enclave and landowners in lowland areas were provided with large amounts of foreign assistance for transforming their estates into modern commercial agricultural enterprises. Much of the economic growth experienced in the lowlands following the agrarian reform was based on the availability of migrant labor from upland areas (109).

The impact of the growing commercial agricultural export sector on rural smallholders in areas such as the Cochabamba department was to recreate the economic imbalance that had characterized their relationship with the mining industry. Agrarian reform and the growth of the commercial agricultural export sector did little to improve livelihoods for small farmers and resulted in large numbers of people migrating to seek employment in cities. This movement continues to swell Bolivia's urban population (87,111).

CAUSES OF EXPANDING COCA PRODUCTION IN BOLIVIA

By the mid-1970s, but before the rapid expansion of coca production, at least 90 percent of rural families in areas of central and southern Bolivia earned at least half of their income from off-farm sources (120). Peasant families, from their bases in rural upland areas, maintained contacts in multiple migratory destinations, and rapidly changed their migration patterns in response to changing opportunities and risks (87,109).

---

[5] This discussion refers generically to *the mining economy* or the *mining sector*. From the beginning of the colonial period through most of the 19th century the mining industry revolved around silver, but beginning in the last quarter of the 19th century, tin grew in importance and became Bolivia's major mineral export. Tin dominated the mining industry until 1985, with the crash in international tin prices and the bankruptcy of the London Metal Exchange (110).

In 1974, international cotton prices collapsed, and cotton producers, who had received substantial national and international assistance in preceding years, found themselves overcommitted to a failing venture. Some continued to be recipients of national support for alternate crops, and some apparently became involved in coca leaf production (20). International financial connections, physical infrastructure, and access to national and international agricultural development assistance facilitated involvement in narcotics by some members of the agricultural elite at this time (76). Following investment by members of the national entrepreneurial classes, coca leaf production increased exponentially, with most of the growth taking place in the Chapare area of the Cochabamba department (109).

When a series of natural and economic disasters dramatically worsened the conditions of rural life during the 1980s, and coca-leaf production rose in response to increasing international demand for cocaine, the nearby Chapare area was incorporated into the migratory strategies of many rural families (table 2-7). Three factors brought about a dramatic deterioration in the living conditions of rural families during the 1980s:

- A severe drought began in 1983 and continued through the 1980s in much of central and southern Bolivia, pushing thousands of smallholders "over the edge" in terms of their ability to earn a living through agriculture. Thousands of families left their homes permanently, and thousands more have either begun to migrate seasonally or have had to increase the amount of time they must spend away from home to provide for family needs. Impoverished rural people in the semiarid upland valleys of the Cochabamba department migrated to the nearby Chapare region and became involved in coca growing.
- International tin prices collapsed in 1985 when the London Metal Exchange stopped

Table 2-7—Reasons for Migration Cited by Chapare Farmers

Reason cited	Number of respondents	Percent of total
Lack of land	74	42%
Seeking employment	39	22
Increase income	33	19
Traveled with family	17	10
Other reasons	13	7
Total	176	100

SOURCE: M. Painter and E. Bedoya, *Socioeconomic Issues in Agricultural Settlement and Production in Bolivia's Chapare Region*, Working Paper No. 70 (Binghampton, NY: Institute for Development Anthropology, 1991b).

trading. Some 27,000 mine workers lost their jobs between August 1985 and August 1986. The *Banco Central de Bolivia* estimated the unemployment rate to be 20 percent by the end of 1985, largely because of the layoff of mine workers. According to the *Central Obrera Boliviana*, the national trade union movement, the figure approached 30 percent by the end of 1986 (45). The impact of the mining collapse on families not directly employed by the mining industry but dependent on it has not been measured. Many families migrated to urban areas, particularly Cochabamba and La Paz. From Cochabamba, many, unable to find work in the city, went to the Chapare.

- Finally, this was a time of general financial collapse. Since the 1970s, different government administrations had relied on external loans and expanding export production, to finance domestic budget deficits and unproductive government spending (134,149). Ultimately, Bolivia was unable to make payments on its substantial foreign debt. In addition, in 1983, the government unlinked the exchange rate of the Bolivian peso from the U.S. dollar. The effects of this *dezdolarización* on the already weakened Bolivian economy were disastrous; the annual inflation rate exceeded 14,000 percent at its peak in 1984. Since only those with access to U.S.

dollars enjoyed any financial protection, many people turned to producing or processing coca leaf as a way to earn hard currency (109).

Official estimates of coca leaf production show a gradual increase from 1963, when production was approximately 4,800 metric tons, and 1975, when it reached 11,800 metric tons. By 1988, coca leaf production was officially estimated at 147,608.3 metric tons (51).

CURRENT MACROECONOMIC TRENDS

Bolivia has a primary export-oriented economy that currently is following a fairly coherent set of economic rules (5). The severe political and economic instability experienced by Bolivia from 1978 to 1985 led to rethinking of the overall economic strategy (44). A drastic stabilization program, implemented by the newly inaugurated Paz Estensoro administration in August of 1985, reduced inflation to 60 percent, limited public spending, increased tax revenues, and brought the fiscal deficit under control (134,149).

Gross domestic product (GDP) growth remained slow throughout the 1980s vis-a-vis population growth, with negative GDP rates occurring between 1980 and 1986, and very slow growth to date. Inflation averaged about 18 percent from 1987 to 1990 (144,149). Furthermore, increasing absolute poverty and sluggish private investment growth continue to plague the economy, although the Bolivian Government has taken some recent policy steps to promote foreign investment (5).

Bolivia has been negotiating its debt since 1986, and had managed to reduce its level of outstanding debt to about 79 percent of GDP (or $3,504 million) by the end of 1990 (149). It has managed to retire most of its commercial debt, and newly contracted debt is being held by bilateral and multilateral official creditors under concessionary terms. Thus, the maturity profile of Bolivia's external debt has improved significantly (149). Despite these considerable improve-

ments, Bolivia's debt burden remains high relative to GDP and exports, and the country has almost no prospects of becoming credit worthy for commercial bank lending for some time to come (5).

CURRENT SOCIOPOLITICAL CLIMATE

Despite severe economic problems, Bolivians have enjoyed uninterrupted, democratic, civilian government rule for the last 10 years. Amongst stronger political candidates, a trend toward coalition building and negotiations has emerged in response to the repeated need for run-offs in past elections. Thus, Bolivia is governed most recently, by a coalition government comprising the centrist and conservative parties (*Movimiento de la Izquierda Revolucionaria* and *Acción Democratica Nacional*, respectively) through an arrangement called the "*Acuerdo Patriotico*" (74).

Nevertheless, Bolivia holds the world record for most government turnovers via coup d'etat (76). The recent transition to democratically elected civilian rule was slow, and remains tenuous in spite of the smooth succession of elections in the 1980s. Prolonged economic instability has weakened government institutions like the judiciary and law enforcement agencies, opening the way for corruption by narcotics interests. Moreover, there have been disturbing signs of decay. At least half of the eligible electorate is turning away from participation at the ballot box, perhaps due to disillusionment with the regressive impact of public policies. Some 80 percent of the population is below the poverty line (74). And, although Bolivia has had a relatively strong human rights record since 1982, there have been moments when the system seems to revert back to military repression (143).

Even under democratic rule, the military continues to wield influence and protect its relative privileges. One legacy of the most recent era of military rule, lasting from 1964 to 1977, is the often drug-related corruption and fraud found throughout the armed forces. Repressive state behavior, coupled with the military's record of political intervention, suggests the potential for subverting democracy via the "militarization" of U.S. counternarcotics policy in the Andes (74).

Some argue that the Bolivian political system lacks the institutional ability to develop effective links between public and private sectors, and that party activists and government officials divert scarce resources and benefits to themselves, friends, and associates (96). In addition, social class and ethnic discrimination place serious constraints on possibilities for broad-based socio-economic development (74,87).

Close to 50 percent of Bolivia's population continues to reside in rural areas, and to derive significant income and food from agriculture (87,113). The peasant sector is responsible for 70 percent of Bolivia's national agricultural production, despite adverse and discriminatory public policies for marketing, credit, investment, transport, export, and rural education (87,103). In exchange for providing cheap food, tax revenues, and a significant part of the labor for lowland commercial agriculture, construction, trade, and commerce, peasant families receive poor housing, negligible health services, meager educational opportunities, rustic transport infrastructure, and almost no effective state assistance for improving their farm operations. Indigenous leader Victor Hugo Cardenas called this structural inequality "internal colonialism" (74).

The social and political inequities in Bolivia create inherent difficulties for state-led rural development. For example, elite groups whose influence often extends to banks, public officials, political parties, foreign aid support, and the media, may monopolize public and private resources earmarked for agricultural production (60). Thus, in the inter-class competition between rural large- and smallholders for resources, the rural elite tend to have the advantage irrespective of the apparent orientation of the national political regime (74).

An elite minority has also benefited disproportionately from public investments in rural infrastructure, agroindustry, technological improvements, and farm price subsidies (150). Figures for the 1970s show that only 5 percent of the subsistence peasant population had access to formal agricultural credit (63). A 1990 Ministry of Agriculture and Peasant Affairs report implied the peasantry had access to only 4 percent of the formal institutional credit available for agricultural production (103).

BOLIVIA'S RURAL SINDICATOS

The rural peasant labor unions, or *sindicatos* have waged the only serious challenge against the prevailing policy environment and entrenched national and regional power structure. The *sindicatos* were organized after the takeover and transfer of lands following the 1952 agrarian reforms (1,49). Subsequently, they have functioned as community development organizations with local, sub-regional (*centrales*), regional (*federaciones*), and national levels with offices and elected leaders (74).

The peasant *sindicato* movement has obliged the government and international interests to take coca-leaf growers concerns into account. Because they have been represented through the union movement, coca growers in Bolivia have repeatedly rejected efforts to organize insurgencies in the Chapare. This situation contrasts sharply with that of Peru's Alto Huallaga coca-growing region, where violence is much more prevalent (74,109).

The implication of the contrast between Peru and Bolivia in this regard is, whether motivated by neo-liberal economic ideology or concerns about the political orientation of the *sindicato* movement, efforts to repress the unions or find ways around their participation in development planning and implementation are badly misplaced. They have been shown to be attuned to the needs of coca producers and, indeed, they have proposed alternative development programs (74).

It is misleading, however, to assume that *sindicatos* are a completely sufficient substitute for true political empowerment. Without locally elected, controlled, and accountable central gov-

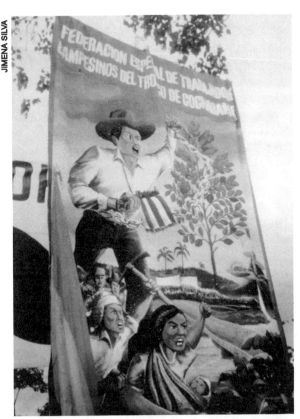

Bolivian sindicatos *help organize rural communities and voice peasants' political and economic concerns at local, regional, and national levels. This banner from a Cochabamba peasant federation depicts a farmer chained to a coca bush.*

ernment institutions, the Bolivian peasant population will continue to be dependent on grassroot and nongoverment organizations for their political voice, and will remain locked out of the central government power structure (87). Opportunities exist for including grassroots social and political organizations in development projects (109). Such involvement likely would strengthen the political and institutional influence of rural dwellers and would further their efforts to secure the political and social justice, equality, and stability they need to overcome the historic, economic roots of involvement in the narcotics industry.

▮ Peru

Recent migration to the Alto Huallaga is only a chapter in a long history of economically induced migrations by Peru's rural peasants. Colonization of the Peruvian Amazon basin began in the 19th century, spurred by increasing rubber exploitation (105). Air transportation to jungle cities, and inland road construction were major contributing factors in the 20th century. Meanwhile, expansion of the *hacienda* system concentrated land ownership, consigning peasants to more marginal lands (9). The upper jungle areas of the Peruvian Andes, such as the Alto Huallaga, were almost exclusively the property of descendants of Spanish settlers, and not until late in the 20th century would social and demographic transformations push the peasant population into these areas (105).

MIGRATION AND ALTO HUALLAGA SETTLEMENT

The economic need to migrate was caused primarily by rapid population growth beginning in the 1940s. When a road through Huánuco, Tingo María, and Pucallpa was opened the same decade, migration increased from the central highlands to the Huallaga area (109). Some commercial estates, including large tea and coffee plantations, were established in the Alto Huallaga, and the central highland departments of Huánuco and Junín became regular suppliers of cheap, seasonal wage labor. Labor-force size depended on foreign exchange earnings: when international prices rose, plantation managers contracted a large number of wage earners; when prices fell, they did not (24). In spite of these early developments, however, most rainforest areas on the Andes' eastern slopes would remain only sparsely populated until the 1970s (105).

The combined effects of high population growth rates throughout Peru, and long-standing political and economic marginalization of the highlands, also led to surges in urban migration. In the 1960s and 1970s, the highland population increased by 20 percent (from 5 to 6 million) and the coastal population increased by 120 percent (from 3,859,000 to 8,513,000). Peruvian peasant farmers, often dependent on outside income for subsistence needs, migrated to the coast to supplement income between growing and harvest seasons. It was in response to the unprecedented burden on coastal city resources that the Peruvian Government introduced policies to redirect migration to the less populous Eastern Andean range (105).

The military regime that took power in 1968 (1968-75) restructured property ownership in most economic and social sectors (100). It also launched radical agrarian reforms, including planned settlement campaigns (25,37,98) and agricultural production cooperatives, some involving the country's most productive land. Nevertheless, reform did not increase most of the rural population's standard of living substantially and, in not incorporating producers outside the boundaries of project areas, it excluded many migrants (25). In the end, even more landless rural residents migrated to urban areas, and by 1972, 45 percent of Lima's population consisted of migrants (105).

A 1973 study of agriculturalists settled in Alto Huallaga from upland areas in the Tingo María, Tocache, and Campanilla regions found that 42 percent had migrated because of acute shortages of land at home, whereas another 26 percent had moved because of the lack of work. Thus, 68 percent of migrants to the region relocated because they could not earn a living at home (40). However, expectations that frontier colonization could solve urban economic and social problems were dashed by the lack of long-term funding, management and guidance, and rampant resource destruction (105). Funds were spent primarily on nonagricultural development, such as urbanization and service sector activity. Most migrants were unfamiliar with the local ecology, appropriate crops, and farming methods, and were left to depend on advice of equally inexperienced authorities (105). Finally, little money went into addressing key agricultural problems such as

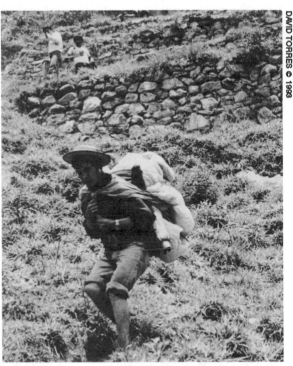

DAVID TORRES © 1993

The shortage of transport infrastructure in most rural Andean and tropical forest regions mitigates in favor of low-tech, low-weight, high-value crops like coca. Local transport of goods still is largely by porters or beasts of burden.

market expansion, or irrigation and farming techniques improvement.

Settlers were economically debilitated by underdevelopment and underproduction. The Alto Huallaga continued to be characterized by low productivity of food crops and minimal use of modern inputs such as fertilizers (109). This placed farmers at a disadvantage relative to those from other tropical valleys. New roads were needed, not to export a bounty of new agricultural products to the rest of the country, but to import food (105).

The profitability of legal crops declined throughout Peru in the 1970s. Agricultural trade was increasingly unfavorable, in part due to international lending policies (e.g., removal of subsidies allowing markets to reflect real demand and supply)(7). Most significantly, production input costs for agricultural crops severely outweighed their market value. Government-instituted cooperatives in the Alto Huallaga, such as the tea and coffee plantations, began disbanding as participants took up coca cultivation. The resulting labor shortage for legitimate agriculture further debilitated the cooperatives and their regions, assuring their demise (109).

The democratic era succeeding the military regimes was based on a new constitution drafted by a constituent assembly popularly elected in 1978. Illiterates (about 40 percent of the population in 1960) were granted voting rights for the first time in 1980. Unfortunately, the 1980s were also marked by the inability of Peru's leaders to cope with the international debt crisis, resulting in the nation's economy spiraling downward.

Under the democratic administration, frontier settlement and tropical forest agricultural production continued to receive the most attention, to the neglect of resource distribution and agrarian development in other regions of the country.[6] A conservative alliance in the Peruvian Congress blocked all reformist measures for the rural highlands proposed in the legislative chamber (109). Longstanding economic policies that did not favor small farmers (e.g., subsidized food imports, maintaining low urban food prices) continued, while the economic crises of 1981 and 1983 increased disparities between agricultural prices and input costs (127). Agricultural policies in the last decade were oriented toward supplying urban areas and have led to deteriorating terms of trade (6). For example, overall production costs increased 2.7 times more than agricultural prices in the Alto Huallaga (10). It was also a period of increasing indebtedness.

Loans from the World Bank, InterAmerican Development Bank, and the U.S. Agency for International Development (AID) financed roads and provided credit for tenant farmers. However, while the government sought a road system that would open the maximum amount of land to settlement (27,109), road construction was not accompanied by economic measures or agricultural policies favoring small producers (142). Economic constraints continue to pose fundamental obstacles to Peru's agricultural development. Long-term economic investments in Peru remain extremely rare, and most come in the form of high interest loans. Without adequate and accessible markets, legal agricultural production is poorly rewarded, particularly in a coca-industry inflated economy. Local banks impose high interest rates that can easily place farmers in debt, forcing them to sell their land and join the migrant labor and squatter populations. Inability to invest in production improvement (e.g., agrichemicals, irrigation) feeds the cycle of economic decline for most farmers of legal crops, further aggravating their debtor status (105).

Economic Developments of the Late-1980s

Peru's GDP per capita declined throughout the 1980s, with an increasing number of Peruvians living in absolute poverty. An unconventional economic strategy was undertaken by the Peruvian Government, between 1985 and 1990, to redistribute income to poorer segments of the population. The Garcia Administration attempted to implement recovery by expanding aggregate demand, instituting price controls, increasing the budget deficit, and deferring external debt service. Domestic supply was expected to expand, while consumption would be fueled by increasing real wages, direct subsidy programs, temporary employment-generating public works in marginal areas, and transfer of disposable income from the public to the private sector. The latter was expected to be accomplished through tax reduc-

---

[6] Resettlement of poor peasants in remote tropical areas of Third World countries often seems to be politically preferable to redistribution of existing agricultural lands. This is because such colonization programs do not threaten politically powerful landowners or other rural elites. It gives the false impression of a ''positive sum game.'' To the extent, nevertheless, that the cleared tropical land ultimately cannot sustain the colonist population, this positive ''sum'' is a political illusion (93).

tion and freezing public sector prices and tariffs, and deferring external debt payments. Use of slack capacity would be guaranteed by closing the domestic market to imported competing goods (88).

The experiment resulted in the most severe economic crisis ever experienced in Peruvian history (5). Peru began to accumulate debt arrears with multilateral financial institutions, and in 1989 its total external debt was about 104 percent of GDP (or $19,156 million) (88,90). The accrued interest obligations on public foreign debt represented about 8 percent of GDP, which was more than tax revenues in 1989 (5.2 percent) (90).

Coca production expanded considerably amid worsening economic conditions in the 1980s. In fact, the coca economy softened the most profound economic and employment crisis in the nation's republican history (109). Coca dollars provide hard currency to finance desperately needed imports and as foreign exchange reserves have been depleted major banks have adopted a tolerant attitude toward coca dollars. The coca economy continues to increase in direct proportion to the decline of the legal economy (90).

Current Macroeconomic Trends

The Fujimori Administration (1990—) has used various strategies to stabilize the Peruvian economy following the years of hyperinflation, real income declines, and budget deficit increases. New legislation has fostered private investment in different economic sectors and the basic economic agenda of the Fujimori Administration has been a return to orthodox economic management and full participation in the world financial community. A "shock treatment" stabilization program and several other policy measures were launched to fulfill these goals, the immediate objective being to stop inflation (5). Although hyperinflation indeed was halted, a second result has been further, severe deterioration of Peruvian standard of living (83). The economic crisis has also taken a heavy social toll on Peru, sharpening perceptions of ethnic and

regional discrimination in an already divided nation, and weakening institutional performance.

When President Fujimori took office, at least two-thirds of the foreign debt was in arrears (5). The stabilization programs and the various reforms implemented to reorder the country's financial situation allowed Peru to start servicing its debt to the multilateral organizations (83). During most of 1990-91, these payments were in the range of U.S. $40 to $60 million a month (100).

The Fujimori Administration slashed government expenditures to gain resources for debt payments. For example, large government outlays for subsidies were halted, freeing prices on foods, medicine, and other staples. In early 1991, Fujimori's finance minister launched a wider array of free-market measures. These included privatization plans for about 30 state companies; the application of free-market rules to the reformed sector of Peruvian agriculture; the adoption of a unified, floating exchange rate; the reduction of import tariffs to an average of 17 percent; and the removal of most nontariff trade barriers (100).

Fujimori's stabilization program exacted a heavy toll on the majority of Peru's already struggling citizens, and no major social emergency programs to ameliorate the harmful economic and social consequences were applied. Social costs of "Fujishock," as the program was called, included increases in the already significant numbers of citizens suffering from critical poverty (specified as a per capita income below $15.50/month) and chronic malnourishment (36).

In light of Peru's historically violent and unstable political situation, private investment in Peru has grown slowly (71,128). A Special Senate Committee report estimated that losses of fixed capital and physical infrastructure related to violence during the period 1980-88 totaled about U.S. $45 billion (67). Although investment has not stopped altogether, its focus has changed in ways that are not conducive to strong economic development. Current investment projects concentrate on: 1) risk-averse activities, such as real estate investments, which have partly replaced investments in transportation equipment and industrial machinery, and 2) new investments in micro-level enterprises, or in small-scale informal sector operations, where overhead costs are low (68).

In practice, Fujimori's economic policies are still undermined by continuing poverty, political concerns, and an uncertain business environment. Even the most adventurous entrepreneurs have had good reason not to undertake productive investment in Peru. Economic balance and growth simply may not be achievable in the medium term if the country's political situation does not stabilize.

CURRENT POLITICAL CLIMATE

Much of the Peruvian populace has been skeptical as to the importance of counternarcotics efforts relative to other domestic crises. In giving precedence to domestic concerns other than the coca industry, the Peruvian Government long has abided with the public sentiment. In opinion polls, the economy consistently is cited as the number one problem, and subversion historically has been the second; drugs were cited as a principal problem by no more than 5 percent of a 1990 Lima sample. Most Peruvians do not consider the drug industry politically advantageous for Peru; however, while the majority support the principle of fighting drugs, few believe that Peru should assume major costs in the effort. Those groups that would be affected most by counternarcotics initiatives hold similar beliefs (100).

Peru's peasant coca producers naturally are leery of counternarcotics efforts. Many peasant leaders have criticized the Fujimori government for failing to consult them on past bilateral counternarcotics agreements, and for bypassing Peru's regional governments, institutions in which producer organizations would have official participation (100). The coca producers contend that they have resorted to coca cultivation only

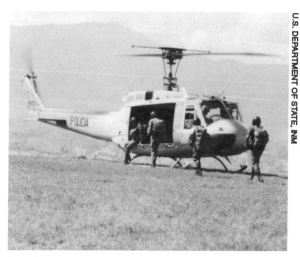

U.S. DEPARTMENT OF STATE, INM

Peru's security forces, like its civilians, are more concerned with chronic political and economic woes than with the drug war. Often poorly paid, security personnel in Peru, Bolivia, and Colombia also are particularly vulnerable to corruption by narcotics dollars.

because no market exists for other crops, and repeatedly stress that their existence is due to demand for cocaine by consuming countries.

Guerrilla movements have had an especially strong presence in Peru's coca-producing areas, primarily the Alto Huallaga Valley. *Sendero Luminoso* historically has been active in the southern sector of the Valley, while the *Movimiento Revolucionario Túpac Amaru* (Tupac Amaru Revolutionary Movement, MRTA) has been vigorous to the north. *Sendero* is said to have received an estimated $20 to $100 million annually in fees (*cupos*) levied on peasant coca producers and drug traffickers (69). Both guerrilla organizations remained powerful in these areas during 1991, thus making on-the-ground counternarcotics initiatives extremely hazardous (e.g., in recent years, 10 workers on the AID/Alto Huallaga Development Project have been killed) (100). No coca was eradicated in Peru in 1990 or 1991, and U.S. and Peruvian efforts at alternative development were not initiated in 1991. Despite the recent capture of numerous *Sendero* and MRTA leaders, the extensive war chest and

---

Box 2-B—The Fujimori Presidency and the April 1992 Coup

Peru's political history is characterized by successions of constitutional and *de facto* regimes (alternating rule about every 5 to 12 years). Historians tell us, however, that the differences among past regimes are nominal; both have been dominated by oligarchical families whose primary concern was exclusion of competitors and disadvantaged sectors from political and economic power. By his actions in April of 1992, Alberto Fujimori seems to have fulfilled a pattern prescribed by history. After more than a decade of democracy, which included his election as president in 1990, Fujimori has instated a government of his own design.

The openness and competitiveness displayed sometimes in Peru's political system were evident in the 1990 election to the presidency of Fujimori, a political unknown until a mere 2 months before balloting. Despite winning the presidency in good part through denouncement of the opposition's proposed economic "shock treatment," Fujimori immediately implemented what many analysts consider an equally draconian economic stabilization program. Fujimori shifted toward a more radical program upon recognizing the need to restore good relations with the international financial community, whom his predecessor had alienated. To open negotiations with the International Monetary Fund (IMF) and the World Bank, Peru had to begin to repay its outstanding debt.

Fujimori's economic reforms ended hyperinflation and renewed prospects for Peru's economic recovery, but also resulted in a severe recession. Given this trade-off, a key concern was the length of time Peruvians would grant Fujimori to achieve economic revival. Critics believe he sought to ensure his government's survival through courting the military, in particular the army, the service that traditionally launches coups in Peru. Upon his inauguration, for example, Fujimori had named an active-duty army general as minister of the interior, and restored army power over the national police. This military alliance was cemented when Fujimori took control of Peru, on April 6, 1992, by dissolving the Peruvian Congress and suspending the Constitution. His pledge to reinstate full democracy after the constitutional reforms—to be arrived at some future date—was approved by popular vote.

Democratic leaders in this hemisphere, and elsewhere, decried the act as an *auto golpe* (self coup). Ensuing events received extensive and negative coverage from the international media: arrests of opposition leaders and journalists, resignations of key Cabinet members, censorship of radio and press reports, and placement of troops throughout Lima. The United States, Germany, Spain and, eventually Canada and Japan, suspended most aid to the Peruvian Government, and the Organization of American States (OAS) issued a stern statement of disapproval.

---

armaments believed to held by the *Sendero Luminoso* in particular, could continue to hamper development efforts in the Huallaga for years to come.

For various reasons, Peru's security forces historically have been unenthusiastic about counternarcotics initiatives. Military officers argue that such initiatives impede their more pressing counterinsurgency demands. Many claim that resentful coca-growers likely would side with insurgents, as would the drug traffickers, thus creating three enemies (100). Finally, in the context of dire fiscal conditions, tolerance of and participation in drug-related corruption have been widespread. Salaries in the Peruvian military often are extremely low and, thus, drug money is tempting. According to some estimates, the majority of drug-trafficking flights depart from official airports. Not only have security forces failed to obstruct traffickers—in some cases they actively have obstructed counternarcotics efforts. Military personnel have shot at helicopters on anti-drug missions, and some believe that government authorities were behind the assassination of Walter Tocas, one of the few coca-growers' leaders to support the May 1991 Anti-Narcotics Agreement (100).

However, from the outset of his takeover, Fujimori argued the necessity. In his address to the Peruvian public April 5, 1992, he claimed that thus far in his term as President, his efforts to revive the economy and to fight *Sendero Luminoso* and the drug trade had been repeatedly undermined by the courts and Peruvian Congress, and that corruption throughout the judicial and political system was to blame. The poor performance of Fujimori's *Cambio 1990* party in the congressional elections had left him with little party support in the Peruvian legislature. The president was put at odds with the congressional representation from his primary opponents, the APRA and FREDEMO parties, whom he blamed thereafter for policy deadlocks.

Although the future of democracy in Peru remains uncertain, the status of Fujimori's government has evolved considerably. Initially, Fujimori would not set dates for presentation of political reforms to Peruvian voters, but increasing international pressure prompted him to accelerate his schedule for the reinstitution of democracy. Instead of first holding a vote on public opinion of his rule by decree, he announced that a plebiscite on creation of a constituent assembly would be held. The elected "Democratic Constituent Congress," of which Fujimori's supporters now hold 43 of 80 seats, is tasked with reforming Peru's now-defunct 1979 constitution.

Fujimori's rapid restoration of some democratic processes has been attributed to concerns about the economic consequences of losing international approval. With much of the government's economic assistance initially cut off, Peru's ability to secure future loans from the World Bank, the IMF, or the Inter-American Development Bank was questionable. Not only would this loss of support jeopardize Peru's present and future programs for debt payment, but would delay indefinitely Peru's economic revival.

At any rate, the capture of *Sendero* leader Abimael Guzman in September 1992, the election of the constituent assembly in November 1992, and continued support from Peru's populace seem to have earned Fujimori tolerance from the international community. Despite concern amongst human rights officials that the leadership of Fujimori's security forces will become abusive in their zeal to root out *Sendero* corroborators (e.g., since April 1992, disappearances and paramilitary activity have increased), the OAS has reestablished relations with the Fujimori government, as have the United States and other foreign countries.

SOURCES: Adapted from C.J. Doherty, "Lawmakers Support Decision to Halt Funding for Peru," *Congressional Quarterly*, 50(15):961, 1992; "Peru and its Neighbors," *The Economist*, 323(7760):44, 1992; "Getting Away with It," *The Economist*, 323(7755):44, 1992; Federation of American Scientists (FAS), *The Sendero File* (Washington, D.C.: FAS Fund's Project for Peru, 1992); G. Gorriti, "Mouse Trap," *The New Republic*, 206(18):14-15, 1992; L. Hockstader, "Peruvian President Takes Case to OAS," *The Washington Post*, May 18, 1992, p. A12; C. McClintock, "Opportunities and Constraints to Source Reduction of Coca: the Peruvian Sociopolitical Context," contractor report prepared for the Office of Technology Assessment, April 1992; Reuters News Service, "Troops Surround Congress and Lima," *The New York Times*, April 7, 1992, p. A1; Reuters News Service, "Peruvian President Schedules New Vote," *The Washington Post*, July 29, 1992, p. A24; L. Robinson, "No Holds Barred," *U.S. News and World Report*, 113(12):49-50, 1992.

CONCLUSION

In 1992, Peru experienced tremendous changes in its social and political situation (see box 2-B). In April 1992, President Alberto Fujimori, with support of the army and police, suspended the Peruvian Constitution and disbanded the Congress in a "psuedo-coup." Additionally, on September 12, 1992, Peruvian police captured the *Sendero Luminoso's* founder and leader Abimael Guzman. With Guzman's imprisonment, Fujimori may succeed in ending what was believed to be an unstoppable campaign for control of Peru. Whether or not the new Fujimori government will respond with similar urgency to the cocaine industry's equally threatening advance, remains to be seen.

■ Colombia

Coca leaf production and consumption in Colombia has not been widespread. Historically, coca use was confined to traditional leaf chewing, mostly by Inca-descended peasants of the southern region, where it was produced legally until 1947 (12). Coca production was banned following lengthy public debate about coca's alleged long-term negative health effects and the role it played in promoting exploitation of Indians by landlords. Coca production was not a public issue again until the late 1970s, when it reappeared in significant quantities, only after development of a cocaine manufacturing industry based on coca leaf imported from Peru and Bolivia (129).

Now, however, Colombian criminal organizations are involved in virtually every aspect of the narcotics trade, from drug plantations and laboratories in Colombia and other South American countries, to smuggling operations and distribution networks at wholesale and street levels in the United States, Canada, and Europe. The entire spectrum of drug exports (marijuana, cocaine, quaaludes, opium) brings nearly U.S. $2.5 to $3 billion a year in profits to Colombia; drugs now rank along with coffee ($2 to $2.5 billion) as the country's principle foreign exchange earner (18). The Medellin and Cali drug trafficking organizations (''cartels'') control the bulk of the Andean region's cocaine traffic. They have used their wealth since the mid-1970s to organize private militias, purchase sophisticated weapons, and bribe, intimidate, and terrorize the Colombian justice and political systems. Their money, firepower, and influence have enabled them to seriously impede the evolution of the Colombian government's counternarcotics program in the last decade.

GROWTH OF THE ILLEGAL DRUG INDUSTRY

Developing appropriate counternarcotics policy in Colombia requires an understanding of why cocaine manufacturing, and the illegal drug industry in general, has developed there. While not a completely sufficient explanation, an important factor behind Colombia's ''international advantage'' in the illegal narcotics industry is that state presence traditionally has been weak. The Colombian Government at times has been unable to control significant areas of the country or enforce its laws, and has been vulnerable to manipulation by interest groups (129).

Like those of its Andean neighbors, Colombia's history is fraught with social and political inequality and instability. Agrarian reform failed

in the early 1970s, largely due to the undermining influence of powerful landed and agro-export interests. Urban reform failed because of the intense opposition of real estate, urban construction, and financial interests. The upper ranks of the educational system remained essentially closed and elitist despite repeated ''reforms'' during the 1960s and 1970s. As land, capital, and credit became more concentrated, and the gap between the rich and poor grew larger, so did the gap between written laws and socially acceptable behavior (17).

Outward signs of Colombia's weakening state were numerous, evidenced by the growing informal economy, and widespread predatory economic behavior and violence. As its economy grew more complex and segmented, the Colombian state took up an increasing number of functions that it performed less and less effectively. Many laws were disregarded, government bureaucracies became inefficient and increasingly unaccountable and unresponsive to the citizenry, and private and public sector corruption grew. As the underground economy expanded, the legitimacy of the regime declined. Drug-related violence and corruption have further undermined the integrity of already weak institutions such as the court system, the police, the customs service, and the military (129).

CURRENT ECONOMIC CLIMATE

The Colombian Government has maintained a resilient and stable economy despite numerous difficulties. Urbanization and income diversification have increased. Colombia did not borrow heavily during the 1970s and, thus, avoided the debt crises that plagued the rest of Latin America (129). With annual GDP growth averaging 3.3 percent from 1981 to 1991, Colombia was also the only country in the region that did not have a year of declining GDP during the 1980s (148). Inflation climbed to 28 percent in 1988 (up from 20 percent in 1984), but dropped to 26 percent in 1990 (47).

Despite positive growth overall, social indicators point to a continuing problem of poverty and lack of opportunity for a large part of the population (47). Colombia's economy is characterized by a high concentration of income and wealth, associated primarily with political privilege and power, and foreign sector booms. Neither innovative entrepreneurship nor accumulation of savings are associated with most private wealth, and property rights are weak (131).

THE COLOMBIAN COCAINE ECONOMY

Drug money's presence and corrupting influence reverberates through the Colombian economy. To estimate the economic impact of the cocaine industry on Colombia and the possibilities for substitution, it is necessary first to determine the order of magnitude of the industry. This requires estimation of domestic consumption and prices, prices of the imported coca paste and chemical products needed to refine cocaine, wholesale export prices, the amounts of the product which are lost to interdiction, and other related factors. The estimation of the Colombian GDP generated by the industry is even more complex because it requires information about value added, and about the income generated outside the country by the Colombian illegal enterprises. While the data to make these estimates can be found, a consensus exists amongst Andean and U.S. experts that they are often extremely weak and inaccurate (129).

Cocaine Economy Data

Although estimates of the size of the cocaine economy vary widely, some trends are apparent. The U.S. wholesale price of cocaine is declining, and the amount produced is increasing. This trend persisted in spite of interdiction and eradication efforts undertaken during the 1980s. In the early 1980s the price of cocaine was high relative to risks involved in the business, so that the incentives to increase output were strong even as prices declined. In this sense, the cocaine output expansion of the 1980s was demand driven (129).

The estimated value of cocaine exports, range between approximately U.S. $1.2 billion to $5 billion depending on the year or source of the estimate. Since Colombian official non-factor service exports fluctuated between the U.S. $4 to $5 billion range, cocaine exports were obviously ''large'' relative to legitimate exports. However, this does not necessarily mean that the cocaine revenues are brought back to the Colombian economy, and it does not measure the impact of the cocaine industry on the economy (129). Rather, cocaine revenue commonly is invested outside of Colombia, enters the black market, or is invested in domestic ventures that provide little benefit to the Colombian people (66).

Consequences of Drug Industry Growth

While the cocaine industry's impact on Colombia's formal economy cannot be measured accurately, the cocaine industry has had a negative impact on the country's welfare, as well as on its economic growth (129).[7]

First, the cocaine boom of the 1980s has made it increasingly difficult to maintain macroeconomic stability. The drug industry acted as a catalyst to growth of the underground economy, which has become relatively large and impossible to track (132). As the government loses information about real exports and imports, capital flows, and investment, the planning and implementation of economic policies becomes formidable (129).

Second, Colombia's growth record was significantly better in the pre-cocaine era than it is in the post-cocaine era. Investment has been distorted as narcotics businessmen choose investments that

---

[7] Colombia may have escaped the debt crisis because of the revenues from cocaine exports. However, the history of the rest of Latin America shows that no relationship exists between a primary resource export boom and the ability to avoid a foreign sector crisis. For instance, all the countries of the region that experienced the oil boom during the 1970s also experienced a debt crisis in the 1980s, in spite of the fact that the oil boom was larger relative to the size of their economies than the illegal drug boom experienced by Colombia during the same period (129).

can be used to launder capital and that have a fast turnover, over those that can produce high, long-term yields (132). The increased violence that accompanies the drug industry also imposes a burden on the rest of the economy as security expenses increase in other business activities, lowering their overall productivity.

Third, the large size of the drug industry has produced a struggle for the control of the country, between old monied elite and the newly emerging drug capitalists. Many elite, though attracted by the capital and foreign exchange that drugs generate, nevertheless do not accept drug businessmen as peers (11,124). This conflict also has been at the core of drug-related violence, and is reflected in government policies that have been predominantly reactive—responding to either external forces (U.S. pressure) or to the assassination of national political figures by the drug groups (129).

Fourth, direct employment in coca growing and cocaine production has been unimportant relative to the size of the labor force of the country and, thus, employment is not among the main impacts studied. Instead, most employment generated is believed to be in the ''security'' branch (e.g., bodyguards, paid assassins, paramilitary), which if anything, has a negative contribution to GDP (129).

Real Estate Construction and Rural Land Investment

Two areas of the domestic economy heavily infiltrated by narcotics investors are real estate and construction. Few sources of nonhousing mortgage funds exist in Colombia; therefore, a substantial proportion of commercial and industrial construction is financed by the informal capital market, short-term bank loans, or personal resources. In recent years, particularly from 1985 on, the amount of new construction financed by mortgage institutions, and the amount of new construction measured by the amount of area for which building permits were issued have deviated markedly. In the absence of formal funding, much

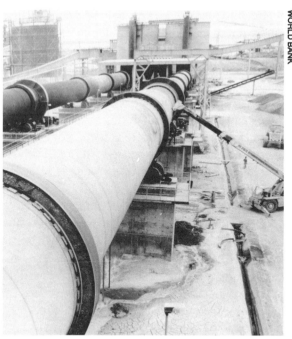

WORLD BANK

The climate for foreign and domestic investment in Colombia is severely undermined by drug- and guerilla-related violence. The personnel and property of important state and private industries increasingly have been targets of political terrorism.

of the new construction in Colombia is attributed to narcotics businessmen, whose investments are estimated at approximately $1 billion a year (65).

Narcotics businessmen have invested heavily in urban real estate and construction and real estate and cattle holdings in certain rural areas of Colombia, particularly in the middle Magdalena valley, the Urabá area in Antioquia and the neighboring Córdoba department, and in the eastern piedmont and prairies. These regions have been settled recently, and frequently have land property rights that are still in question (119). Furthermore, they were regions of significant guerrilla activity before narcotics investors moved in (123). Narcotics investors have appropriated their own dairy and cattle plantations, as well as private paramilitary security forces which compete with local guerrilla forces for the rights to ''protect'' area estates (131).

The involvement of narcotics businessmen in these regions has had a technologically modernizing but socially backward effect (129). Their resources have allowed them to increase the capital intensity of production processes, and introduce new technologies for increasing productivity in beef and dairy. Simultaneously, the paramilitary groups have discouraged political participation among local peasants. Violent land counter-reform has led to increased land concentration, even in areas chosen for official land reform programs. Ironically, rural wages have increased in those areas, perhaps as a result of the higher productivity, and the emigration of rural workers pressed by the increased violence (123).

INCREASING NARCOTICS-RELATED VIOLENCE IN THE 1980s

The narcotics trafficking organizations brought urban and rural violence in Colombia to new heights in the late 1970s and throughout the 1980s, in the form of brutal assaults on the state, guerrilla action, and conflicts between rival drug organizations. Authorities responded with stepped-up military and police repression, which often served only to intensify the country's spiralling violence, multiply human rights abuses, and threaten further the stability of Colombia's democratic regime. In the ensuing cycles of government crack-downs, narcotics-related terrorist retaliations, and uneasy truces, Colombian leadership repeatedly nurtured and then abdicated their country's role as the frontline in Washington's "war" on drugs.

Included in the U.S.-supported counternarcotics effort, along with militarization and eradication (see Chapter 3), was a bilateral treaty for extradition of nationals directly between Colombia and the United States. The rationale was that such a treaty would deter drug lords, reduce narcotics trafficking, improve bilateral relations, and alleviate the Colombian legal process from the burden of mounting drug-related offenses. Implicit in the agreement, however, was the U.S. Government's lack of confidence in the Colombian justice system. Nevertheless, the Treaty of Extradition was sanctioned in Colombia in November 1980, and ratified by the United States in late 1981 (17).

When the Betancur Administration took office in 1982, it refused to honor the extradition treaty, preferring to try Colombian traffickers in Colombian courts (41). Nevertheless, when successful police interdiction efforts against the Medellin "cartel" prompted the assassination of Betancur's Justice Minister in April 1984, the President signed an extradition order for Medellin leader, Carlos Lehder (17).

Betancur further invoked state-of-siege powers in 1984, announcing a "war without quarter," which led to an unprecedented number of arrests, raids, and seizures. The success of these preliminary efforts, however, seemed to confirm U.S. Government officials' suspicions that Colombian authorities had more information about drug smugglers' operations than they routinely acted upon (17). Major "cartel" figures avoided the crackdown by fleeing Colombia. Several subsequently offered to negotiate a truce with the Colombian Government, conditional upon their exemption from extradition. Rather than bargain, President Betancur escalated the war. With U.S. Government backing, the Colombian Government extradited 10 Colombians, stepped up eradication programs, and seized more illegal drugs than all previous administrations combined (41).

The campaign was costly, however, for continuing violence between 1981 and 1986, resulted in the murder of more than 50 Colombian judges. It is widely believed in Colombia that the Medellin "cartel" paid guerrillas to seize the Palace of Justice in November 1985. The struggle ended in the deaths of 17 Colombian Supreme Court justices, all the guerrillas involved, and numerous military and police personnel (41).

Not long after President Barco took office, in 1986, a massive wave of army and police raids yielded almost 800 arrests, including three traffickers targeted for extradition. In February 1987, the government captured and extradited Medellin kingpin Carlos Lehder. Despite the fanfare surrounding Ledher's capture and extradition, the flow of cocaine from Colombia and the wave of drug-related violence in the country were not stemmed. Furthermore, during the same period, eight of nine Colombian guerrilla groups broke the truces they had negotiated with the preceding administration, and, thus, began a new cycle of violent retaliation from the guerrilla and drug organizations (17,41).

The "cartels" mounted an all-out war against extradition, in which they aimed at government officials and judges, in particular. After Medellin assassins killed the Colombian Attorney General, in 1988, the Colombian President instituted state-of-siege measures, built up police forces, and appointed 5,000 new judges and assistants. More violence followed, including the assassination, in 1989, of Liberal politician and 1990 presidential candidate Senator Carlos Galán. Between August 1989 and January 1990, 263 bombs were set off throughout Colombia, killing 209 people, and in late 1989 and early 1990, the Medellin "cartel" began a kidnapping campaign aimed at the Colombian elite. Most of the 420 police deaths in 1991 were related to counternarcotics efforts or narcotics-related terrorism (17).

These nationwide terrorist attacks made apparent the narcotics traffickers' ability to disrupt normal life throughout the country. In mid-December, members of the Colombian Congress attached a proposal for a national referendum on extradition to the Barco Administration's constitutional reform bill. President Barco ultimately withdrew the constitutional reform package altogether, but continued to face pressure to end the violence through talks with drug "cartel" members. Barco denied involvement in any such negotiations and, in January 1990, ordered the extradition of another Colombian trafficker. However, after January 1990, extradition efforts were reduced, and narcotics-related terrorism subsided noticeably (17).

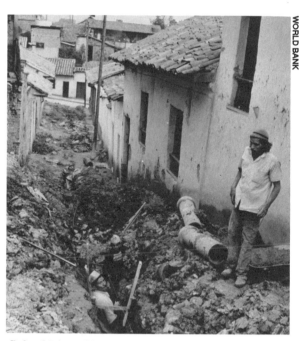

WORLD BANK

Colombia's public infrastructure serves a greater portion of its population than does Peru's or Bolivia's. Recently, however, these services have been threatened by mismanagement and neglect: drought-induced electricity shortages in 1992 wreaked havoc throughout Colombia and heightened political tensions.

The extradition policy dilemma faced in the 1980s is illustrative of two distinct facets comprising Colombia's narcotics problem: domestic violence and terrorism on the one hand, and international trafficking on the other. The security of the Colombian state most directly is threatened by narcotics-related terrorism, not drug trafficking (17). Barco's forceful reaction to the wave of violence that led to the murder of Senator Galán was motivated by the need to defend state security from a clear and present danger. Narcotics-related terrorism was viewed as an urgent Colombian problem that required an immediate response by the government. The international narcotics business, in contrast, was seen as a broader and more complicated problem that could not be solved quickly nor unilaterally by Colombian authorities and policy actions (17). Under the current administration a new constitution, ratified in 1991, again halted extraditions.

CURRENT POLITICAL CLIMATE

Strengthening and redefining the role of the state in Colombian society is a prerequisite for success of any narcotics-control policy. One significant step begun by the previous administration (Barco 1986-1990) and continued by the current one, was the institution of constitutional reform, which included strengthening the judiciary system and reforming the legal system. The Gaviria Administration also focused its efforts on accelerating the opening of the economy to foreign trade and investment, and broadening the political legitimacy and popular support of the state. In August 1991, the maximum tariff for most imports was reduced to 23 percent. On many other items, tariffs were reduced to zero, severely undermining Colombia's once thriving contraband trade (17).

However, the economic *aperatura* (opening) has not been problem-free: interest rates have stayed high and the process has encouraged the re-entry of drug money. Another tax reform, granting amnesty to those who had illegally acquired assets and who had income abroad, was implemented in late 1991, to complement the elimination of the exchange control system (129). Foreign exchange reserves in 1991 alone grew by almost U.S. $2 billion, of which 60 percent is believed to be drug money (17).

Since the Gaviria Administration took office in August 1990, the dynamics of the drug problem in Colombia once more have come full circle. For a time, the narcotics-related terrorism of the late 1980s subsided, and many major figures of the Medellin "cartel" were in jail. Of the country's principle guerrilla groups, all but two had negotiated peace treaties with the government and were actively engaged in legal political activities. However, in mid-1992, widespread guerrilla and narcotics-related violence resumed. To the chagrin of the Colombian government, their most prominent state prisoner, Medellin drug leader

Pablo Escobar, escaped. Terrorist attacks in rural and urban areas by Colombian guerrilla groups had been on the rise, and Escobar's escape coincided with a resurgence of narcotics-related terrorism. In November, 1992, the Colombian Government instituted a 90-day state of emergency (55).

CONCLUSION

The Colombian President proposed steps at the Cartagena II Drug Summit, held in San Antonio in early 1992, to improve international cooperation to halt the flow of precursor chemicals for cocaine processing, control arms trafficking, curb international money laundering of drug profits, and improve judicial and law enforcement cooperation in the area of counternarcotics intelligence gathering and evidence sharing. Additionally, the Colombian Government has made efforts to democratize, and in general, to promote an economy in which profits are not associated with privilege and predatory capitalism. Unfortunately, reforms of this nature bear fruits in the medium and long term, and face many obstacles in the short run. As in Bolivia, entrenched economic and political groups that benefit from the current conditions will oppose any significant changes. Cooperation in foreign trade, economic assistance, and several types of technical assistance are needed (17).

Many Colombians believe that the influence of Colombia's drug "cartels" has continued to spread through the economic and political systems; and recent events like Escobar's escape suggest that drug trafficking activities continue largely unchecked in Colombia. When these problems are set in the context of Colombia's reduced economic growth, trend toward declining economic productivity, continuing widespread rural poverty, and infrastructure bottlenecks to the expansion of legal export agriculture, it is clear the Colombian Government and citizens face serious threats to social and political stability in the 1990s. Colombia remains one of the most violent countries in the hemisphere (e.g., murder is the leading cause of death in males aged 15 to

44, and overall second leading cause for all Colombians) and there has been no overall reduction in the number of Colombians killed in political and criminal violence (17,18).

Finally, the illegal drug industry in Colombia has continued to diversify. Although illegal drug cultivation in Colombia is not an especially profitable business, social and political factors, not economic imperatives, constitute the main impediments to the implementation of government-sponsored alternative development strategies. The conditions in some areas, such as the impoverished and badly neglected Southern Cauca regions, where marijuana is grown, add increasing urgency to the search for alternative development options for Colombia's rural poor.

Until viable economic alternatives are created for the poorer peasantry in rural areas, coca cultivation and, now, the opium poppy trade are likely to spread, bringing with them increasing levels of violence and corruption. Furthermore, most of the opium fields are believed to be in areas under the influence of the guerrillas groups with which the government has yet to negotiate peace. Partly because of the growing heroin industry, many observers doubt that peace talks will be successful soon. Even if a peace treaty is negotiated, a high risk exists that many factions of the two rebel groups could continue fighting as bandits or terrorists, using funds derived from their links in the heroin trade (17).

THE COCA ECONOMY

Nowhere, perhaps, is the social and economic importance of the coca industry more significant than at the local supply, or micro-level. Small-scale coca growers and coca-leaf processors and traffickers are the trade's principal dependents. Predictably, they remain at the bottom of the illegal industry's pay scale, and they are the least well represented actors in supply reduction ef-

forts. Many international narcotics policymakers suggest that if the monetary value of coca could be sufficiently diminished, coca growers would voluntarily leave the coca trade for alternative crops (135). This overlooks many, less-direct circumstances that are promoting and perpetuating coca cultivation. The size and importance of the coca economy among small-scale industry-related producers, processors, and transporters clearly determine opportunities and constraints to source reduction at the microeconomic level.

■ Difficulties Establishing the Size of the Coca Economy

Gathering agricultural data for any crop in the Andean region is difficult for a variety of reasons, including: 1) diversified geography and topography, 2) variation in types of agricultural units, agricultural farming systems, and productivity levels, 3) wide dispersion of agricultural units, and 4) inadequate funding and personnel to develop official agricultural data. The remote nature of production regions, their inaccessibility, and dangerous trafficker or guerrilla presence further compound data gathering problems (5).

Establishing annual coca industry price estimates is hampered by frequent market price adjustments at the macro-economic level, and because the coca industry is so segmented, price variation often can be traced to a regional level as well. Variation may depend on a industry participants' ''business connections.'' For example, growers, processors, or transporters from unconnected or unestablished regions likely will receive lower prices.[8] Thus, to arrive at a reasonably accurate price estimate, researchers would be required first to pool the prices posted from innumerable markets, and then to adjust these prices relative to the size of each particular market segment (131).

---

[8] An example of region- and, even, individual-specific price variation, found in Peru, results from *Sendero Luminoso*'s use of quotas. The *Sendero* charges quotas from transporters and peasant growers according to various criteria. The quotas in *Sendero*-controlled regions, have a direct adverse impact on the incomes of local producers, as well as an adverse, albeit indirect impact on local market prices (15).

Estimates of the size of the coca economy also vary with different assumptions regarding yield, geographical scope, number of hectares involved, different prices at different stages and, in particular, overall inaccurate knowledge about the underground "industry." This latter factor forces analysts to make arbitrary assumptions which may or may not reflect the changing reality of the cocaine industry (5). Researchers have labored since the early 1980s to calculate and report the size of the population employed and/or estimate the value of coca earnings by participants in the various stages of its cultivation and transformation. These numbers vary over years and across surveys. It is enormously difficult to collect accurate information for such figures.

■ Importance of Coca Production at the Microeconomic Level

A former Finance Minister of Bolivia stated that if the narcotics industry were to disappear overnight, the result would be rampant violence and unemployment. Indeed, as a relatively stable source of income and employment, the cocaine industry has cushioned the blow of poverty for many in the Andes. The cocaine industry provided work for between 750,000 and 1.1 million people in Bolivia, Peru, and Colombia according to some 1988 employment estimates (58).

The cocaine industry comprises a large assortment of workers, who have assumed a variety of occupational and socio-economic niches. The three principal categories of the locally employed are:

- Those involved in coca cultivation, whether as plantation and land owners, farmers and their families, migrant laborers, or fertilizer and pesticide merchants;
- Those involved in coca paste and cocaine processing, such as laboratory owners, their hired "chemists," pit laborers, and armed guards, and those who trade in leaf-processing and paste-processing materials and chemical ingredients;

Table 2-8—Percentage of the Mid-1990 Wholesale Value of a Kilogram of Cocaine Received at Successive Stages of Activity

Stage	Bolivia	Colombia	Peru
Coca leaf	.43%	NA[a]	1.80%
Coca paste	2.12	NA	2.01
Cocaine base	3.29	3.29	2.53
Cocaine hydrochloride . . .	10.70	5.80	19.50
Miami wholesale level cocaine hydrochloride (U.S. $20,500/kg)	100%	100%	100%

[a] Colombian organizations or cooperative ventures process coca leaves directly into cocaine base. Leaves are not usually sold separately.

SOURCE: Adapted from U.S. Department of Justice, Drug Enforcement Administration, "From the Source to the Street: Mid-1990 Prices for Cannabis, Cocaine, and Heroin—Special Report," *Intelligence Trends* (Washington, DC: U.S. Department of Justice, 1990).

- Participants in the transport of coca, processing ingredients, and paste and cocaine, including local manufacturers, suppliers, traders, and haulers, international dealers and associated transport vehicle and small aircraft owners and operators, airfield security guards, bribed government abettors, and directly and indirectly employed legal and financial advisers (75).

No more than 1 or 2 percent of the final coca revenue is enjoyed by coca growers. Instead, coca-product prices increase substantially at each marketing stage, with value added more so for the risk involved than for actual processing or transportation costs (131). In producing the smallest proportion of raw coca, but refining and transporting the highest proportion of cocaine bound for the United States and elsewhere, Colombians historically have obtained the lion's share of the illegal drug profits (table 2-8) (129).

Some trafficker networks establish close ties with coca growers in specific regions, and provide them with seeds, tools, suppliers' credits, and other forms of assistance that obligate the farmers to sell their crops exclusively to the traffickers sponsoring them. The traffickers use these patron-client relations to wield considerable social and political control in some coca-growing regions. Like the insurgent groups with whom they may compete in Colombia and Peru, traffickers are able to limit the state's ability to execute alternative development projects in coca growing areas. The traffickers have brought jobs and higher income to otherwise impoverished zones of some Colombian and Peruvian rural communities long-neglected by the government. As a result, traffickers in some of these areas commonly are sheltered and protected from police and other authorities (17).

SIZE OF THE COCA-COCAINE INDUSTRY

Conservative employment estimates in early 1990 for Peru's illegal coca industry (based on a survey of 60,000 families) suggested that 200,000 people, or 3 percent of the total population of Peru, may be directly employed by coca activities (50). The figure would be higher if indirect employment were considered (6). In Bolivia, an estimated 120,000 people labored in the drug industry in 1990, or about 1.7 percent of the total population (50). However, a wide range of estimates are available concerning most aspects of the coca economy's size and value (table 2-9). Given Peru's and Bolivia's cocaine industry employment estimates, the number of Colombian's employed is negligible, an arbitrary estimate being about 50,000, or no more than 0.2 percent of Colombia's total population (130). Nevertheless, the U.S. Department of State estimates suggest that there were 40,100 hectares of coca in Colombia in 1990; this represents 18.8 percent of the total area cultivated in the Andean countries. Colombia produces about 13.7 percent of the coca leaf volume, a share that has been increasing continuously during the last decade (129).

EARNINGS AT THE MICRO-ECONOMIC LEVEL

Although information on coca farmers' earnings are scattered and commonly anecdotal, the contrasts between annual income from illegal coca production and any other source of income

Table 2-9—Range of Estimates of the Importance of Coca in Bolivia (1989) and Peru (1988)

	Bolivia	Peru
Coca production value (*millions $U.S.*)	313-2,300	869-3,000
Coca exports (*millions $U.S.*)	132-850	688-2,100
Total income (*millions $U.S.*)	246-442	743-1,200
Total employment (*thousands*)	207-463	145-700
Area of coca production (hectares)	35,000-55,400	115,530-166,500
Share of coca economy relative to legitimate[a] (*percent*)		
GDP	6-19%	2-11%
Exports	15-98	14-78
External debt	7-25	3-18

[a] For Bolivia: totals for 1989 were GDP, U.S.$4,494 million; exports, U.S.$868 million (includes goods and services); and total external debt, U.S.$3,420.2 million. For Peru: totals for 1988 were GDP, U.S. $28,200 million; exports, U.S.$16,494 million; and external debt, U.S.$2,691 million.

SOURCES: Adapted from E. Alvarez, "Opportunities and Constraints to Reduce Coca Production: The Macroeconomic Context in Bolivia and Peru," contractor report prepared for the Office of Technology Assessment, March 1992; R. Henkel, "The Cocaine Problem," *Bolivia After Hyper Inflation: The Restructuring of the Bolivian Economy* (Tempe, AZ: Arizona State University, Center for Latin American Studies, 1990); R. Henkel, "Coca Cultivation, Cocaine Production, and Peasants in Bolivia," presented at the annual meeting of the Association of American Anthropologists, Washington, DC, November 1989; U.S. Department of State, Bureau of International Narcotics Matters, *International Narcotics Control Strategy Report* (Washington, DC: U.S. Department of State, 1991).

are marked. AID estimated in 1989 that $375 million in coca profits went to small-scale cultivators, paste producers, and wage laborers, whereas legal crops brought in no more than $50 million (89). U.S. Government sources report that coca-leaf prices remained fairly stable, at an average of $3 to $4/kilogram, throughout the 1980s (89). While an average Bolivian worker's income was approximately U.S. $600 a year, a Chapare coca farmer's earnings were up to U.S. $5,500 a year (28).

The earning opportunities for migrant and day laborers are also impressive. For example, in Peru migrant farmers were earning U.S. $16 a day picking coca, whereas rice field laborers collected only $3 a day (133). Similar disparities also occur in urban wages. For instance, in 1986, a seasonal coca plantation worker in Monson or Uchiza, Peru, might earn a daily minimum wage of U.S. $2 or $3, respectively, in addition to room and board. These wages were significantly higher than the U.S.$1.60 daily minimum wage paid to the unskilled industrial laborers in Lima (106). Figures in 1989 were reported as follows: day laborers could expect about U.S. $12 a day ($3,600/year); and cultivators/owners a gross of U.S. $3900/hectare a year. On average, coca laborers could earn from 2.5 to 8 times more than other laborers; and coca farmers and coca field owners, from 3 to 11 times more than their law abiding counterparts (89). Although coca production employs a predominantly unskilled class of laborers, they may receive 20 times more than public employees, and 3 to 5 times what they would earn in their home departments (50).

Information on wages is sketchier for small-time participants in other sectors of the coca and coca-product industry. Nevertheless, the following breakdown of the highly lucrative kerosene trade in Bolivia illustrates the increase of value as it enters the black market. In 1985, a 5-liter daily ration of kerosene was routinely resold on the black market for about 20 times its original value. In the Chapare, its black market price could again double or triple (75). Meanwhile, the salary for paste transport was usually U.S. $2.00 per arroba (approximately 11 1/2 kilograms), resulting in an average day's earnings of about U.S. $8, an amount 500 percent greater than the average $1.60 minimum wage for a Lima laborer (106).

CONCLUSION

As sociocultural, political, and economic circumstances in the Andean region suggest, differing U.S. and Andean interests that have long hindered cooperation on the drug front are not likely to be resolved soon. Bilateral cooperation on anti-drug policies is hinged less on straightforward agreement than on rhetoric, tension, and protracted negotiation (100).

Coca generates high incomes because it is illegal, (i.e., the market has to pay a premium to the producers involved for the risk associated with it). Coca-leaf products, in addition, are high value/low volume commodities that cover high transportation costs particularly where transportation is primitive. Legal crops cannot command a comparable premium under these conditions. Thus, coca has been incorporated as part of a portfolio of crops, in which it is the chief cash crop (5).

Because of the coca economy's size, it may not be realistic to believe that alternative crops will be enough to substitute for coca in the short or even the medium run. Coca remains the best alternative for many farmers and, if its price declines, growers always have the option of simply leaving the leaves on the bush until the price improves. Interdiction activities have helped lower the price of coca in the past, but without adequate demand control, industry participants are assured that higher prices eventually will return (4).

Other important considerations for long-term coca substitution include:

- *Creating secure economic opportunities*— Growers already obtain the smallest piece of the cocaine industry pie. While artificially created coca-price declines such as those created by interdiction activities cause some growers to find other sources of income to offset their losses (coca paste and base processing, in some cases), they do not provide long term solutions. The need to diversify agricultural activity is recognized by growers (5). Crop substitution and alternative development may not have to replace coca income on a dollar-for-dollar basis, if they create a safer and more stable social and economic environment.

- *Diminishing comparative advantage*—The Bolivian, or Huánuco, variety of coca has a high cocaine alkaloid content and grows successfully in the Chapare and Alto Huallaga. However, features that further contrib-

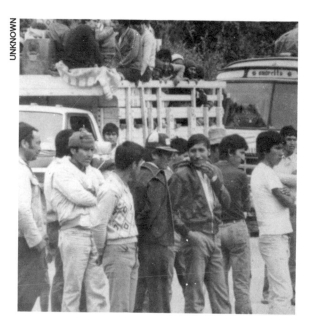

In a seemingly timeless tradition, young, unemployed men migrate to the Bolivian Chapare to find work in the coca trade.

ute to the ''comparative advantage'' of producing coca in these areas are twofold: 1) their ecological conditions, and 2) their remoteness. The latter, creates difficulties first for policing illegal activity and second for profitability of other livelihoods. Although it would be undeniably useful to drug traffickers, developing and improving transportation infrastructure in the Chapare and Alto Huallaga areas would, in particular, improve the profit potential of alternative crops and resources *vis-à-vis* coca by facilitating their internal and external movement and marketability.

- *Reinforcing the role of the state*—In general, strengthening the state's presence and role in producing public goods and services would contribute to alternative development. There are a number of things the Andean countries can do to increase the standard of living of agricultural producers that the coca industry does not. The national government, through help from the international community, could provide potable water, access to basic health care, electricity, and better schools. These are basic preconditions for almost any type of successful economic development.

- *Fostering equity and political stability*—Alternative development strategies that target populations at the bottom of the scale of income distribution need to be applied to the agricultural sectors of Bolivia, Peru, and Colombia. The neglected rural peasant populations long have been a major target group for the guerrilla organizations' membership expansion, as well as being primary illegal drug cultivators. Increased stability in the Andean states likely will require improvements in the standard of living of rural populations.

The U.S. and Andean Governments have differed with respect to the correct ratio of ''sticks'' (repression of drug production and trafficking) to ''carrots'' (economic support and development assistance). Drug policymakers across the board have thus far been unable to fashion a realistic, consensus-based, multilateral, long-term approach to address demand and supply sides of the drug equation effectively. Although difficult, no other approach is likely to offer anything but temporary and partial victories on specific battle fronts in an overall failing effort. Profound changes are probably needed in the economic and social structure and public policy of the United States and Latin America, yet these changes are unlikely to be achieved quickly and cheaply, and certainly not by law enforcement and military tactics alone (17).

CHAPTER 2 REFERENCES

1. Albó, X., and Barnadas, J.M., *La Cara Campesina e Indígena de Nuestra Historia* (La Paz, Bolivia: UNITAS, 1985), In: Healy, 1992.
2. Alford, D., ''The Geoecology and Agroecosystems of the Northern and Central Andes,'' contractor report prepared for the Office of Technology Assessment, March 1991.

3. Allen, C., *The Hold Life Has: Coca and Cultural Identity in an Andean Community* (Washington, DC: Smithsonian Institution Press, 1988), In: Reeve, 1991.

4. Alvarez, E., economist, State University of New York, Albany, NY, personal communication, May 1992.

5. Alvarez, E., "Opportunities and Constraints to Reduce Coca Production: the Macroeconomic Context in Bolivia and Peru," contractor report prepared for the Office of Technology Assessment, March 1992.

6. Alvarez, E., "Reasons for the Expansion of Coca Exports in Peru," U.S. Congress, Senate Permanent Subcommittee on Investigations, Committee on Governmental Affairs, *Cocaine Production, Eradication, and the Environment: Policy, Impact, and Options*, Proceedings of a Seminar Held by the Congressional Research Service—February 14, 1990, Senate Print 101-110 (Washington, DC: U.S. Government Printing Office, 1990), pp. 67-79.

7. Alvarez, E., *Política Económica y Agricultura en el Perú, 1969-1979* (Lima, Peru: Instituto de Estudios Peruanos, 1983), In: Painter and Bedoya, 1991a.

8. Antognini, J., Research Leader, Tropical Science and Research Lab, U.S. Department of Agriculture, "Remarks," U.S. Congress, Senate Permanent Subcommittee on Investigations, Committee on Governmental Affairs, *Cocaine Production, Eradication, and the Environment: Policy, Impact, and Options*, Proceedings of a Seminar Held by the Congressional Research Service—February 14, 1990, Senate Print 101-110 (Washington, DC: U.S. Government Printing Office, 1990), p. 3.

9. Aramburú, C., "Problemática Social en las Colonizaciones." *Población y Colonización en la Alta Amazonía Peruana* (Lima, Peru: Consejo Nacional de Población [CNP] y Centro de Investigación y Promoción Amazónica [CIPA], 1984), In: Painter and Bedoya, 1991a.

10. Aramburú, C., Alvarado, J., and Bedoya, E., *La Situación Actual del Crédito en el Alto Huallaga* (Lima, Peru: INANDEP, 1985), In: Painter and Bedoya, 1991a.

11. Arango, M. (ed.), *Impacto del Narcotráfico en Antioquía, 3rd Ed.* (Medellin, Colombia: n.p., 1988), In: Thoumi, 1992.

12. Arango, M., and Child, J., *Narcotráfico: Imperio de la Cocaína* (Mexico City, Mexico: Editorial Diana, 1987), In: Thoumi, 1992.

13. Ardila, P., "Beyond Law Enforcement: Narcotics and Development," The Panos Institute, February 1990, pp.1-8.

14. Armstead, L., *Illicit Narcotics Cultivation and Processing: The Ignored Environmental Drama*, United Nations Intenational Drug Control Programme, May 1992.

15. Arroyo, A., and Medrano, O., "Huallaga in Flames," *CARETAS*, August 13, 1992, pp. 30-37, In: *Terrorism*, JPRS Report, JPRS-TOT-92-029-L (Washington, DC: Foreign Broadcast Information Service/Joint Publication Research Service, 1992).

16. Arthur, H., Houck, J., and Beckford, G., *Tropical Agribusiness Structures and Adjustments—Bananas*, Harvard University, School of Business Administration (Boston, MA: 1968), In: Alford, 1991.

17. Bagley, B., "Coca Eradication and Crop Substitution in Colombia," contractor report prepared for the Office of Technology Assessment, April 1992.

18. Bagley, B., "Colombia and the War on Drugs," *Foreign Affairs*, 67(1):70-92, 1988.

19. Barraclough, S., *Agrarian Structure in Latin America* (Lexington MA: DC Heath and Co., 1973), In: Alford, 1991.

20. Bascopé Aspiazu, R., *La Veta Blanca: Coca y Cocaína en Bolivia* (La Paz, Bolivia: n.p., 1982), In: Painter and Bedoya, 1991a.

21. Basile, D.G., *Tillers of the Andes: Farmers and Farming in the Quito Basin*, Studies in Geography, No. 8 (Chapel Hill, NC: University of North Carolina, Department of Geography, 1974), In: Alford, 1991.

22. Bastien, J., *Healers of the Andes: Kallawaya Herbalists and Their Medicinal Plants* (Salt Lake City, UT: University of Utah Press, 1987), In: Reeve, 1991.

23. Bastien, J., *Mountains of the Condor: Metaphor and Ritual in an Andean Ayllu* (St. Paul, MN: West Publishing Co., 1978), In: Reeve, 1991.

24. Bedoya, E., "Intensification and Degradation in the Agricultural Systems of the Peruvian Upper Jungle," P.D. Little and M.M. Horowitz (eds.), *Lands at Risk in the Third World* (Boulder, CO: Westview Press, 1987).

25. Bedoya, E., *La Destrucción del Equilibrio Ecológico en las Cooperativas del Alto Huallaga*, Serie Documento CIPA No. 1 (Lima, Peru: 1981), In: Painter and Bedoya, 1991a.

26. Beek, K.J., and D.L. Baramo, "Nature and geography of South American soils," E.J. Pittkau, et al. (eds.), *Biogeography and Ecology in South America* (The Hague, the Netherlands: Dr. D.W. Junk Publishers, 1968), pp. 82-112, In: Alford, 1991.

27. Belaúnde, F. *Peru's Own Conquest*. (Lima, Peru: American Studies Press, 1965), In: Painter and Bedoya, 1991a.

28. Bird, B., "Christians Who Grow Coca." *Christianity Today* 33(12):40-43, 1989.

29. Bolton, R., "Andean Coca Chewing: A Metabolic Perspective," *American Anthropologist* 78(3):630-634, 1976, In: Reeve, 1991.

30. Bray, W., and Dollery, C., "Coca Chewing and High Altitude Stress: A Spurious Correlation," *Current Anthropology* 24(3):269-282, 1983, In: Reeve, 1991.

31. Brush, S.B., "The Natural and Human Environment of the Central Andes," *Journal of Mountain Research and Development* 2(1):19-38, 1982, In: Alford, 1991.

32. Brush, S., *Mountain, Feild, and Family: The Economy and Human Ecology of an Andean Valley* (Philadelphia, PA: University of Pennsylvania Press, 1977), In: Alford, 1991.

33. Buenaventura, M., "Victims of the Drug Trade," U.S. Congress, Senate Permanent Subcommittee on Investigations, Committee on Governmental Affairs, *Cocaine Production, Eradication, and the Environment: Policy, Impact, and Options*, Proceedings of a Seminar Held by the Congressional Research Service—February 14, 1990, Senate Print 101-110 (Washington, DC: U.S. Government Printing Office, 1990), pp. 143-148.

34. Burchard, R., "Una Nueva Perspectiva Sobre la Masticación de la Coca." J. Boldó e I. Clement (eds.), *La Coca Andina: Visión Indígena de una Planta Satanizada*. (Mexico City, Mexico: Instituto Indigenista Interamericano, 1986), In: Reeve, 1991.

35. Burchard, R., "Coca y Trueque de Alimentos," G. Alberti and E. Mayer (eds.), *Reciprocidad e Intercambio en los Andes Peruanos* (Lima, Peru: Instituto de Estudios Peruanos, 1974), In: Reeve, 1991.

36. Burgos, H., "Adiós a las Aulas: del Ajuste Económica al 'Shock' Educativo," *QueHacer*, No. 73:36-56, 1991.

37. Caballero, J.M., and Alvarez, E., *Aspectos Cuantitativos de la Reforma Agraria (1969-1979)* (Lima, Peru: Instituto de Estudios Peruanos, 1981), In: Alvarez, 1992.

38. Camino, A., "Coca: del Uso Tradicional al Narcotráfico," D. García-Sayán (ed.), *Coca, Cocaína, y Narcotráfico: Laberinto en los Andes* (Lima, Peru: Comisión Andina de Juristas, 1989), pp. 91-108, In: Reeve, 1991.

39. Carter, W.E., Parkerson, P., and Mamani, M., "Traditional and Changing Patterns of Coca Use in Bolivia," F. Jerí (ed.), *Cocaine 1980: Proceedings of the Interamerican Seminar on Coca and Cocaine*. (Lima, Peru: Pacific Press, 1980), In: Reeve, 1991.

40. CENCIRA, "Diagnóstico Socio-Económico de la Colonización Tingo María-Tocache-Campanilla," (Lima, Peru: 1973), In: Painter and Bedoya, 1991a.

41. Claudio, A., "United States-Colombia Extradition Treaty: Failure of a Security Strategy," *Military Review* 71:69-77, 1991.

42. Clawson, D.L., "Genetic Diversity of Staple Food Crops in Subsistence Tropical Agriculture," 79th Annual Meeting of the Association of American Geographers, Los Angeles, CA, 1981, In: Alford, 1991.

43. Clawson, D.L., and Crist, R.E., "Evolution of land-use patterns and agricultural systems," *Journal of Mountain Research and Development* 2(3):265-272, 1982, In: Alford, 1991.

44. Conaghan, C., Malloy, J., and Abugattas, L., "Business and the 'Boys': The Politics of Neoliberalism in the Central Andes," *Latin American Research Review* 25(2):3-30, 1990, In: Alvarez, 1992.

45. Crabtree, J., Duffy, G., and Pearce, J., *The Great Tin Crash: Bolivia and the World Tin Market* (London, England: Latin America Bureau, Research and Action, Ltd., 1987), In: Painter and Bedoya, 1991a.

46. Crist, R.E., and Nissly, C.M., *East from the Andes* (Gainesville, FL: University of Florida Press, 1973), In: Alford, 1991.

47. Cuellar, F.H., "Incidencia del cultivo de coca en la economía Colombiana y comparación con los casos de Perú y Bolivia," (Santafe de Bogotá, Colombia: Instituto Interamericano de Cooperación para la Agricultura, 1991).

48. Dandler, J., "Campesinado y Reforma Agraria en Cochabamba (1952-1953): Dinámica de un Movimiento Campesino en Bolivia," F. Calderón and J. Dandler (eds.), *Bolivia: La Fuerza Histórica del Campesinado*, (Cochabamba, Bolivia: Centro de Estudios de la Realidad Ecónomica y Social and UNRISD, 1984), In: Painter and Bedoya, 1991.

49. Dandler, J., "Sindicalismo Campesino en Bolivia," *Cambios Estructurales en Ucaren, 1935-52* (Cochabamba, Bolivia: Centro de Estudios de la Realidad Económica y Social, 1983), In: Healy, 1992.

50. DeFranco, M. and Godoy, R., "Economic Consequences of Cocaine Production in Bolivia: Historical, Local, and Macroeconomic Perspectives," Harvard University (Boston, MA: 1990).

51. Dirección Nacional de Reconversión Agrícola (DIRECO), *Programa de Reconversión Agrícola* (Cochabamba, Bolivia: Ministerio de Asuntos Campesinos y Agropecuarios, Subsecretaría de Desarrollo Alternativo, DIRECO, 1988), In: Painter and Bedoya, 1991a.

52. Doherty, C.J., "Lawmakers Support Decision to Halt Funding for Peru," *Congressional Quarterly* 50(15):961, 1992.

53. Dourojeanni, M., "Impactos Ambientales del Cultivo de Coca y la Producción de Cocaína en la Amazonía Peruana," F.R. Leon and R. Castro de la Mata, (eds.) *Pasta Básica de Cocaína: Un Estudio Multidisciplinario* (Lima, Peru: Centro de Información y Educación Para la Prevención del Abuso de Drogas, 1989) pp. 281-299.

54. Duke, J., "Crop Diversification in Lowland Bolivian Hills," *Hill Lands*, Proceedings of the 1976 International Symposium, West Virginia University (Morgantown, WV: 1979), pp. 331-335.

55. "Emergency, Emergency," *The Economist* 325 (785):45, 1992.

56. "Peru and its Neighbors," *The Economist* 323(760): 44, 1992.

57. "Getting Away with It," *The Economist* 323(755): 44, 1992.

58. "The Cocaine Economies, Latin America's killing fields," *The Economist*, October 8, 1988, pp. 21-24.

59. Eidt, R.D., "The climatology of South America," E.J. Pittkau, et al. (eds.), *Biogeography and Ecology in South America* (The Hague, the Netherlands: Dr. D.W. Junk Publishers, 1968), pp. 54-81, In: Alford, 1991.

60. Estudios Andres Ibanez, *Tierra, Estructura Productiva, y Poder en Santa Cruz* (La Paz, Bolivia: Estudios Andres Ibanez, 1983), In: Healy, 1992.

61. Feder, E., *The Rape of the Peasantry* (New York, NY: Doubleday and Co., 1971), In: Alford, 1991.

62. Federation of American Scientists (FAS), *The Sendero File* (Washington, DC: FAS Fund's Project for Peru, 1992).

63. Fondo Internacional de Desarrollo Campesino, Centro de Estudios Para el Desarrollo Laboral y Agrario, "Propuesto Para Una Estrategia de Desarrollo Rural de Base Campesino," *Informe Especial de Programmación de Bolivia, vol. 1 y 2* (La Paz, Bolivia: 1985), In: Healy, 1992.

64. Fuchs, A., "Coca Chewing and High-Altitude Stress: Possible Effects of Coca Alkaloids on Erythropoiesis," *Current Anthropology* 19(2):277-282, 1978, In: Reeve, 1991.

65. Giraldo, F., "Narcotráfico y Construcción," *Economía Colombiana* N. 226-227:38-39, 1990, In: Thoumi, 1992.

66. Gómez, H.J., "El Tamaño del Narcotráfico y Su Impacto Económico," *Economía Colombiana* N. 226-227:8-17, 1990, In: Thoumi, 1992.

67. Gonzales, J.A., President, Peruvian-U.S. Chamber of Commerce of Florida, Inc., "Prepared Statement," Hearings, House Ways and Means Committee, Sub-Committee on Trade, 25 July 1991.

68. Gonzales de Olarte, E., *Una Economía Bajo Violencia*, Working Paper No. 40 (Lima, Peru:

Instituto de Estudios Peruanos, 1991), In: Alvarez, 1992.

69. Gonzales Manrique, J., "Peru: Sendero Luminoso en el Valle de la Coca," D. Garcia-Sayán (ed.), *Coca, Cocaína, y Narcotráfico: Laberinto en los Andes* (Lima, Peru: Comisión Andina de Juristas, 1989), In: McClintock, 1992.

70. Gorriti, G., "Mouse Trap," *The New Republic* 206(18):14-15, 1992.

71. Gorriti, G. *Sendero. Historia de la Guerra Milenaria en el Perú* (Lima, Peru: Apoyo, 1990), In: Alvarez, 1992.

72. Hanna, J., "Coca Leaf Use in Southern Peru: Some Biosocial Aspects," *American Anthropologist* 76(2):281-296, 1974, In: Reeve, 1991.

73. Harris, O., and Albó, X., *Monteras y Guardatojos: Campesinos y Mineros en el Norte de Potosí* (La Paz, Bolivia: CIPCA, 1984); originally published 1974, In: Painter and Bedoya, 1991a.

74. Healy, K., "The Bolivian Sociopolitical Context for Rural Development," contractor report prepared for the Office of Technology Assessment, 1992.

75. Healy, K., "Coca, the State, and the Peasantry in Bolivia, 1982-1988," *Journal of Interamerican Studies and World Affairs*, Special Issue, 30(2-3):105-126, 1988.

76. Healy, K., "The Boom Within the Crisis: Some Effects of Foreign Cocaine Markets on Bolivian Rural Society and Economy," D. Pacini and C. Franquemont (eds.), *Coca and Cocaine: Effects on People and Policy in Latin America*, Cultural Survival Report #23 (Peterborough, NH: Transcript Printing Company, 1986), pp. 101-143.

77. Heath, D.B., "Land Reform and Social Revolution in Eastern Bolivia," H.C. Beuchler, C. Erasmus, and D.B. Heath (eds.), *Land Reform and Social Revolution in Bolivia* (New York, NY: Praeger Publishers, 1969), In: Painter and Bedoya, 1991a.

78. Heaton, L., *The Agricultural Development of Venezuela* (New York, NY: Praeger Publishers, 1969), In: Alford, 1991.

79. Henkel, R., "The Cocaine Problem," *Bolivia After Hyper Inflation: The Restructuring of the Bolivian Economy* (Tempe, AZ: Arizona State University, Center for Latin American Studies, 1990).

80. Henkel, R., "Coca Cultivation, Cocaine Production, and Peasants in Bolivia," presented at the annual meeting of the Association of American Anthropologists, Washington, DC, November 1989.

81. Hockstader, L., "Peruvian President Takes Case to OAS," *The Washington Post*, May 18, 1992, p.A12.

82. Hurtado, O., *Political Power in Ecuador*, Mill, N. (trans.) (Albuquerque, NM: University of New Mexico Press, 1980, In: Alford, 1991.

83. Instituto Cuanto, *Ajuste y Economía Familiar: 1985-1990* (Lima, Peru: 1991), In: Alvarez, 1992.

84. James, D.E., "The Evolution of the Andes," *Scientific America* 229(2):60-69, 1973, In: Alford, 1991.

85. Jerí, F.R., "Coca Paste and Cocaine Abuse in Peru: Associations, Complications, and Outcomes in 389 patients," in E. Morales (ed.) *Drugs in Latin America*, Studies in Third World Societies #37 (Williamsburg, VA: College of William and Mary, 1986) pp. 149-162, In: Reeve, 1991.

86. Jerí, F.R., *La Epidemia de Pasta de Coca en America del Sur*, Campana Educativa Sobre Estupifacientes (La Paz, Bolivia: n.p., 1982), In: Reeve, 1991.

87. Kraljevic, I.J., "Migration, Social Change and the Coca/Cocaine Economy in Bolivia." contractor report prepared for the Office of Technology Assessment, February 1992

88. Lago, R., "The Illusion of Pursuing Redistribution Through Macropolicy." R. Dornbusch and S. Edwards (eds.), *The Macroeconomics of Populism in Latin America* (Chicago, IL: The University of Chicago Press, 1991), In: Alvarez, 1992.

89. Laity, J., "The Coca Economy in the Upper Huallaga," (Lima, Peru: U.S. Agency for International Development, 1989).

90. Larrain, F., and Sachs, J.D., "International Financial Relations," C.E. Paredes and J.D. Sachs (eds.), *Peru's Path to Recovery* (Washington, DC: Brookings Institution, 1991), In: Alvarez, 1992.

91. Larson, B., *Colonialism and Agrarian Transformation in Bolivia: Cochabamba 1550-1900*

(Princeton, NJ: Princeton University Press, 1988), In: Painter and Bedoya, 1991a.

92. Lauer, W., "Ecoclimatological Conditions of the Paramo Belt in the Tropical High Mountains," *Journal of Mountain Research and Development* 1(3-4):209-221, 1981, In: Alford, 1991.

93. Ledec, G., and Goodland, R., "Epilogue: An Environmental Perspective on Tropical Land Settlement." D.A. Schumann and W. Partridge (eds.) *The Human Ecology of Tropical Land Settlement in Latin America* (Boulder, CO: Westview Special Studies in Latin America and the Caribbean, 1989), In: Painter and Bedoya, 1991a.

94. Lerner, R., and Ferrando, D., "El Consumo de Drogas en Occidente y Su Impacto en el Peru," D. Garcia-Sayán (ed.) *Coca, Cocaína, y Narcotráfico: Laberinto en los Andes* (Lima, Peru: Comisión de Juristas, 1989), In: Reeve, 1991.

95. MacNeish, R.S., "The Beginnings of Agriculture in Central Peru," C. Reed (ed.), *Origins of Agriculture* (The Hague, the Netherlands: Mouton Publishers, 1977), In: Alford, 1991.

96. Malloy, J., and Gamarra, E., *Revolution and Reaction: Bolivia, 1964-85* (New Brunswick, NJ: Transaction Books, 1988), In: Healy, 1992.

97. Martin, R., "The Role of Coca in the History, Religion, and Medicine of South American Indians," *Economic Botany* 24(4):422-438, 1970, In: Reeve, 1991.

98. Martinez, H., *Las Colonizaciones Selváticas en el Perú* (Lima, Peru: UNAMS, 1983), In: Painter and Bedoya, 1991a.

99. Mayer, E., "The Uses of Coca," E. Morales (ed.), *Drugs in Latin America*, Studies in Third World Societies #37 (Williamsburg, VA: College of William and Mary, 1986), In: Reeve, 1991.

100. McClintock, C., "Opportunities and Constraints to Source Reduction of Coca: the Peruvian Sociopolitical Context," contractor report prepared for the Office of Technology Assessment, April 1992.

101. McElroy, A., and Townsend, P.K., "Profile: Coca Chewing and Health in the High Andes," *Medical Anthropology in Ecological Perspective* (Boulder, CO: Westview Press, Inc., 1989), pp. 189-192.

102. Milliones, O., "Patterns of Land Use and Associated Environmental Problems of the Central Andes: an Integrated Summary," *Journal of Mountain Research and Development* 2(1):49-61, 1982, In: Alford, 1991.

103. Ministerio de Agricultura y Asuntos Campesinos-FAO-PNUD, *Lineamientos de Política Agropecuaria*, Manuscript (La Paz, Bolivia: n.p., 1990), In: Healy, 1992.

104. Molina, E., and Little, A.V., "Geoecology of the Andes: the Natural Science Basis for Research Planning," *Journal of Mountain Research and Development* 1(2):115-144, 1981, In: Alford, 1991.

105. Morales, E., *Cocaine: White Gold Rush in Peru* (Tuscon, AZ: University of Arizona Press, 1989).

106. Morales, Edmundo, "Coca and Cocaine Economy and Social Change in the Andes of Peru," *Economic Development and Cultural Change* 35(1):143-161, 1986.

107. Murra, J., "El 'Control Vertical' de un Máximo de Pisos Ecologicos en la Economía de las Sociedades Andinas," J. Murra (ed.), *Visita de la Provincia de León de Huánuco (1562). Iñigo Ortiz de Zuniga, Visitador, tomo II* (Huánuco, Peru: Universidad Nacional Hermilio Valdizán, 1972) pp. 429-476, In: Alford, 1991; and Reeve, 1991.

108. Painter, M., *Upland-Lowland Production Linkages and Land Degredation in Bolivia*, IDA Working Paper No. 81 (Binghamton, NY: Institute for Development Anthropology, 1991).

109. Painter, M., and Bedoya, E., "Institutional Analysis of the Chapare Regional Development Project (CRDP) and the Upper Huallaga Special Project (PEAH)," contractor report prepared for the Office of Technology Assessment, July 1991a.

110. Painter, M., and Bedoya, E., *Socioeconomic Issues in Agricultural Settlement and Production in Bolivia's Chapare Region*, IDA Working Paper No. 70 (Binghamton, NY: Institute for Development Anthropology, 1991b).

111. Pérez Crespo, C. A., *Why Do People Migrate? Internal Migration and the Pattern of Capital Accumulation in Bolivia*, IDA Working Paper No. 74, Cooperative Agreement on Settlement and Natural Resource Systems Analysis (Bing-

hamton, NY: Institute for Development Anthropology, 1991).

112. Plowman, T., "Coca Chewing and the Botanical Origins of Coca (*Erythroxylum* ssp.) in South America," D. Pacini and C. Franquemont (eds.), *Coca and Cocaine: Effects on People and Policy in Latin America*, Cultural Survival Report #23 (Peterborough, NH: Transcript Printing Company, 1986), pp. 5-33.

113. Population Reference Bureau, *1992 World Population Data Sheet* (Washington, DC: Population Reference Bureau, 1992).

114. Posner, J., Antonini, G., Montanez, G., Cecil, R., and Grigsby, M., "A Classification of the Steeplands in the Northern Andes," *Journal of Mountain Research and Development*, 2(3):273-280, 1982, In: Alford, 1991.

115. Raymond, J.S., "A View from the Tropical Forest," R. Keatinge (ed.), *Peruvian Prehistory: An Overview of Pre-Inca and Inca Society* (Cambridge, England: Cambridge University Press, 1988), In: Reeve, 1991.

116. Reeve, M.E., "Traditional Roles and Uses of Coca Leaf in Andean Society." contractor report prepared for the Office of Technology Assessment, July 1991.

117. Reuters News Service, "Peruvian President Schedules New Vote," *The Washington Post*, July 29, 1992, p. A24.

118. Reuters News Service, "Troops Surround Congress and Patrol Lima," *The New York Times* April 7, 1992, p. A1.

119. Reyes, A., "Geografía de los Conflictos Sociales y de la Violencia en Colombia," presented at "Political Crisis in Colombia: Violence, Mobilization, and Restoration of Legitimacy" Symposium, Center for Iberian and Latin American Studies, University of California, San Diego (La Jolla, CA: December, 1989), In: Thoumi, 1992.

120. Riordan, J., *An Assessment of the Southern Valley Region of Bolivia*, Farm Policy Study Analytical Document No. 1A (La Paz, Bolivia: U.S. Agency for International Development, 1979), In: Painter and Bedoya, 1991a.

121. Robinson, L., "No Holds Barred," *U.S. News and World Report* 113(12):49-50, 1992.

122. Sandagarda, A., "Sociocultural Aspects of Coca Use," F. Jerí (ed.), *Cocaine 1980: Proceedings of the Interamerican Seminar on Coca and Cocaine*, (Lima, Peru: Pacific Press, 1980), In: Reeve, 1991.

123. Sarmiento, L., and Moreno, C., "Narcotráfico y el Sector Agropecuario en Colombia," *Economía Colombiana* N. 226-227: 29-37, 1990, In: Thoumi, 1992.

124. Sarmiento Palacio, E., "Economía del Narcotráfico," C.G. Arrieta, et. al., (eds.), *Narcotráfico en Colombia: Dimensiones Políticas, Económicas, Jurídicas, e Internacionales* (Bogotá, Colombia: Tercer Mundo Editores, 1990), pp. 47-96.

125. Steward, J. (ed.), *Handbook of South American Indians, Volume 2: The Andean Civilizations*, Smithsonian Institute, Bureau of American Ethnology Bulletin 143 (New York, NY: Cooper Square Publishers, 1963), In: Reeve, 1991.

126. Steward, J., and Faron, L., *Native Peoples of South America* (New York, NY: McGraw-Hill, 1959), In: Reeve, 1991.

127. Stocks, A., *Fragile Lands Development and the Palcazu Project in Eastern Peru*, IDA Working Paper No. 34 (Binghamton, NY: Institute for Development Anthropology, 1988), In: Painter and Bedoya, 1991a.

128. Thorp, R., and Bertram, G., *Peru 1890-1977* (New York, NY: Columbia University Press, 1978), In: Alvarez, 1992.

129. Thoumi, F., "Colombia: Opportunities and Constraints to Source Reduction of Coca and Cocaine," contractor report prepared for the Office of Technology Assessment, April 1992.

130. Thoumi, F., economist, Arlington, VA, personal communication, August 1991.

131. Thoumi, F., "Institutional Crisis and Economic Policy Reform Challenges in Colombia," California State University, Chico, Department of Economics (Chico, CA: 1990).

132. Thoumi, F., "Some Implications of the Growth of the Underground Economy in Colombia," *Journal of Interamerican Studies and World Affairs*, Special Issue, 29(2):35-53, 1987.

133. Tullis, F.L., "Cocaine and Food: Likely Effects of a Burgeoning Transnational Industry on Food Production in Bolivia and Peru," *Pursuing Food Security: Strategies and Obstacles in Africa, Asia, Latin America, and the Middle East*

(Boulder, CO: Lynne Rienner Publishers, Inc., 1987) pp. 247-283.

134. Ugarteche, O., *El Estado Deudor. Economía Política de la Deuda: Perú y Bolivia 1968-1984* (Lima, Peru: Instituto de Estudios Peruanos, 1986), In: Alvarez, 1992.

135. U.S. Congress, Office of Technology Assessment, "Biological Control of Coca," workshop held Jan. 23, 1992, Washington, DC.

136. U.S. Congress, Office of Technology Assessment, *Beneath the Bottom Line: Agricultural Approaches to Reduce Agrichemical Contamination of Groundwater*, OTA-F-418 (Washington, DC: Government Printing Office, November 1990).

137. U.S. Department of Justice, Drug Enforcement Agency, "From the Source to the Street: Mid-1990 Prices for Cannabis, Cocaine, and Heroin—Special Report," *Intelligence Trends* (Washington, DC: U.S. Department of Justice, 1990).

138. U.S. Department of State, Bureau of International Narcotics Matters (INM), *Narcotics: The Environmental Consequences* (Washington, DC: U.S. Department of State, 1991).

139. U.S. Department of State, Bureau of International Narcotics Matters (INM), *International Narcotics Control Strategy Report* (Washington, DC: U.S. Department of State, 1991).

140. Urioste, M., *Segunda Reforma Agraria: Campesinos, Tierra, y Educación Popular* (La Paz, Bolivia: Talleres CEDLA, 1987), In: Painter and Bedoya, 1991.

141. van den Berghe, P., and Primov, G., *Inequality in the Andes: Class and Ethnicity in Cuzco* (Columbia, MO: University of Missouri Press, 1977), In: Alford, 1991.

142. Verdera, F., "Estructura Productiva y Ocupacional en la Selva Alta." *Población y Colonización en la Alta Amazonía Peruana* (Lima, Peru: CNP-CIPA, 1984), In: Painter and Bedoya, 1991a.

143. Washington Office on Latin America (WOLA), "Resurgence of Human Rights Violations in Bolivia," *Latin America Update*, 16(1):2, 1991, In: Healy, 1992.

144. Webb, R., and Fernandez Baca, G., *Perú en Numeros 1991* (Lima, Peru: Instituto Cuanto, 1991), In: Alvarez, 1992.

145. Webster, S., "An Indigenous Quechua Community in Exploitation of Multiple Ecological Zones," *Actas y Memorias del XXXIX Congresso Internacional de Americanistas, vol. 3* (Lima, Peru: 1971), pp. 174-183, In: Alford, 1991.

146. Willey, G.R., *An Introduction to America Archeology, Vol. 2* (Englewood Cliffs, NJ: Prentice Hall, 1971), In: Alford, 1991.

147. Winterhalder, B.P., and Thomas, B.P., *Geoecology of Southern Highland Peru: a Human Adaptation Perspective*, Occasional Paper No. 27 (Boulder, CO: University of Colorado, Institute of Arctic and Alpine Research, 1978), In: Alford, 1991.

148. World Bank, *World Tables 1992* (Baltimore, MD: The Johns Hopkins University Press, 1992).

149. World Bank, "Bolivia from Stabilization to Sustained Growth," Draft (Washington, DC: World Bank, 1991), In: Alvarez, 1992.

150. World Bank, *Country Study: Bolivia, Agricultural Pricing and Investment Policies, 1984* (Washington, DC: World Bank, 1984), In: Healy, 1992.

151. Zuidema, T., "The Lion in the City: Royal Symbols of Transition in Cuzco," G. Urton (ed.), *Animal Myths and Metaphors in South America* (Salt Lake City, UT: University of Utah Press, 1985), In: Reeve, 1991.

History of Selected Narcotics Supply-Reduction Efforts | 3

T he majority of coca leaf used to produce cocaine and other coca derivatives is grown in Peru and Bolivia (i.e., nearly 90 percent), whereas Colombian involvement largely centers on cocaine trafficking. Difficulty with controlling U.S. demand has fueled interest in reducing foreign production of narcotic crops such as coca. An examination of past opium poppy reduction efforts may provide some insights into ongoing coca supply reduction activities in the Andean nations.

INTRODUCTION

Institutions involved in the narcotics supply-reduction effort include: the U.S. Department of State, Bureau of International Narcotics Matters (INM) and Agency for International Development (AID); the U.S. Department of Justice, Drug Enforcement Administration (DEA); the U.S. Department of Defense (DOD); and the United Nations International Drug Control Programme (UNDCP), which includes what was once the United Nations Fund for Drug Abuse Control (UNFDAC). These organizations and agencies use a variety of strategies to reduce or stop cultivation of illegal crops, including identifying viable substitute crops, providing training and assistance for national military enforcement and interdiction, and offering economic incentives for eradication.

International treaties and agreements developed over the past 80 years concentrated on identifying the narcotics abuse problem and encouraging controls by consuming countries. Later treaties integrated supply and demand control efforts (box 3-A). However, effectiveness of recent treaties is not clear, and one reason is the inadequacy of narcotics data for assessing narcotics control measures. Irrespective of data shortcomings, narcotics traffick-

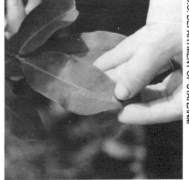

U.S. DEPARTMENT OF STATE/INM

Box 3-A—Selected Narcotics Control Treaties and Legislation

The Hague Opium Convention of 1912

The Hague Convention of 1912 was the first attempt at international oversight of narcotics production and trade (3). Treaty members outlined a system of production and trade regulations designed to curtail abuse of opium, its derivatives, and cocaine. Key points included farm-level production controls, processing controls, and international-trade controls (6). However, disputes over target narcotics and producing countries, and implementation mechanisms plagued the Convention resulting in a fairly ineffectual and narrow final text. Ultimately, the treaty required all parties to enact legislation allowing only medical use of opium, its derivatives, and cocaine.

The Harrison Act of 1914

The Harrison Act of 1914 marked the first attempt to regulate the distribution of narcotics in the United States and establish national narcotics record keeping. The Act included taxes and accounting of narcotic-containing "medicines." It had a profound effect on pharmaceutical and medical professions in the United States and spurred a reduction in the psychotropic drug content of "over-the-counter" medicines. The act's impact was further underscored by the emergence of black markets and higher prices for narcotics.

The Geneva Opium Convention of 1925

The League of Nations organized the Geneva Opium Convention of 1925 to discuss the regulation of international drug trade. This Convention addressed an earlier proposal that crop substitution programs be developed for opium-producing countries in order to help them limit production to legitimate needs (14). The resulting treaty required all raw materials and finished products in international trade to be licensed, but did not address production levels (6).

The Geneva Convention to Limit the Manufacture and Regulate the Distribution of Narcotic Drugs of 1931

This Convention limited any country's ability to manufacture narcotic drugs beyond the levels adequate to supply international medical needs as established by an international board. Consequently, many factories involved in opiate manufacture were closed. Analysts of the Convention suggest that this act led traffickers to establish their own laboratories.

Conference for the Suppression of the Illegal Traffic in Dangerous Drugs of 1936

In an effort to increase the effectiveness of interdiction activities, the treaty called for international cooperation of member countries in curtailing trafficking, and providing evidence and information leading to narcotics seizures.

The Opium Protocol of 1953

The 1953 Opium Protocol limited the number of countries that could legally produce opium poppies, created government licensing of poppy cultivation, and established government monopolies over all opium purchases. It made no reference to cocaine.

The Single Convention on Narcotic Drugs of 1961

In 1961, all of the international drug treaties/conventions since the Geneva Convention of 1925 were combined into the Single Convention on Narcotic Drugs. Whereas previous treaties dealt almost exclusively with the production and distribution of opium, the Single Convention extended the cultivation and licensing provisions of the 1953 Opium Protocol to coca and marijuana. It also included a specific provision requiring participating countries to phase out the practice of coca-leaf chewing by 1989, 25 years from the treaty's effective date. The United Nations Fund for Drug Abuse Control (UNFDAC) was established to replace the League of Nations as the body responsible for oversight and enforcement of international narcotics regulation.[1]

---

[1] The UNFDAC is now integrated with the formerly separate International Narcotics Control Board and Division of Narcotic Drugs into a single organization—the United Nations International Drug Control Programme.

ing and abuse laws continue to be the primary counternarcotics approaches based on the assumption that they are a clear deterrent to present and potential drug traffickers and users. The focus of international narcotics control remains on how to improve enforcement of international and domestic regulations.

The United States has worked with security forces in the Andean region to reduce coca production. However, the public and the media have often viewed the efforts as heavy-handed and intrusive. The Bolivian response to U.S. military intervention, for example, has been no more favorable than their view of development-related eradication. One expert in Bolivia goes so far as to assert the "DEA has replaced the CIA [Central Intelligence Agency] in unpopularity" (10). Despite coordination efforts, conflicting goals of development and narcotics control have created difficulties for development personnel.

OPIUM-REDUCTION ACTIVITIES

Aggressive international drug control policies began in the early 1970s with the establishment of Inter-Agency Task Force One charged with identifying targets for supply-reduction efforts. Mexico was a key target because of opium poppy (the source of heroin) and marijuana production. Search-and-seizure border operations were undertaken, yet quickly abandoned for political reasons (i.e., contradicting the "good neighbor policy") (9). Heroin abuse subsequently was elevated to a national security problem, and the U.S. Government began investigating potential heroin supply-reduction tactics.

Turkey was identified as the most politically advantageous country for heroin supply-reduction efforts. The proximity of the country to European smuggling routes and laboratories convinced U.S. officials that Turkey was a key player in the heroin problem, despite the fact that only 4 percent of U.S. supply came from Turkey (31). U.S. supply-reduction goals were embraced by the Turkish military regime that gained power in

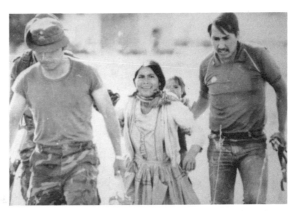

A disproportionate number of those arrested and imprisoned for illegal, coca-related activities are peasants. Eradication and crop substitution policies further heighten distress and conflict in coca-growing communities by forcing those least able to control the circumstances of their coca-trade dependency to risk impoverishment or imprisonment or both.

1971 (26). A ban on opium poppy cultivation was announced in 1971, declaring that all poppy production would be forbidden by 1972 (31). This move was followed by U.S. technical and monetary assistance to promote alternative production systems.

The Turkish program was deemed a success by the U.S. Government and the American public, and the heroin problem was briefly reduced. However, supplies from Mexico, Southeast Asia's Golden Triangle, Afghanistan, and Pakistan quickly filled the gap (15).

Within 2 years, the Turkish Opium Ban was revoked for several reasons. The Turkish population felt that undue control was being exerted and insufficient compensation offered for the adverse effects of opium reduction on the Turkish economy and populace. Contributing to this sentiment was U.S. purchase of opium derivatives from other countries. Dwindling political support led Turkish politicians to pledge their allegiance to poppy growers and this quickly became a major theme in the 1973 election (30). The U.S. Government responded by cutting off monetary assistance (23,28).

Pakistan became a primary opium supplier in the 1970s, complete with clandestine laboratories and trafficking organizations (29). The government of Pakistan complied with international drug treaties because of internal concerns over increasing addiction problems. Having met with little success in their own programs, the Pakistanis were willing to accept and support U.S. supply-reduction efforts.

Four major U.S.-supported projects were attempted in Pakistan, including:

- *The Buner Agricultural Development Project, 1976*—Crop substitution in key poppy production areas combined with eradication (26), sponsored by the U.N. Fund for Drug Abuse Control;
- *Malakand Area Development Project, 1981*—Incorporated economic assistance for narcotics control organizations and enforced eradication (26), sponsored by the U.S. Department of State, Bureau of International Narcotic Matters;
- *Tribal Areas Development Project, 1982*—Focused on infrastructure development, education, and voluntary eradication (27), sponsored by the U.S. Agency for International Development; and
- *Northwest Frontier Area Development Project, 1983 (ongoing)*—Combined eradication and development; components included introducing various high-yield crops, providing short-term relief, improving irrigation, and teaching farmers about long-term agricultural options (26). Vocational training is provided for those wishing to leave agricultural livelihoods, sponsored by the U.S. Agency for International Development.

Although enforcement of opium poppy eradication is considered a critical aspect of the opium supply-reduction policy, AID acknowledged that its most successful projects were those that combined development with enforcement, and permitted eradication to occur gradually and in conjunction with the emergence of new income opportunities. This method offered the local leadership and citizenry a greater role in assuring their financial security (26).

COCA REDUCTION EFFORTS: THE ANDEAN STRATEGY

Coca has been cultivated in the Andes for centuries, and the plant has traditional cultural significance. Although the governments of Bolivia and Peru allow some legal production of coca for traditional use, they have attempted to support U.S. efforts to eliminate all production above traditional and medical needs.

The governments of Bolivia, Colombia, and Peru have worked to reduce their supply of coca and cocaine using differing methods, according to specific regional problems and anticipated outcomes. Projects undertaken in Colombia, for instance, largely focus on interdiction because of Colombia's cocaine trafficking role. Conversely, approaches in Bolivia and Peru (the major leaf producers) incorporate development as well as enforcement approaches. Past mandatory eradication efforts in Bolivia and Peru have been suspended, in favor of encouraging voluntary eradication and identifying alternative crops for coca cultivators. Bolivia, and the Chapare region in particular, has been the primary focus in recent years as security declined in Peruvian coca-producing regions.

■ Bolivia and Coca Substitution Projects

Initial AID development efforts took the form of the Agricultural Development in the Coca Zones Project (ADCZP) (1975). ADCZP sought to identify alternative crops and evaluate them for production and marketing feasibility. However, viable alternatives were slow coming, and the project reached its deadline with its goal unfulfilled. Bolivia's economic concerns and coca's heritage presented some barriers to acceptance of the AID project (26).

The Department of Regional Development of the Organization of American States (OAS) worked with the Bolivian government between 1978 and 1980, to formulate an ambitious development strategy for the Chapare that included identifying investment opportunities for immediate implementation. First and foremost, the strategy provided a framework for coordinating the activities of some 54 international, national, regional, and private institutions promoting development in the Chapare at the time (17). The OAS plan remains the standard from which all subsequent Chapare development activities have been drawn, and included seven areas: 1) technology transfer; 2) provision of agricultural credit; 3) promotion of agroindustry; 4) zonal market development; 5) secondary road construction; 6) electrification; and 7) installation of potable water systems (19).

OAS foresaw a controversy that would characterize much of the discussion surrounding the Chapare and other coca-growing regions in the decade to come: that development would promote the production of coca leaf along with other economic activities. Recognizing farmer interest in coca leaf was in large measure the due to lack of other economic options, OAS acknowledged that coca leaf production might expand in response to development investment over the short-to-medium term. However, it felt that only as economic development opened opportunities to earn a reliable income through other activities, would the importance of coca leaf and cocaine diminish (19).

The U.S. Department of State's Bureau of International Narcotic Matters (INM) funded the first effort specifically intended to reduce coca cultivation in Bolivia. The project, *Proyecto de Desarrollo y Sustitución* (Development and Substitution Project, PRODES), was to investigate the feasibility of crop substitution and produce a project proposal for implementing crop substitution through AID. The 1980 Bolivian coup halted PRODES activities and U.S. assistance was suspended (26). Drug related activities escalated

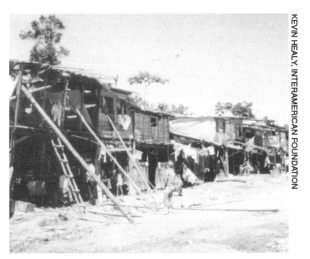

Many coca-growing regions lack sufficient infrastructure (e.g., roads, electricity, irrigation) for alternative development. How to improve infrastructure without unduly benefiting local narcotics traffickers presents a policy dilemma.

under the military regime. When democratic control was restored in 1982, the new government was unable to assert authority in the Chapare.

ORIGIN OF THE CHAPARE REGIONAL DEVELOPMENT PROJECT

The Chapare Regional Development Project (CRDP) was initiated in August 1983 as an agreement between the Bolivian Government and AID. New development efforts began in 1984 as control was regained in the region. It quickly became apparent that the CRDP effort could not proceed under its original design (21). Two practical problems confronted the CRDP and catalyzed the redesign effort:

• State control over the Chapare was and remains tenuous. Bolivian government presence in the Chapare is limited to a small group of development specialists and to a repressive police force, both funded largely by the United States. Effective efforts would require a continuous development presence in the Chapare.

• The overall production systems of Chapare farmers, and the relationships of those systems to the physical capacity of different parts of the Chapare to support sustained agricultural production were largely neglected. This problem had two dimensions. The one most fully appreciated before the redesign was that the cropping systems being promoted probably would not be sustainable in most parts of the Chapare. This raised the specter that, should crop substitution be successful, it could be the cause of an environmental disaster. The second dimension, was that potential alternate crops to coca leaf were assessed primarily in terms of the technical feasibility of cultivating them in the Chapare. Little attention was paid to where and if farmers would be able to sell their new crops (19).

A strategy to improve economic conditions in upland areas—the origin of most Chapare settlers and coca laborers—was developed by AID. The redesign was formalized in 1987 and incorporated the framework that continues expanding today— a combination of crop substitution in the Chapare and improving resource management activities in the Associated High Valleys (AHV) (cf: 17,19). The amendment recognized that the solution to the problem of widespread involvement in the production of coca leaf in the Chapare was not to be found exclusively in the tropical lowland valley itself (figure 3-1).

Migration created chronic labor scarcity in highland areas, and affected family capacity to manage on-farm resources effectively. Consequently, long-term agricultural production and livestock management strategies were neglected in favor of short-term gains. The resulting decline in agricultural productivity progressively intensified migratory pressures (19).

The Campero and Mizque provinces of southern Cochabamba Department were selected as the areas in which the AHV component would be implemented initially, based on a study by the *Corporación de Desarrollo de Cochabamba* (Regional Development Corporation of Cochabamba,

CORDECO). The study suggested the areas had potential to become a center of economic growth and a secondary area of population attraction (13). Through this effort, AID/Bolivia and Bolivian implementing agencies expected to gain experience relevant to an expanded AHV component.

THE REDESIGNED CHAPARE REGIONAL DEVELOPMENT PROJECT

The redesigned CRDP suffered from political and institutional difficulties that diffused development efforts. Fighting political and institutional brushfires consumed a great amount of development personnel time. The link with narcotics control created a dual goal for development personnel, drawing resources toward nondevelopment activities. Similar difficulties were faced by the Bolivian institutions involved in the CRDP—the *Subsecretaría de Desarrollo Alternativo y Sustitución de Cultivos de Coca* (Subsecretariat for Alternative Development and Coca Substitution, SUBDESAL), the *Programa de Desarrollo Alternativo Regional* (Regional Program for Alternative Development, PDAR), and the *Instituto Boliviano de Tecnología Agropecuaria* (Bolivian Institute of Agriculture and Livestock Technology, IBTA). Lack of staff continuity impeded CRDP progress in the late 1980s. These problems and others resulted in ineffectual implementation of CRDP activities (12,18,20). The CRDP likewise suffered criticism in Campero and Mizque because it had created expectations that were not being fulfilled, and results in the Chapare were equally modest. Activities largely concentrated on continuing agricultural research programs, although this research was frequently criticized in government circles and among unions representing coca growers as having little impact on Chapare farmers (18,22).

AID/Bolivia

The AID/Bolivia has been criticized as an overly passive manager, potentially unable to obtain the respect due the entity that finances existence of the two Bolivian institutions responsible for the CRDP. Problems that have limited the effectiveness of the CRDP, include unnecessary bureaucratic awkwardness among participating institutions, a lack of connection between the objectives of individual CRDP activities and overall project goals, and use of CRDP resources to respond to parochial political party interests inconsistent with project goals (19).

AID officials suggest that several factors have hindered their ability to solve management problems confronting the CRDP:

- Staffing and other resources are inadequate to participate in day-to-day project management. This is exacerbated by the complexity of CRDP and associated bureaucratic procedures.
- The project is highly visible because of its link to narcotics, resulting in AID/Bolivia officials spending large amounts of time on nondevelopment related activities.
- Avenues exist to "bypass" the AID/Bolivia management structure with little avenue for AID recourse (19).

Figure 3-1—Evolution of the Cochabamba Regional Development Project

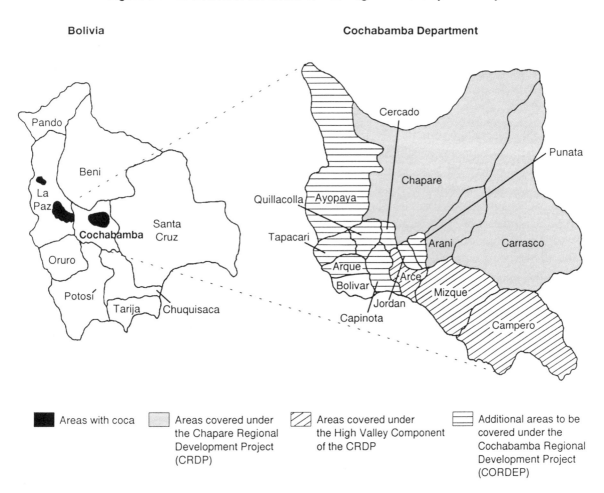

Bolivia

Cochabamba Department

■ Areas with coca ☐ Areas covered under the Chapare Regional Development Project (CRDP) ▨ Areas covered under the High Valley Component of the CRDP ☰ Additional areas to be covered under the Cochabamba Regional Development Project (CORDEP)

SOURCE: Adapted from Development Alternatives, Inc., (DAI), *Cochabamba Regional Development Project (CORDEP)—Bolivia*, Technical Proposal (Bethesda, MD: DAI, 1992).

Subsecretaría de Desarrollo Alternativo y Sustitución de Cultivos de Coca

The SUBDESAL was responsible for direction of the CRDP, and it had authority to change fundamental directions in the project without approval or coordination with implementing institutions. Directional changes made by SUBDESAL have been criticized for complicating implementation. In addition, the SUBDESAL heads up the council charged with coordinating the participation of international assistance organizations.[1] The SUBDESAL is the principal source of information for the ministers comprising the council, and primary interpreter of their wishes regarding implementation of drug policy. However, specific lines of authority and responsibility were not defined, sometimes leading to arbitrary and internally contradictory uses of power that prejudiced implementation of the redesigned CRDP (19).

Programa de Desarrollo Alternativo Regional

The PDAR has major responsibility for implementing development projects in the Chapare, like the CRDP, and coordinating the activities of state agencies and nongovernmental organizations (NGOs) that would be responsible for the bulk of implementation activities in the AHV.[2]

The PDAR would provide resources and administrative support to the state agencies and NGOs already involved in development activities to provide alternatives to migrating to the Chapare. The coordinating role was assigned for several reasons, including: 1) the substantial burden that its implementing role in the Chapare was expected to entail; 2) the large number of state agencies and NGOs involved in rural development activities in upland Cochabamba (4); 3) the desire to maximize the immediate impacts of the AHV by tapping into existing efforts; and 4) the desire to promote participation in activities that supported the CRDP by as wide a range of Bolivian institutions as possible (19).

However, despite its strong technical abilities, PDAR has not been effective at planning, implementing, and evaluating individual projects in light of overall CRDP goals. This reflects the scarcity of skilled planners in Bolivia, and a reluctance to engage in this type of planning and implementation because of its potential to remove some flexibility for executive auspices. Consequently, while PDAR carries out a number of activities, the contribution of these activities to the goals of CRDP is insufficient. It has been suggested that the lack of AID/Bolivia authority may foster such poor administrative practices (19).

Instituto Boliviano de Tecnología Agropecuaria

Instituto Boliviano de Tecnología Agropecuaria (Bolivian Institute of Agriculture and Livestock Technology, IBTA) is the inheritor of agricultural research begun under PRODES, and, thus, has acquired long-term tropical agriculture research experience. It has assembled what is widely regarded as an excellent team of agricultural scientists and technicians, and has conducted important research on a wide range of crops in the Chapare that might provide farmers with alternatives to coca-leaf production. However, research has focused primarily on technical feasibility and yield maximization, rather than product marketability. The IBTA–Chapare long

---

[1] Additional confusion was introduced when SUBDESAL threw the United Nations Fund for Drug Abuse Control (UNFDAC) into the midst of the AID-funded institutions with no clarification of what their respective roles were to be (19).

[2] PDAR has undergone several name changes. At the time of the redesign of the CRDP, in 1987, the entity was called the *Subsecretaría para el Desarrollo del Trópico Boliviano* (Secretariat for Development of the Bolivian Tropics, SDTB) under the Ministry of Planning and Coordination. In July 1987, SDTB was placed under SUBDESAL authority and renamed the *Programa de Desarrollo Alternativo de Cochabamba* (Cochabamba Program for Alternative Development, PDAC). In January 1990, this was changed to the *Programa de Desarrollo Alternativo Regional*, reflecting concern with regional development problems that extended beyond the boundaries of Cochabamba department (19).

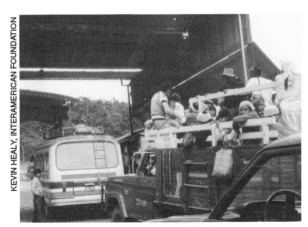

The poor, unemployed, and landless from neighboring communities often migrate to centers of coca-related activity. Thus, counternarcotics projects must also target areas of out-migration to reduce the lure of coca-related income. Here, vehicles pass a checkpoint before entering the Bolivian Chapare.

maintained that marketing issues were outside of their purview and that PDAR should be responsible for addressing these.[3] However, past PDAR efforts on market issues had been inadequate (19).

THE CHAPARE REGIONAL DEVELOPMENT PROJECT SINCE 1989

Significant improvements were made in this bleak picture in mid-1989. PDAR staff and technical abilities increased during this period. A new government assumed power in August 1989, and with it came increased commitment to CRDP activities (18). PDAR initiated 29 "immediate impact projects" in the Campero and Mizque provinces, which engendered considerable enthusiasm and participation by rural communities. During 1990, the number of projects carried out in the AHV increased to at least 40, and additional increases were projected for 1991. Institutional arrangements and responsibilities were defined (19).

Since 1989, SUBDESAL also has undergone several changes that improved the ability of the

CRDP to implement projects (18). SUBDESAL was placed in a chain of command with the Minister of Peasant Affairs and Agriculture clearly at the top, and a clear relationship between national policy objectives and the planning and implementation of local activities was established (25). Furthermore, some redefinition of the division of labor between SUBDESAL and PDAR occurred.

Increased attention also has been placed on marketing aspects in the CRDP (24). Technical assistance to PDAR and producer groups is now being strengthened, particularly in marketing. Irrespective of where market issues are addressed, an integrated production-to-market approach is needed for crop substitution efforts in the Chapare to be successful. Research might be prioritized by market availability for potential alternative crops. Thus, market identification and research would be closely integrated with agricultural research and extension.

Still, the CRDP was criticized for being unable to: address the development issues underlying participation of rural populations in coca production, conduct the necessary planning and coordination to repeat past successes and reduce or eliminate failures, or develop individual activities to reinforce one another to produce the multiplier effect needed for results to be long-term and significant beyond the local level. Problems continued to confront the major institutions involved in the CRDP (cf: 12,17,19). The CRDP was recently replaced by CORDEP (Cochabamba Regional Development Project), and CORDEP's relationships with Bolivian Government agencies have been modified or redefined (figures 3-1 and 3-2), in part to address the kinds of problems referred to above.

■ Peru and Coca Substitution Projects

In the early eighties, the Peruvian Government, in cooperation with the United States, created

---

[3] Nevertheless, IBTA–Chapare has, on the other hand, on several occasions invited input from international advisors on marketing issues, and is taking a larger role in this matter under CORDEP (19).

Figure 3-2—Cochabamba Regional Development Project Organizational Structure

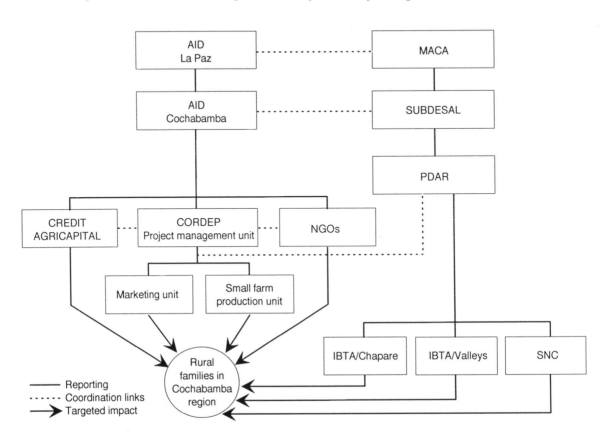

AID = Agency for International Development.
CORDEP = Cochabamba Regional Development Project.
IBTA = Instituto Boliviano de Tecnología Agropecuaria (Bolivian Institute of Agriculture and Livestock Technology).
MACA = Ministerio de Asuntos Campesinos y Agricultura (Ministry of Agriculture and Campesino Affairs).
NGO = Nongovernmental organization.
PDAR = Programa de Desarrollo Alternativo Regional (Regional Program for Alternative Development).
SNC = Servicio Nacional de Camines (National Road Service).
SUBDESAL = Subsecretaría de Desarrollo Alternativo y Sustitución de Cultivos de Coca (Subsecretariat for Alternative Development and Crop Substitution for Coca).

SOURCE: Development Alternatives, Inc., (DAI), *Cochabamba Regional Development Project (CORDEP)—Bolivia*, Technical Proposal (Bethesda, MD: DAI, 1992).

several special projects to develop the upper jungle, among them, the *Proyecto Especial Alto Huallaga* (Alto Huallaga Special Project, PEAH) (figure 3-3). The general objectives of this set of projects were to:

- Increase regional agricultural productivity;
- Occupy upper and lower jungle areas;
- Economically matriculate the region by means of the Marginal Highway; and
- Maintain regional ecological equilibrium, rational exploitation of natural resources, and improvement in the living standards of the population (8).

PROYECTO ESPECIAL ALTO HUALLAGA

PEAH had peculiar characteristics that distinguished it from the other projects because of the need to address the problem of coca expansion. The Peruvian Government and AID/Peru designed a Project Paper for the execution of PEAH. The project design included research, extension, and training components; highway maintenance; and credit development components (19).

The Project Paper incorporated control and development strategies. It proposed massive coca eradication under direction of the *Proyecto de Control y Reducción de los Cultivos de Coca en el Alto Huallaga* (Project for the Control and Reduction of Coca Cultivation in the Alto Huallaga, CORAH) and a development plan to increase legal agricultural production in the region under the responsibility of PEAH. The second objective, however, was subordinate to the former (8). While the development objective is considered in some sections of the Project Paper as an independent one, in reality, both objectives were interrelated and even explicitly articulated.[4] PEAH management assumed that eradication would oblige farmers to turn to legal production,

irrespective of the economic and historical processes that gave coca production in the Alto Huallaga its importance (19).

Several features of a national social, political, and economic nature were neglected and contributed to the failure of CORAH and PEAH. Some more notable of these include:

- The narrowly defined project area that excluded producers outside identified boundaries;
- The assumption that producers inside boundaries would remain after eradication irrespective of economic dysfunctions associated with legitimate agricultural production in the region;
- Failure to anticipate a violent reaction to eradication by the population, and subsequent expansion of subversive violence;
- Lack of development components appropriate to the producing areas (e.g., despite the suitability of the region for tropical forest production, a forestry component was lacking); and
- Failure to recognize the historical labor scarcity problem (8).

Labor shortages are one of the worst consequences of coca expansion in Alto Huallaga, and constitute an authentic bottleneck for the promotion of technical assistance and the extension of areas under legal crops (19). Those farmers who originally were unwilling to enter into coca production finally did so in the face of the pressure from increased production costs.

The Project Paper was amended in 1986 to emphasize agricultural extension above research and training, and also include a community development component. The principal objective of the extension component was to increase the

---

4 For example, the Project Paper said that regional development should minimize the negative social effects of coca eradication, and that eradication and economic development formed two sides of the same coin, with economic development efforts depending on progress in eradication. The paper did not treat regional development as an end in itself and did not formulate significant proposals for an integrated program of economic development to include all farmers in the region, not just coca producers (8). Also, it did not consider how coca eradication might negatively affect possibilities for development.

Figure 3-3—Location of Proyecto Especial Alto Huallaga

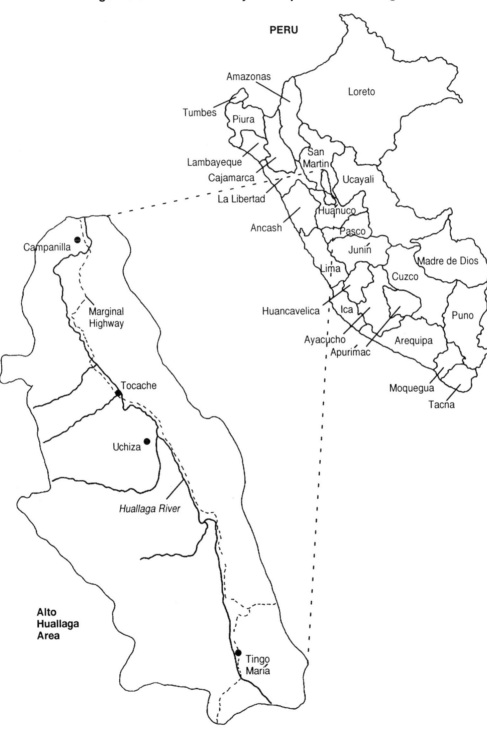

SOURCE: Adapted from ECONSULT, *Final Report on the Evaluation of AID Project No. 527-0244—Development of the Alto Huallaga Area* (Lima, Peru: ECONSULT S.A., 1987).

rate of adoption of new production technologies developed through agricultural research. The lack of a relatively stable market for most legal crops hindered extension efforts and made it difficult for legal crops to be as attractive to farmers as coca. In light of the importance of family labor, a stable market has always been important in making a legal crop an attractive alternative to coca. Family labor reduces price sensitivity and increases incentives to distribute labor inputs over longer periods (19).

The introduction of the community development subcomponent was a positive decision, resulting in a qualitative change in attitude among the farmers affected by the actions implemented by social promoters. Agricultural clubs and women's clubs, established and supported by the component, were capable of managing new cultivated plots and proved efficient in installing nurseries for cocoa and citrus plants and in rearing small livestock. Similarly, the community development subcomponent successfully carried out a range of activities including road construction, park beautification, and latrine construction. The community development operations were placed in the context of regional agricultural development that took into account the most important problems of coca expansion. Even though it was a positive step, community development was not placed within the principal objective of stimulating legal agriculture in the Alto Huallaga (19).

■ Colombian Narcotics Control and Eradication Projects

Only a small amount of coca is produced in Colombia (i.e., roughly 13 percent); its clandestine laboratories and an efficient trafficking network pose greater concerns. Therefore, narcotics control policies have focused on disruption and deterrence of drug processing and trafficking, often by military and police countermeasures. Furthermore, because relatively few Colombians grow coca, U.S.-assisted eradication programs have a narrower social and economic impact and,

thus, have been more politically feasible than is the case in Bolivia or Peru.

1978-1982

Early Colombian counternarcotics efforts began in the 1970s, aimed at marijuana trade on the Atlantic Coast. The marijuana industry permeated the economic and political fabric of the Guajira region, and with corruption and violence reaching anarchic proportions, the government feared loss of control in the area (1). Then, as now, the Colombian Government was under pressure to adopt U.S. counternarcotics policies in return for assistance. Two policies of fundamental importance in Colombian supply-reduction efforts were interdiction and eradication (1). (See also Extradition, in chapter 2.)

In November 1978, Colombia's President responded by instituting a National Security Statute, authorizing military participation in national governance and law enforcement. The Colombian Government then initiated *Operación Fulminante*, a U.S.-assisted, militarization- and manual eradication-based effort to curb the marijuana trade and regain control of the Guajira. Approximately 10,000 troops were deployed. Results of that campaign were mixed, and did not suggest success (1,2). For example:

- Although marijuana trade was reduced, it was not halted.
- To the extent that enforcement efforts were successful, they tended merely to displace production and trade activities to other parts of the country (the "balloon effect"), rather than eliminate them.
- The Colombian military was susceptible to corruption.
- Traffickers proved able to reestablish activities quickly as military presence withdrew.
- Supply-sided eradication and interdiction campaigns were not coupled with parallel demand-reduction programs, thus reducing prospects of disrupting narcotics trafficking.

- The costs to the local population were high and deeply resented, and lacking rapid headway, the general public quickly concluded that repressive counternarcotics measures were not in Colombia's best interest, despite U.S. Government praise for the operation.

From the Colombian military's perspective, the guerrilla challenge was more important, and from the civilian perspective, increasing political violence and social unrest were of greater concern (2). In March 1980, the Colombian army announced that it was abandoning its anti-marijuana efforts in the Guajira region.

During this period, the Colombian Government commissioned a study on using herbicides to eradicate marijuana. However, Colombia's National Council of Dangerous Drugs (*Consejo Nacional de Estupificantes*) determined by consensus not to apply herbicides (1).

1982-1986

A new narcotics directive was established under President Betancur: no extradition on nationalist grounds, no militarization because of domestic considerations, and no herbicidal eradication for environmental reasons. Yet, despite its seemingly unaggressive agenda, the new administration quickly initiated an ambitious, DEA-backed interdiction effort. Furthermore, when narcotics traffickers retaliated by assassinating the Justice Minister, the new government promptly reversed its no-extradition and no-herbicide policies (1,5).

As had occurred with anti-marijuana operations, the narcotics trafficker's quickly adopted new tactics for evading interdiction. Processing was reverted to mobile, small-scale operations, and the powerful cartel bosses negotiated new trade routes and alliances through other countries. They also increased their use of bribery, murder, kidnapping, and other terrorist activities to protect themselves, and assure the loyalty of their employees (2).

Betancur initiated programs for herbicidal eradication of marijuana in 1984, and coca in 1985. Both programs were protested by the public, and neither achieved long-term success. Marijuana production declined only temporarily, and, again, many growers responded to the threat of eradication by reducing their plots, moving operations to less air-accessible canyons, and growing marijuana alongside legal crops (1).

1986-1990

In the mid-1980s, the Colombian Government faced conflicting images: though praised for cracking down on narcotics trafficking, it did not seem to have restricted the flow of cocaine. Moreover, the Colombian justice system had been decimated by drug-related violence, and the new administration faced the same daunting panorama of threats (e.g., guerrilla insurgencies, drug-related corruption and killing, and rampant human rights abuses).

Marijuana and coca eradication programs continued, but the returns on these efforts, particularly for marijuana, began to decline relative to increases in the number of hectares under cultivation. Explanations for the declining rates included: 1) shifting of marijuana cultivation to other regions; 2) increasing profitability of other illegal drug markets, such as hashish and poppies; 3) declines in U.S. Government assistance; and 4) diverted government effort to militarization and extradition aspects of narcotics policy, as well as ongoing counter-insurgency concerns (1).

1990-PRESENT

Although production of narcotic plants has never weighed heavily in Colombia's involvement in narcotics industry, evidence indicates expansion of these activities. A January 1992 *Departamento Administrativo de Seguridad* report stated that Colombia had some 25,000 hectares of opium poppies under cultivation, while the U.S. Government estimated 10,000 hectares (16). The Colombian Government began eradicating opium poppy fields with glyphosate in 1992, despite protests from the peasant population (16).

Coca eradication as a Colombian narcotics control policy has had short-term effects, although little chance to have a large impact. Growth of coca cultivation came *after* Colombians were deeply involved in the cocaine trade and, thus, the supply of coca leaves in the country grew in response to the growth of the cocaine industry. Most of the income obtained by Colombians from the coca and cocaine trade comes from the manufacturing and international distribution of cocaine and the drug "cartels" have already large investments in and out of the country. Thus, policies to disrupt illegal drug manufacturing and marketing, and to make it more difficult to use the capital accumulated, are likely to have a greater overall impact on the Colombian cocaine industry than eradication programs (1).

■ National Narcotics Enforcement and Effects on Development

In addition to the inherent difficulties faced by development projects in Bolivia and Peru, enforcement practices in both countries sometimes have compounded the task of generating local support for activities. Rather than fostering alternative means of livelihood, even limited eradication has notably impeded execution of some agricultural extension and community development efforts (8). Some experts suggest that competing goals of narcotics control and development generally contribute to this situation. Repressive actions on the part of some U.S.-sponsored institutions may be the single largest constraint on the success of U.S.-sponsored developments efforts (19).

Unidad Móvil de Patrulla Rural (Mobile Rural Patrol Unit, UMOPAR) has primary responsibility for narcotics control activities in Bolivia. The organization has been accused of brutality against peasants involved in coca production as well as providing protection for narcotics traffickers on occasion (11). Analysts suggest that increasing militarization of the "drug war" generally and U.S. sponsorship of UMOPAR particularly may constitute the largest constraints on success of U.S.-sponsored development efforts in Bolivia. Partly as a response to the problems with UMOPAR, the Bolivian Government, with U.S. sponsorship, has created a new counternarcotics force, the *Fuerza Especial en la Lucha Contra el Narcotráfico* (Special Force in the Struggle Against Drug Trafficking, FELCN), which began operations in late June 1991. Because of the corruption problems associated with UMOPAR, plans call for the FELCN to be "insulated" from the rest of the Bolivian police force. How this insulation is to be accomplished remains unclear. It is also unclear how the addition of a second counternarcotics unit will address the problems of abusive and violent behavior on the part of police that have undermined development efforts (19).

The effectiveness of Peru's PEAH in working with coca farmers also was hampered by its association with repressive police action. This situation was provoked by the fact that CORAH received logistic support from the *Unidad Móvil de Patrullaje Rural de la Guardia Civil del Perú* (Mobile Rural Patrol Unit, Peruvian Civil Guard, UMOPAR of Peru). The coercive method used by the CORAH with the support of UMOPAR produced resistance by the affected coca farmers (8). The process of eradication also caused an important sector of rural and urban populations to fail to discriminate or distinguish between these three different institutions. Drug dealers and the *Sendero Luminoso* have taken advantage of this fact to distort the program of PEAH. This problem should also be analyzed in terms of the PEAH concept and its relation to the eradication process implemented by CORAH. While it is true that PEAH was designed to promote regional legal agricultural development, the emphasis on the need to assist former coca farmers constituted a risk inherent in the institutional life of the project. The violent image of CORAH and UMOPAR of Peru evidently affected PEAH's image not only

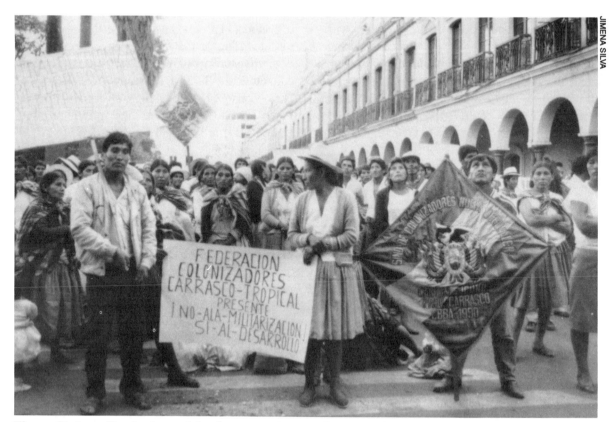

The conflicting militarization and development assistance objectives of past counternarcotics programs have undermined their effectiveness and often generated lasting resentment among target populations. Here, demonstrators in Cochabamba, Bolivia, carry a poster that reads, "No to militarization! Yes to development!"

among coca producers, but also among other economic sectors, increasing the resentment of the farmers against CORAH as well as PEAH (19).

CONCLUSION

Crop substitution and eradication efforts are inherently slow. Coordination among development and enforcement organizations is critical; coordination can help ensure that they will not adversely affect one another in pursuit of their individual goals. In the past, they have worked in different areas with varied degrees of success. Development groups generally work to improve the region's standard of living, whereas enforcement agencies work to impede production of illegal crops and their derivatives.

Colombia poses an interesting political problem because it is not a major coca producer and does not depend on U.S. development assistance. It is possible that Colombia's involvement will change if supply is reduced, but concomitant demand reduction will be necessary to avoid the "balloon effect."

Development organizations can maintain their original philosophies while working with enforcement agencies. "Phased eradication" has been most successful for crop substitution and eradication projects in the past, and existing U.S. organizations are well-equipped to adopt such a strategy.

AID and INM [Bureau of International Narcotics Matters] have fundamental differences in their bureaucratic ethos and staff orientation. The former is essentially a development agency and its staff has expertise in overseas development. AID personnel tend to view the problem of narcotics control from a long-term development perspective and give priority to economic and social factors that affect coca production. INM has a narcotics control orientation and its staff is experienced in enforcement work. They tend to have a short-term perspective and believe enforcement must begin early in the project. These different attitudes can sometimes create barriers to cooperation and coordination efforts (26).

A proper blend of development assistance and enforcement and domestic and international agencies is needed. However, separation of enforcement and assistance activities should be clear at all levels. Determining the relative importance of each of these components, however, is problematic. Trust and education will probably prove to be the most important factors for success.

Ideally, public pressure for elimination of the drug problem should not be met with fewer options. Rather the effective translation of knowledge, scientific and historical, should enable the public to avoid over-simplification, and to exert influence based on more rational understanding (26).

CHAPTER 3 REFERENCES

1. Bagley, B., "Coca Eradication and Crop Substitution in Colombia," contractor report prepared for the Office of Technology Assessment, April 1992.
2. Bagley, B., "Colombia and the War on Drugs," *Foreign Affairs*, fall 1988, pp. 70-92.
3. Brunn, K., Pan, L., and Rexed, I., *The Gentlemen's Club—International Control of Drugs and Alcohol* (Chicago, IL: University of Chicago Press, 1975).
4. Carafa, Y., Arellano, S., and Uribe, M., *Tratamiento de la Temática de la Mujer en los Valles del Sur de Cochabamba* (La Paz, Bolivia: U.S. Agency for International Development, 1987), In: Painter and Bedoya, 1991.
5. Claudio, A., "United States-Colombia Extradition Treaty: Failure of a Security Strategy," *Military Review*, 71:69-77, 1991.
6. Cusack, J.T., "The International Narcotics Control System: Coca and Cocaine," D. Pacini and C. Franquemont (eds.), *Coca and Cocaine: Effects on People and Policy in Latin America*, Cultural Survival Report #23 (Peterborough, NH: Transcript Printing Company, 1986), pp. 65-71.
7. Development Alternatives, Inc. (DAI), *Cochabamba Regional Development Project (CORDEP)—Bolivia*, Technical Proposal (Bethesda, MD: DAI, 1992).
8. ECONSULT, *Final Report on the Evaluation of AID Project No. 527-0244—Development of the Alto Huallaga Area* (Lima, Peru: ECONSULT S.A., 1987).
9. Epstein, E.J., *Agency of Fear* (New York, NY: G.P. Putnam's Sons, 1977).
10. Healy, K., "Coca, the State, and the Peasantry in Bolivia, 1982-1988," *Journal of Interamerican Studies and World Affairs*, 30:105-127, 1988.
11. Jones, J.C., *Farmer Perspectives on the Economics and Sociology of Coca Production*, IDA Working Paper No. 77 (Binghamton, NY: Institute for Development Anthropology, 1990).
12. Jones, J.C., *Institutional Analysis of the Programa de Desarollo Alternativo Regional (PDAR)*, Working Paper (Binghamton, NY: Institute for Development Anthropology, 1991), In: Painter and Bedoya, 1991.
13. Kent, R., *Regional Planning and the Subsecretariat for the Development of the Bolivian Tropics* (La Paz, Bolivia: U.S. Agency for International Development, 1987).
14. McNicoll, A., *Drug Trafficking: A North-South Perspective* (Washington, DC: North-South Institute, 1983).
15. Musto, D.F., *The American Disease: Origins of Narcotics Control* (New Haven, CT: Yale University Press, 1987).
16. "Many in Colombia Resisting Use of a Strong Herbicide on Poppies," *New York Times*, Feb. 17, 1992, A5.
17. Organization of American States (OAS), Secretariat for Economic and Social Affairs, *Integrated Regional Development Planning: Guidelines and Case Studies from the OAS Experience*, Depart-

ment of Regional Development (Washington, DC: OAS, 1984), In: Painter and Bedoya, 1991.

18. Painter, M., *Institutional Analysis of the Chapare Regional Development Project (CRDP)*, Working Paper No. 59 (Binghamton, NY: Institute for Development Anthropology, 1990), In: Painter and Bedoya, 1991.

19. Painter, M., and Bedoya, E., ''Institutional Analysis of the Chapare Regional Development Project (CRDP) and the Upper Huallaga Special Project (PEAH),'' contractor report prepared for the Office of Technology Assessment, July 1991.

20. Painter, M., and Rasnake, R.N., ''Human Dimensions of the War on Drugs,'' *IDA: Development Anthropology Network* 7(2):8-16, 1989, In: Painter and Bedoya, 1991.

21. Pool, D.J., Adams, C., Boonstra, C., and Morris, G.L., *Evaluation of the Chapare Regional Development Project* (Gainesville, FL: Tropical Research and Development, Inc., 1986), In: Painter and Bedoya, 1991.

22. Rasnake, R.N., and Painter, M., *Rural Development and Crop Substitution in Bolivia: USAID and the Chapare Regional Development Project*, Working Paper No. 45 (Binghamton, NY: Institute for Development Anthropology, 1989), In: Painter and Bedoya, 1991.

23. Spain, J.W., ''The United States, Turkey, and the Poppy,'' *Middle East Journal*, summer 1975, pp. 295-301.

24. Stevenson, B., *''Post-Harvest Technologies to Improve Agricultural Profitability in Bolivia and the Andean Region,''* contractor report prepared for the Office of Technology Assessment, May 1992.

25. Subsecretaría de Desarrollo Alternativo y Sustitución de Cultivos de Coca (SUBDESAL), *Marco Institucional Para Desarrollo Alternativo y Sustitución de Cultivos de Coca* (La Paz, Bolivia: SUBDESAL, Ministerio de Asuntos Campesinos y Agricultura, 1990), In: Painter and Bedoya, 1991.

26. U.S. Agency for International Development, *A Review of AID's Narcotics Control Development Assistance Program*, AID Evaluation Special Study No. 29 (Washington, DC: Agency for International Development, 1986).

27. U.S. Agency for International Development, *Tribal Areas Development Project*, Special Second Evaluation, PD-AAZ-101 (Washington, DC: USAID, 1988).

28. U.S. Congress, General Accounting Office, *Rescission of the Opium Growing Ban by Turkey*, Report to the Congress B-173123 (Washington, DC: U.S. Government Printing Office, Sept. 9, 1974).

29. U.S. Department of State, Bureau of International Narcotics Matters (INM), *International Narcotics Control Strategy Report 1985* (Washington, DC: U.S. Government Printing Office, 1985).

30. U.S. Congress, House of Representatives, Committee on Foreign Affairs, Special Ad Hoc Subcommittee on International Narcotics Problems, *Politics of the Poppy,* Report of a Special Study Mission to Turkey: March 14-16, 1974, House of Representatives Print 93-n.a. (Washington, DC: U.S. Government Printing Office, 1974).

31. Zentner, J.L., ''The 1972 Turkish Opium Ban: Needle in the Haystack Diplomacy?'' *World Affairs* 136(1):36-40, 1973.

Renewable Resource-Based Alternatives to Coca Production | 4

T he geography and topography of the Andean region provide diverse ecological settings with a broad range of natural renewable resources. Developing and implementing sustainable management of these renewable resources could help improve food and fiber production for national consumption and for export markets. Today, agricultural, forest, wildland and wildlife, and aquatic resources are all exploited to some extent. However, use of improved production and management technologies could expand these activities and generate increased economic benefits. In terms of coca substitution programs, greatest attention has been given to agriculture and some promising crops and cropping systems.

INTRODUCTION

Agroecosystems in the Andean coca-producing regions differ markedly from the highly mechanized lowland agriculture practiced, for example, on the great plains of North America. Rather, agriculture tends to be small-scale and distant from markets or political or financial support, and extremes of topography preclude extensive mechanization in most cases. The small returns for most farmers impede acceptance of new and potentially risky technology. High-input approaches to farming, characterized by the green revolution, are less applicable in these settings.

Moreover, the diversity of Andean environments does not favor regional agricultural and agronomic planning. For example, almost 50 percent of Bolivian and Peruvian land area is steep slopes and highlands. Only about 10 percent of the total surface area of each country is suitable for row crop agriculture. Frequent floods, droughts, and severe soil erosion make agricultural production difficult in many areas.

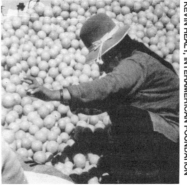

KEVIN HEALY, INTERAMERICAN FOUNDATION

The most fertile agricultural soils are alluvial deposits in the valleys. Physical environmental features (e.g., soils, slope, erosion potential) can change character markedly over short distances. Climatic features (e.g., precipitation patterns, winds, temperature) may vary with distances (especially altitudes) and time (season). This variability means that a site-specific approach must be applied to defining realistic technical solutions for coca substitution. Unfortunately, little site-specific information exists on climate, soils, or topography for some parts of the Andes and the prospects are minimal for gaining this information in certain coca producing areas (e.g., Alto Huallaga).

Intricate patterns of land uses and land tenure have evolved over the years as a result of disparate cultural forces. Current agriculture in the region is a mixture of pre-Columbian, Spanish, and contemporary practices, many of which are incompatible with one another. This situation further complicates development of alternative crops and cropping systems. Nevertheless, significant efforts have been invested in identifying crops and crop combinations that might improve the value of agricultural activities in the Andean region. Largely, these efforts have focused on export agriculture rather than enhancement of the domestic food supply system. Difficulties in moving these commodities to the international market, as well as in providing sufficient quantity and quality of product, have constrained alternative crop efforts to date.

In addition to agricultural resources, forest, aquatic, and wildlife resource exploitation could offer alternative livelihoods. Tropical forest resources have received increased global attention over the last several decades. Tropical timber exports were key in national economies in the mid-1900s and continue to command high prices in the international market. Constraints to continued or increased exploitation largely arise from concerns over conservation of biological diversity and potential adverse global environmental effects. Indeed, consumer boycotts of tropical

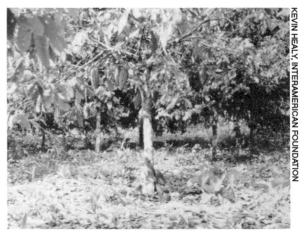

*Simple processing and storage requirements make cocoa (*Theobroma cacao*) an attractive alternative in remote areas. Shown here is cocoa production in the Alto Beni, Bolivia.*

KEVIN HEALY, INTERAMERICAN FOUNDATION

hardwoods for these reasons are becoming more common. Nevertheless, there are opportunities for sustainable timber production and forest conservation and protection in the Andean region (71).

Tropical wildlife has been an important domestic and export resource in South America for at least 400 years (70,72) and has been economically important. Unsustainable exploitation, however, increased concerns over species loss and led to international treaties and trade agreements to protect rare, threatened, and endangered species (i.e., Convention on International Trade in Endangered Species). More recently, international conservation organizations have focused on sustainable development of wildlife resources. Potential markets include hides and fibers, pet, meat, and other animal products (e.g., bone), and technologies exist for managing a variety of amphibians, reptiles, fishes, birds, and mammals to provide these commodities. Nature-based tourism associated with protection and conservation of wildlife and wildland resources offers another opportunity for increasing economic returns from conservation activities (6).

Freshwater aquatic resources, largely fisheries in lakes, rivers, and streams, currently occupy a small share of national food production systems.

Estimates suggest that current harvest is far below optimum sustainable yield for many species. A paucity of data on the extent of Andean freshwater resources hinders analysis of the potential contribution they could make to national food production and economies. Yet, use of improved postharvest handling, storage, and transportation of fishery products alone could increase their contribution. Additional opportunities lie in implementation of improved capture, resource restoration, and aquaculture technologies (101).

Opportunities exist for improving crop substitution programs and increasing their acceptability to local populations. Some crops, production and processing technologies, and markets are available. New crops that might improve the economics of agricultural production have been identified. However, further research will be needed to identify appropriate cultivars, production techniques, and market potential. If substitution programs expand the range of resources exploited, sustainable development technologies for forest, wildland and wildlife, and aquatic resources will be needed.

AGRICULTURAL RESOURCES[1]

Coca is grown mostly in the humid tropic regions of the Andean countries of Bolivia, Peru, and Colombia. While little variation in temperature is evident among the coca growing zones, precipitation variation is obvious (table 4-1). The difficulties faced by agriculture in such areas are well known (49,55,98). Many problems are related directly to high rainfall and temperature regimes that promote nutrient leaching, poor soil

Table 4-1—Temperature and Rainfall of Major Coca Production Zones

	Mean annual temperature (C)	Rainfall (mm)
Bolivia		
Chapare	23 - 25	2,500 - 5,000
Colombia		
Amazon[a]	22 - 26	2,500 - 5,000
coffee belt	20 - 24	1,000 - 1,900
Peru		
Alto Huallaga	22 - 26	2,500 - 3,500
Central Hullaga	21 - 25	1,400 - 1,900
Central Urubamba	21 - 25	2,000 - 2,500
Ene	23 - 25	1,700 - 1,900
Gran Pajonal	21 - 25	1,700 - 1,900
La Convencion	22 - 24	n.d.
Mayo	21 - 25	n.d.
Pachitea[a]	23 - 25	2,000 - 3,500
Palcazu[a]	23 - 25	4,000 - 8,000
Pichis[a]	23 - 25	2,500 - 3,500
Tambo	23 - 25	1,700 - 1,900
Yurimaguas[a]	23 - 25	2,000 - 2,500

[a] Little diurnal temperature variation.
n.d. = no data.

SOURCE: H. Villachica, C. Lescano, J. Lazarte, and V. Chumbe, "Estudio de oportunidades de inversion en desarrollo e industrializacion de cultivos tropicales en Pucallpa," Perfil de proyecto para la planta de coloantes naturales yu para la planta de conservas de palmito, Convenio FUNDEAGRO, Region Ucayali, Lima Peru, 1992.

composition, low fertility, and rapid growth of pest problems. All of these features can lead to increasing dependence on external inputs (e.g., pesticides, fertilizers, fuels) and affect the types of agricultural opportunities available to farmers.

Distinct changes in the agricultural sector resulting from the expansion of the cocaine economy complicate efforts to improve agricultural profitability. As production of coca leaf became agronomically and economically attrac-

---

[1] This section was drawn largely from the following contracted background papers:

H. Villachica, "Crop Diversification in Bolivia, Colombia, and Peru: Potential to Enhance Agricultural Production," contractor report prepared for the Office of Technology Assessment, April 1992.

S. Gliessman, "Diversification and Multiple Cropping as a Basis for Agricultural Alternatives in Coca Producing Regions," contractor report prepared for the Office of Technology Assessment, February 1992.

B. McD. Stevenson, "Post-Harvest Technologies to Improve Agricultural Profitability," contractor report prepared for the Office of Technology Assessment, March 1992.

A. Chavez, "Andean Agricultural Research and Extension Systems and Technology Transfer Activities: Potential Mechanisms To Enhance Crop Substitution Efforts in Bolivia, Colombia, and Peru," contractor report prepared for the Office of Technology Assessment, December 1991.

tive, many farmers abandoned livestock raising and other crop production systems. Some local traditional agriculture systems were abandoned as well. Larger areas were deforested, more coca planted, and less time and energy were invested in traditional agriculture. This increasingly affluent agricultural sector developed a dependence on imported purchased food and experienced a shift in aspirations.

While the agricultural sectors in Bolivia, Peru, and Colombia are diverse, some similarities among producers and farm size are evident in primary coca producing regions. Producers tend to be semi-commercial (i.e., producing subsistence crops along with some cash crops including coca), production units are small (e.g., 20 hectare units or less are common); and production systems tend to be labor intensive. The remote nature of the producing zones means that inputs may be costly and difficult to obtain and markets (other than at the "farm-gate") are difficult to reach. Coca plays a key role in farm income.

Crop substitution strategies must work on two fronts. Development of new production options for the coca producing regions must be complemented by development in areas from which migrant coca growers and laborers come. National and international assistance and research organizations support efforts to identify and expand opportunities for new crops that can replace coca in the agricultural economy (105). Primary categories through which agricultural profitability might be increased in the coca growing regions of the Andean nations include:

- Diversifying production,
- Intensifying production,
- Improving production efficiency, and
- Increasing the value of products through processing (chapter 5).

Current crop substitution efforts focus on diversifying production by incorporating high value crops. However, attention is being given increasingly to the latter categories.

Despite the potential for improving production through innovative cropping systems, the acceptability to producers comprises an important concern. Social and economic advantages must accompany improved systems. Crop diversification, increased market options, reductions in direct costs and risks, and increased opportunities for involvement for all members of the family or community become critical components of acceptable alternative systems.

■ Diversifying Agricultural Production

Diversifying agricultural production by incorporating high-value crops into production systems offers one approach to expand alternatives for agricultural populations and allows an incremental evolution from a coca-based production system to one based on legitimate markets. Indeed, this approach is the basis of traditional crop substitution efforts, and ongoing research focuses on identifying high-value traditional and nontraditional crops suitable to local agricultural production systems.

Inherent in the diversification strategy is the ability of farmers to continue to provide for their basic needs during the development stage of the new production system. For example, many cropping systems require 3 to 5 years of effort prior to realization of profit (105,122). Coca could be maintained as a cash source during this period although it seems counter to substitution program goals. However, such an approach could offer an alternative to costly agricultural subsidies.

Research has focused on a variety of crops that could be suitable for local, regional, national, and international markets. Largely this research is market driven and focuses on grains, industrial crops, fruits and nuts, and spices. Blending of these crops into traditional food production systems is another important feature of these efforts. In this way, producers continue to provide for basic food and fiber needs while developing opportunities to generate cash through marketing.

Table 4-2—Cropping Patterns of the Chapare, Bolivia

Crop	Hectares (thousands)	Percent	Percent of total
Annuals			
Corn	3.3	9.0%	2.7%
Rice	20.0	54.3	16.8
Yuca	13.3	36.1	11.2
Perennials			
Banana	19.8	24.0	16.6
Citrus	6.5	7.9	5.46
Coca	55.9	67.8	46.9
Other	0.3	0.3	2.5

SOURCE: Development Alternatives, Inc., "Environmental Assessment of the Chapare Regional Development Project, Bolivia," DAI, Bethesda, MD, 1990, In: Stevenson, 1992.

The range of potential commodities that could offer agricultural alternatives is restricted to a certain extent by the environmental features of coca growing areas. Box 4-A describes some crops identified as potential alternatives. Although the list is not exhaustive, it illustrates the range of crop types that might be considered and blended into existing production systems.

Most crop substitution strategies in the Chapare region of Bolivia involve some combination of soil-conserving perennial crops and annual cash crops for immediate returns (table 4-2). Research in annual crops concentrates on maize, rice, beans, and yuca; the perennials program is focused on citrus, coffee, cocoa, and pepper. Other research deals with production and management of cattle, pigs, and poultry.

Efforts are also underway to examine essential oils (e.g., eucalyptus, pyrethrum oils); natural plant chemicals (e.g., xanthophyll); spices (e.g., *piper nigrum);* tropical fruits (e.g., pineapple, passionfruit, bananas, carambola); and nuts (e.g., macadamia). Pineapples and bananas seem to be promising in terms of fresh export and there has been some success with shipments to Argentina and northern Chile. Nontraditional crops of turmeric (*Curcuma domestica*) and ginger (*Zingiber officinale*) demonstrate export potential and production is underway at a trial level. Several other

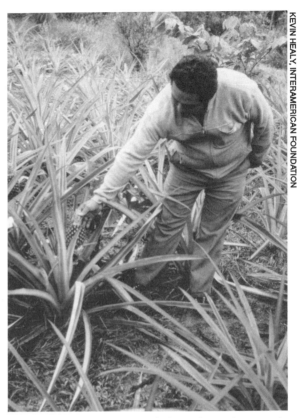

Pineapple is being produced as an alternative crop in the Chapare, Bolivia. Private sector investment in a local processing facility for Chapare and Santa Cruz pineapples may promote the value of production.

crops from the areas may have potential for increased profitability, including garlic, onions, peanuts, anise, cumin, and perennial fruit crops. Although export potential for many of these crops is low, improved postharvest practices could contribute to higher quality and greater economic returns.

A number of agricultural products are being industrialized, including: tea, banana, kudzu, yuca, mint, and lemon grass. In addition, a coffee production and processing industry is being developed in the Chapare. The scale of existing production and the 5-year potential for production increases for these crops are shown in table 4-3. Achieving this potential will require investment in producing plant material, promoting the crops

Box 4-A—Alternative Crops

Alternative crop research poses an immense problem because of the numerous, and sometimes competing, requirements associated with identifying legitimate crops that can compete with a "black market" activity. Not only must crops be suitable to agroecological conditions, they must possess qualities that make them socioculturally acceptable and economically attractive. This is a tall order for any research activity. Research in the Andean countries has focused on annual grain crops, industrial crops, commercial fruits, nuts, and specialty crops (e.g., spices, fibers, dyes). The following briefly describes some of these crops.

Annatto (*Bixa orellana*): Annatto (also Achiote) is a native plant from the Amazon region. The plant chemical bixin is extracted from the seeds and has commercial value as a natural dye. Peru currently supplies 40 percent of the international bixin market. Substitution efforts in Bolivia have begun to work on increasing Annatto production. Primary production concerns include the highly variable yields and bixin content of seeds (2.5 to 3 percent), appropriate planting densities, difficulties in blending annatto with other crops because of its fast-growing nature (although some success has been noted in annatto/cowpea combinations), and high hand labor requirements. Plant breeding efforts are focusing on increasing yields and the bixin content of seeds (up to 4 percent) and developing cultivars suitable to low-fertility, acid soils. High hand labor requirements might be addressed through harvest and threshing mechanization. Improved processing techniques could provide products with higher bixin content (increasing from 30 to 35 percent to 90 to 95 percent). The trend toward natural dyes may increase market opportunities for annatto production. Annatto seems to be relatively free of pests and disease problems.

Araza (*Eugenia stipitata*): Araza is a tropical fruit tree native to the Amazon region, although it is not yet widely cultivated. While the tree is tolerant of acid, low-fertility soils, best production is observed in well-managed and properly fertilized fields. Primary production concerns include the relative lack of agronomic technology for cultivation, planting densities and field management to obtain optimum production, and fertilizer requirements. Improved production techniques, including promising ecotypes and associated nursery and field management needs, are current research areas. Fruit production begins 1 year after transplanting with final height reached by 6 to 7 years, although this is affected by soil fertility. Araza's slow growth rate allows intercropping with crops such as cassava or turmeric, thereby generating benefits during the field development stage. However, there is no international market for araza currently. The high acid content precludes fresh consumption but it can be used for juice, dried fruit, and ice cream flavoring.

Bananas (*Musa sp.*): Bananas currently are produced in coca-growing zones and some success with export has been noted in Bolivia. Banana is a traditional crop in the Andean region and thus adoption is not a key concern. Further, since farmers already are familiar with banana production they could be more responsive to extension efforts to improve production. Primary production concerns include need for evenly distributed rainfall, high sunlight requirements, fertilizer requirements, need for low wind conditions, and soil condition (deep with high organic matter content). Research is needed on improved varieties to enter export markets, appropriate planting densities, improved propagule selection, careful field management (e.g., weeding and thinning) to sustain production, and postharvest technologies. A number of pests and diseases affect bananas; however, chemical and management techniques exist to control the most devastating of these.

Black Pepper (*Piper nigrum*): Black pepper is being cultivated to some extent in or near coca-growing regions in the Andean countries. Pepper is a climbing shrub and requires a support to grow on. Either posts or trees may be used as supports and production techniques exist for both systems. National research institutes are working to improve production technology, and potential exists for technology transfer from current producing countries. Key needs include improved cultivars (for increased yield and pest resistance), propagation, and seedling management. Production concerns include field preparation, soil condition (e.g., well-drained, aerated, high organic matter content), fertilizer needs, and high labor requirements during establishment and harvest phases. Systems have been developed that intercrop pepper with ginger or cassava during the early growth stages, and additional work in China indicates potential for pepper, rubber, and tea systems. Primary pests include fungi and nematodes and while chemical controls are available, they are costly. Despite high labor requirements for production, primary processing is relatively simple and generally involves sun-drying and threshing.

Brazil nut (*Bertholletia excelsa*): Brazil nut trees are not found in most coca-growing zones and a somewhat lengthy development period may hinder plantation development. Under cultivated conditions, nut production may begin in 8 to 10 years after planting or if trees are grafted this may be shortened to 6 years. Production concerns largely center on the need for well-drained soils and the lengthy period from initialization to production. Brazilian researchers have developed techniques for brazil nut production and cropping systems. Further work conducted in Peru indicates some potential for mixed systems of brazil nut, cassava, rice, and tahiti lime. In fact, intercropping with other fruit trees may increase nut production by maintaining pollinator populations during the time the nut tree is not flowering. Testing is still in initial stages and there are no accurate estimations of potential income. Areas where the tree currently exists and coca is expanding, or areas where it is likely to expand, may provide the best possibilities for introducing this type of production system.

Cardamom (*Elettaria cadamomum*): Cardamom, a high-value spice, is not native to the Andean region, although it has been identified as a potential alternative crop. Shade is important for cardamom growth but the plant will produce in poorly drained soil. This combination may offer an opportunity for farmers to crop some of their lower quality production areas. Propagation by rhizome allows cardamom production within 3 years, but the susceptibility of rhizomes to mosaic virus detracts from this approach. Seed is being used increasingly, however, development time increases to 5 years and seeds lose their viability quickly. Cardamom has been incorporated in some Colombian cropping systems in an effort to diversify coffee and it is being introduced in Bolivia and Peru. Constraints to expansion include the lack of a local market and that the international market currently is satisfied by Asian and Central American production.

Citrus (Orange, Mandarin, Tangelos): Citrus production requires rather specific soil and climatic conditions. However, it is suitable for the Chapare, Alto Huallaga, Upper Mayo, and Colombian piedmont. Orange production largely would be directed to the juice market, while mandarin and tangelo production have potential for fresh markets. Intercropping systems incorporating citrus are used widely in current production areas. Primary production concerns include soil conditions (e.g., well-aerated, deep soils), market size, and processing options for small communities. Pests and diseases are well known—ants, aphids, fruit flies, root rot, tristeza, and exocortis. Tolerant varieties are available and other management methods exist to prevent viral infections.

Cocoa (*Theobroma cacao*): Cocoa is cultivated in coca-growing areas of Peru and, to a lesser extent, in Colombia and Bolivia. Research undertaken in Colombia, Brazil, Ecuador, and Costa Rica has focused on improved cultivars, nursery management, planting densities, cropping systems, agrichemical needs, and postharvest processing. Additional research needs include: matching varieties to ecological zones, seed production and availability, shade management for new fields, and intercropping systems for cocoa and other subsistence or economic crops. Evenly distributed rainfall and soil pH factors are primary production concerns for cocoa. Cocoa is affected by several diseases—witches broom, black pod, and monilia. Cultivation and harvest practices can combat witches broom and black pod infestation (i.e., tree pruning, frequent harvest), while monilia currently is only controlled through pesticide applications.

Coffee (*Coffea arabica*): Coffee seems to offer the closest economic alternative to coca in some regions and production methods and cultivars exist for shade and sun coffee. However, coca-growing regions that do not experience sufficient diurnal temperature variation may not be suitable since coffee requires such shifts for ripening. Primary production concerns include soil drainage, nursery management, and pest- and temperature-resistant cultivars. Coffee is affected by a number of pests and diseases (e.g., insects, nematodes, fungi), although

(continued on next page)

Box 4-A—Continued

the cherry borer and yellow rust pose the primary problems. Pesticides and tolerant varieties are available to reduce the adverse impact of pest infestations on production. Research supported by the Colombian National Coffee Growers Association (NCGA) has contributed significantly to solving a number of production problems.

Macadamia (*Macadamia integrifolia* and *Macadamia tetraphylla*): Macadamia production typically requires well-drained fertile soils with high organic matter content. Low temperatures can reduce nut production and the tree is very susceptible to freezing. This aspect may pose some difficulty for expansion in the Chapare, where seasonal winds can bring temperatures as low as 6 degrees C. Production concerns focus on the need for appropriate fertilizer regimes to sustain production. Current low grafting success (i.e., only 15 to 20 percent) has hindered expansion in Bolivia and Peru, although efforts are ongoing to promote macadamia production. The tree is suitable for interplanting with annual crops or coffee or other trees during early years and thus could be integrated in existing production systems. Pests and diseases that attack macadamia include the black bee, ants, nut borers, rats, root diseases, and fungi; yet control measures are available, although in some cases expensive. Interest in production is increasing because of ongoing substitution programs. However, market is largely international and thus will require concomitant infrastructure development.

Passion fruit (*Passiflora edulis*): Passion fruit is a fast growing tropical vine and fruit production may begin as early as 8 to 10 months after transplanting from the nursery. While two varieties exist, the *flavicarpa* variety seems to be more suitable to the temperature conditions of the Andean region. Seed production is prolific and thus does not pose a constraint to increased production. The fast growth rate, however, affects passion fruit's suitability for intercropping systems, although it may be associated with short-season cassava, turmeric, pineapple, or as a nurse species for establishing another crop. Primary production concerns include high cost of posts to allow the vine to climb, pruning and fertilizing to sustain production, and need for hand labor. Insects and worms are the primary pests although control measures have been identified. Fungal pathogens can be controlled by appropriate field management that ensures good soil drainage. Although internal and external market conditions are good, improved field management techniques and harvest and processing opportunities could increase the profitability of passion fruit production.

Peach palm (*Bactris gassipaes*): Peach palm is native in many of the coca-growing regions of the Andean countries. The tree is cultivated for fruit and palm heart with the latter being more economically attractive. Primary production concerns include need for well-distributed rainfall and dry periods, fertilizers, and near access to processing facilities. Harvests can be made within 18 to 20 months after planting. The palm has a high rate of sucker production allowing for 3 to 4 harvests per year. Instituto Nacional de Investigación Agraria y Agroindustrial (INIAA) in Peru has been working on production technology since 1985, including seedling types, transplanting techniques, and appropriate planting densities. Peach palm can be integrated with other crops at lower densities, but shading by the palm may preclude certain species; cassava can be planted prior to the palm to provide shade and income until the palm outshades it. Few problems with pests or diseases are noted and currently most can be controlled through good field management efforts (e.g., cultivation). Peach palm has been identified as one of the most promising alternative crops. However, efforts would be needed to expand the currently small world market for palm hearts.

Pineapple (*Ananas comosus*): Traditional pineapple production is largely dependent on hand labor and although traditional varieties tend to have low yields, fields may produce for 6 to 10 years. Improved yield cultivars have been developed, however the production period length is shortened significantly (i.e., $1\frac{1}{2}$ to 3 years). Production concerns include improved cultivars (smooth cayenne), planting densities, fertilizer programs, soil preparation, and flower induction to increase yield and speed time to first harvest. The shallow rooting system makes pineapple extremely susceptible to competition and higher planting densities make it difficult to intercrop successfully. Numerous pests and diseases affect pineapple production, although chemical and cultural controls exist. Some of these problems may be reduced by using traditional varieties resistant to fungi although there is a trade-off with yields.

Rice (*Oryza sativa*): Increased rice production opportunities largely lie in import substitution. Research has identified high-yielding cultivars for certain production systems (e.g., alluvial and flooded systems), although varieties appropriate to upland coca zones are scarce. Primary production concerns include agrichemical requirements, field preparation (e.g., land bevelling which is costly and if done improperly can pose problems for water management), improved water management, and equipment. Fungal diseases pose the largest pest problems for rice production, and fungicides to treat these diseases are costly. Development of disease-resistant varieties could improve opportunities for expanded rice production.

Silk: Mulberry/silk production systems are being promoted in Colombia as an alternative to coca. Production technologies are well-known and easily available and technical assistance and credit opportunities exist for silk production in Colombia. Primary production concerns include the susceptibility of silkworms to agrichemicals requiring an organic production approach, establishment of "casetas" to house the silkworms, and availability of transportation to processing sites. Silk markets are well-established and, with quality cocoons, should be open to Andean production.

SOURCE: H. Villachica, "Crop Diversification in Bolivia, Colombia, and Peru: Potential to Enhance Agricultural Production," contractor report prepared for the Office of Technology Assessment, April 1992. P. Conway, "Silk For Life—Project Proposal," Silk for Life, Madison, Wisconsin, January 1991.

through extension programs, establishing post-harvest and marketing infrastructure, increasing availability of credit and private investment, and expanding market opportunities through product promotion in local and foreign markets (105).

Instituto Boliviano de Tecnología Agropecuaria— Chapare (IBTA-Chapare) research focuses on identifying profitable agricultural options suitable to the producers and markets in the Chapare. These efforts indicate that a variety of agroecologically suitable production options are available. Yet, factors such as credit and market availability seem to determine the acceptability of identified options. Thus, setting specific research priorities will continue to be difficult until marketing studies are completed for some of the identified alternatives (e.g., perennial tree crops). Lack of farmer representation in the project and lack of transition production systems[2] further constrain setting realistic research and extension priorities (22). Nevertheless, on-farm research and the production systems approach are valuable methodological tools arising from the Chapare project (box 4-B).

Considerable agricultural research has been conducted in Peru's Amazonia, covering agroecological conditions from the tropical highlands to the lowlands. Research programs and projects have addressed production problems in a variety of crops (e.g., rice, maize, grain-legumes, oilseeds, tobacco, coffee, cocoa, tropical fruits, and palms) as well as tropical soils management, tropical pastures, livestock production systems, and forestry. Research programs conducted in the 1980s increased yields and reduced production costs for rice, maize, potatoes, and beans, thus opening new technology options for the average producer in Peru. These programs yielded a substantial number of new varieties and cultivars adapted to diverse agroecological conditions and cropping techniques (79).

Several research centers located in the Amazonian and Orinoquian regions of Colombia have been active in developing high-yielding cultivars, and applying improved technology and management practices to support agricultural expansion. For example, high-yielding soybean varieties led to a 5-fold production area increase since 1985

---

[2] Transition systems are based on gradual reduction of coca cultivation and involve development of production schemes that integrate coca with legitimate crops. This approach offers security to risk-averse farmers during the lag time between planting alternative crops and receiving economic benefits.

Table 4-3—Current Production and Potential Increase of Some Alternative Crops in the Chapare, Bolivia

Crop	Current planted area (ha)	Mature crop production average (mt/ha)	Total production in the region (mt)	Value of product (FOB Chapare) (U.S.$)	Potential developed areas (ha)	Potential (5 yr) increase in total area (ha)	Value of increased production (U.S.$) (1991 prices)
Achiote	135	1.00	20.0	20,000	23,200	1,000	1,000,000
Bananas–Total	14,000	13.00	2,000.0	160,000	28,000	1,000	
Export	2,000					500	727,000
National	12,000		174,000.0	3,300,000	500	142,000	
Industry			40,000.0				
Citrus	20,000	40.00	800,000.0	12,000,000	27,000	1,000	600,000
Coffee	74	0.80	59.2	17,500	6,750	200	47,000
Ginger	8	13.00	106.0	42,000	2,000	50	264,000
Passion Fruit					5,620		
Export	21	10.00	15.0	4,000	300	810,000	270,000
National			75.0	2,100		100	
Industry			120.0	32,500			
Pepper	18	0.80	4.0	4,000	5,070	100	80,000
Pineapple–Total	274	13.50	582.0		3,100	500	891,000
Export	150			128,000			
National			978.0	110,000		500	2,700,000
Industry/losses			1,082.0	146,000			
Tea	55	5.50	302.5	49,000	7,500	200	178,000
Turmeric	44	10.00	120.0	12,229	1,500	500	510,000
Yuca	5,000	19.00	95,000.0	4,400,000		1,000	873,000
Total	53,779			20,446,229	109,740	7,450	9,092,000

KEY: FOB = Freight on board/shipping point; mt = metric ton.

SOURCE: B. McD. Stevenson, "Post-Harvest Technologies to Improve Agricultural Profitability," contractor report prepared for the Office of Technology Assessment, March 1992.

Box 4-B—Examples of Successful Bolivian Research and Extension Efforts

The most dynamic agricultural region in Bolivia is the eastern plains, with 50 percent of national agricultural land. Only 20 percent of the population, concentrated mostly around Santa Cruz, occupy this region. This area is likely to provide the most immediate agricultural expansion in Bolivia, and some successes can already be cited. Soybean production, for example, has jumped from 67,000 hectares in 1985 to almost 150,000 hectares in 1988, accompanied by an average productivity increase of 20 percent. A new high-yielding cultivar (Totai) developed by Centro de Investigación Agrícola Tropical (CIAT) has been instrumental to this development. CIAT's work on other aspects of soybean production is outlined in a manual widely distributed among extension workers. CIAT soybean recommendations are based on field trials and open discussion of results.

Bolivia's positive experience with soybean improvements can be attributed to several factors: Bolivia took full advantage of foreign technical development (in this case, genetic material and agronomic practices from Brazil) and the active involvement of private interests and collective action. CIAT used practical and effective methods of technical diffusion; and extensionists from private entities were trained and backed by CIAT to solve specific technical problems and to reach farmers with sound technical recommendations.

Another example of effective research and extension work in the Santa Cruz area is seen in CIAT and the Asociación de Productores de Oleaginosas y Trigo (ANAPO) 5-year plan for expanding wheat production to reduce wheat imports. This plan is supported by the recent removal of wheat import subsidies and P.L. 480 wheat sales. The Bolivian Government also will allocate revenues from P.L. 480 wheat imports to support research and extension and to finance seed production and marketing. An agreement between ANAPO and Santa Cruz's mill industry guarantees a minimum price for local wheat.

First year production under the plan (40,000 metric tons) was double the plan goal for that year, and saved the Bolivian economy an estimated $8 million in wheat imports. Bolivia's success with wheat, as with soybeans, can be attributed in part to technology and experience borrowed from neighboring countries. The specific wheat variety used (Cordilleraz) came from Paraguay; ANAPO traded soybean seed for wheat seed of this variety. For its part, CIAT has developed a comprehensive technology package for wheat production and is training extensionists.

Another success story is that of the Instituto Boliviano de Technología Agropecuario (IBTA) research in quinoa. New varieties with low saponin content have led to a wider consumption of this traditional product. IBTA also has produced barley varieties widely adopted in highland production areas. These and other of IBTA's research successes are in the form of specific projects financed by external sources. As such, they have been isolated from IBTA's financial and institutional instability.

Finally, a long-term joint effort by the Bolivian Government, Cooperación Técnica Suiza (COTESU), and Centro Internacional de la Papa (CIP) to increase potato production throughout Bolivia with high-quality seed has been reaping results. Proyecto de Investigación de la Papa (PROIMPA) takes a multidisciplinary approach to this goal. Specific project areas include plant genetics, entomology, phytopathology, nematology, postharvest physiology, seed production technology, and socioeconomics. A complementary Dutch-supported project, Proyecto de Semilla de Papa (PROSEMPA), is aimed at strengthening local and regional capacities to produce commerical high-quality potato seed. PROSEMPA is basically a technology transfer/extension effort directly relevant to producers' problems and market realities.

SOURCE: A. Chavez, "Andean Agricultural Research and Extension Systems and Technology Transfer Activities: Potential Mechanisms to Enhance Crop Substitution Efforts in Bolivia, Colombia, and Peru," contractor report prepared for the Office of Technology Assessment, December 1991.

and yield increases. Other crops being examined for expansion include rice, oil palm, mace, sorghum, cassava, and tropical fruits. In addition, research on tropical pasture and soil management is performed at the Macagual Regional Research Center in the Amazonian region. Results from the Orinoquia could be transferred to other areas of the Colombian Amazon, although such an effort would require greater investment in extension activities (22).

■ Intensifying Agricultural Production

Diverse, multiple cropping[3] systems have a history in the Andean coca growing regions and thus provide a likely starting point for intensifying agricultural production (46). Sustainable[4] systems that preserve the natural renewable resource base and provide long-term environmental and economic benefits to farmers are needed (box 4-C).

MULTIPLE CROPPING

Traditional multiple cropping systems make use of locally available resources and provide for local consumption needs while also contributing to regional or national markets. The key feature of multiple cropping systems is the intensification of production to include temporal and spatial dimensions (box 4-D). Production focuses on long-term sustainability of the system. The continued productivity of traditional multiple cropping systems provides the kind of social and ecological stability that modern monoculture systems have not achieved.

Multiple cropping can have a definite advantage over monoculture systems (46,40,57,128) (e.g., total crop yield can be greater than that achieved in monoculture systems). In some cases, the yield of one crop may be lower than under monoculture, but the yield of the companion crop

---

Box 4-C—Criteria for Measuring Agroecosystem Sustainability

- Low dependence on external, purchased inputs.
- Use of locally available and renewable resources.
- Beneficial or minimal direct or indirect negative impacts.
- Adapted to or tolerant of local environmental conditions.
- Focus on long-term productivity.
- Conservative of biological and cultural diversity.
- Incorporate traditional knowledge, skills, and aspirations.
- Adequate production to provide for local consumption and exportable goods.
- Integrates components at all organizational levels (i.e., crop, farm, local, regional).

SOURCE: S. Gliessman, "Diversification and Multiple Cropping as a Basis for Agricultural Alternatives in Coca Producing Regions," contractor report prepared for the Office of Technology Assessment, February 1992.

---

is sufficiently greater to offset any loss. Land Equivalent Ratios—the amount of land needed in monoculture to produce a yield equal to that achieved through intercropping of two or more crops—developed for a number of common tropical crops indicate that greater production may be achieved through intercropping compared to monoculture (57,111) (figure 4-1). Of course, crop complementarity and proper crop mixtures must be determined to achieve such results.

Multiple cropping systems mimic the energy and nutrient cycling processes of natural ecosystems. Characteristics common to natural and multiple cropping systems include:

- Return of organic matter to the soils (enhancing nutrient cycling, improving fertility, and reducing needs for external inputs);

---

[3] *Multiple cropping*, *mixed cropping*, and *polyculture* are terms used to describe agricultural systems that incorporate spatial and temporal dimensions in production. For the purposes of this discussion, such systems will be referred to as multiple cropping.

[4] *Sustainable* refers to the ability of an agroecosystem to improve or maintain production over many generations despite long-term ecological constraints and disturbances or social and economic pressures (3).

Box 4-D—Classification of Types of Multiple-Cropping Systems

Multiple cropping is the intensification of cropping in time and space dimensions generally defined by growing of two crops in the same field within the same year. This type of cropping may be further defined as intercropping or sequential cropping.

Intercropping: Growing of two or more crops simultaneously in the same field. Crop intensification is in time and space dimensions. However, under this system, potential for competition and growth interference exists during all or part of the growth period. Thus, crop complementarity is a key concern in developing production systems. Varieties of intercropping include:

- *Mixed intercropping*—growing two or more crops simultaneously with no distinct row arrangement,
- *Row intercropping*—growing two or more crops simultaneously with one or more crops planted in rows,
- *Strip intercropping*—planting crops in strips wide enough to permit independent cultivation but close enough for them to interact agronomically, and
- *Relay intercropping*—growing crops simultaneously for some part of each others life cycle. Typically, the second crop is planted after the first has reached a certain growth stage but before the first crop is ready for harvest.

Sequential cropping: growing two or more crops in sequence on the same field each year. The succeeding crop is planted after the first crop has been harvested. There is only temporal intensification and no intercrop interference or interaction. Sequential cropping may be further defined based on the number of crops incorporated in the crop year (e.g., double, triple, quadruple, and ratoon cropping).

SOURCE: S. Gliessman, "Diversification and Multiple Cropping as a Basis for Agricultural Alternatives in Coca Producing Regions," contractor report prepared for the Office of Technology Assessment, February 1992.

- Soil conditioning (e.g., improving soil moisture storage, increasing soil biota populations, soil stabilization);
- Plant diversity;
- Suitability to varied soil, topographic, and altitude conditions; and
- Efficient resource capture due to the varied rooting geometries, canopy patterns, and beneficial associations with other ecosystem components (e.g., nitrogen fixing soil bacteria).

Under the moist tropical conditions of most coca production zones, farmers produce a variety of crops per year under a sequential cropping system. This requires timely harvests, appropriate cultivars, and proper sequencing to minimize potential negative interactions. It can be expanded to form a continuum from strict sequential cropping to relay intercropping for additional beneficial effects. Indeed, much of the agronomic research conducted in the Andean nations has focused on the potential for beneficial associations among early planted crops and later crops. These early crops improve microclimatic conditions so that growth of later, often more economically important, crop species is enhanced (122). Such advantage reaches its greatest point when mutualistic or symbiotic relationships occur that permit plants in mixtures to do better than when planted alone (45). The ideal mixture provides income and food for the family.

Largely, coca farmers are smallholders and produce a composite of subsistence crops and coca. Risk aversion is a key feature of these production systems. There are numerous socioeconomic advantages of multiple cropping systems compared with monoculture systems for the humid tropic regions, including:

- Reduced risk from market changes, pest infestation, and climatic variability;
- Greater energy cycling (reducing the need for costly external inputs);

Figure 4-1—Land Equivalent Ratios

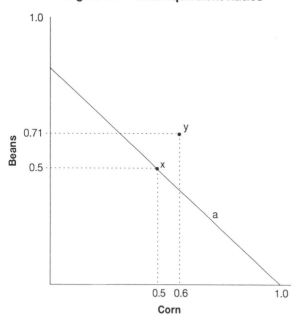

In this example, one hectare of land is planted half in corn and half in beans. The expected yield based on monoculture projections falls on line **a** at point **x**. In many cases, however, the yield of each crop is greater than expected (point **y**). The observed production at point **y** shows that under monoculture 0.71 hectares and 0.6 hectares would be required for monoculture bean and corn production respectively. Therefore, the total amount of land needed to produce an equivalent amount under monoculture would be the sum of the two, or 1.31 hectares. The Land Equivalent Ratio, then, is 1.31—translating to roughly a one-third increase in production under intercropping as compared with monoculture production.

SOURCE: Adapted from: D.C.L. Kass, "Polyculture Cropping Systems: Review and Analysis," *Cornell International Agriculture Bulletin* 32:1-69, 1978; B.C. Trenbath, "Biomass Productivity of Mixtures," *Advances in Agronomy* 26:177-210, 1974; C.A. Francis, *Multiple Cropping Systems* (New York, NY: McMillan, 1986).

- Harvest periods throughout the year (providing better annual distribution of income and farm labor needs/opportunities);
- Faster returns (earnings) from combining short-, medium- and long-term crops; and
- A diversity of products (reducing the need for purchased supplies such as fuelwood and construction materials).

Multiple cropping systems are more complex than monoculture systems, having greater agro-nomic and biological diversity and a greater need for hand labor. In coca zones where labor is expensive, therefore, these systems might be economically handicapped. Improved yields are highly dependent on appropriate system structure. A large body of traditional knowledge of multiple cropping systems remains in the Andean countries and could provide a research and extension resource for improving multiple cropping systems.

AGROFORESTRY

Incorporating trees in multiple cropping systems—agroforestry—is a traditional tropical and subtropical agricultural practice. The objective of most agroforestry systems is to generate diverse products, reduce external input requirements, and sustain resource productivity (44).

Agroforestry systems may be designed to produce trees with crops, trees with livestock, or trees with crops and livestock. The level of complexity increases along the continuum. Generally, little soil disturbance is involved once the agroforestry system is developed. The environmental benefits of agroforestry are well-identified and the principal limitations to widespread use are largely economic, social, and technological.

Home gardens have the greatest complexity but also offer the greatest product diversity. A widely used agroforestry system in tropical areas, home gardens are broadly defined as a piece of land with definite boundaries usually near a house, occupying an area generally between 0.5 and 2.0 hectares (2,21,78). They are an integrated system of humans, plants, animals, soils and water, with trees playing key roles in ecology and management. Home gardens tend to be rich in plant species, usually dominated by woody perennials, and generally have multistoried canopies (1,23). A mixture of annuals and perennials of different heights form layers of vegetation resembling a natural forest structure. The high diversity of species permits year-round harvesting of food, fuelwood, medicinal plants, spices, and ornamental plants (24,47,48).

STEPHEN GLIESSMAN

Home gardens are a common feature of tropical agriculture. This diversified home garden agroforestry system in Costa Rica generates multiple products including banana, papaya, and pineapple.

Much of the coca production region is characterized by brush fallow and poor second-growth forest that could be used for agroforestry. The U.S. Agency for International Development (AID) sponsored research in the Chapare region suggests that many of the promising agricultural alternatives to coca are nontraditional tree crops, such as macadamia and peach palm and long-cycle perennials such as passion fruit and black pepper (4). Incorporating these economic crops into an agroforestry system could provide increased economic and environmental benefits for producers.

Agroforestry systems are being developed by *Instituto Nacional de Investigación Agraria y Agroindustrial* (INIAA) in Peru incorporating cassava or beans, fruit trees, and timber species (*Schizolobium amazonicum* or *Guazuma crinita*). This combination allows producers to use their low fertility soils unsuitable to production of other crops. Although the income generation capability of this system is low in the initial years, when the timber species becomes harvestable (6 to 8 years) it could generate as much as U.S. $1,500/ha with harvests being made every 3 years (122). Hand labor and investment requirements for this system are low. However, potential for pest infestations is likely to be higher in the

mature timber monoculture and could create additional maintenance costs.

Potential also exists for interplanting timber species in coca fields to diversify production. While coca cultivation would benefit timber growth, it also would provide a source of income for the farmer until the trees are harvestable. Ultimately, the trees will shade out the coca and reduce production. Such a "natural" eradication scheme initially may need to be coupled with other incentives (e.g., subsidies to maintain the forest until maturity) to encourage adoption.

Despite the apparent benefits of multiple cropping systems, little research has focused on optimizing plant densities. Incomplete understanding of the ecological processes of these systems complicates identifying ideal combinations and patterns. Applied research on crop combinations, patterns, and planting densities could be promoted under existing alternative cropping research, for example, through IBTA-Chapare. Demonstration activities could be undertaken to provide examples for local farmers and perhaps increase system adoption. In addition, research at each demonstration site could identify specific environmental differences among production zones and promote adaptive work to optimize production systems.

▋ Improving Production Efficiency

Improving production efficiency, by reducing costs of required inputs or increasing output, can increase economic returns to producers. Production efficiency can be improved through use of proper fertilizer regimes, pest control systems, improved soil and water management practices, and improved cultivars. However, inadequate infrastructure, extension and technology transfer, and agricultural credit constrain use of improved practices.

Lack of infrastructure causes production inputs to be costly and difficult to obtain. Many cropping systems previously described focus on reducing needs for external inputs; nonetheless, some inputs are needed to sustain agricultural land use. The infrastructure problem is being addressed by a number of multilateral and bilateral agencies in the forms of road development, irrigation projects, and energy production systems. However, lag time between project initiation and realization of benefits is likely to be lengthy.

Extension of improved production practices (e.g., Integrated Pest Management, cropping system management) is hindered further by inadequately developed national agricultural systems and concerns over personal security. While extension occurs, it is small scale relative to the overall need (see chapter 5).

NUTRIENT MANAGEMENT

Addition of nutrients to a cropping system is an accepted axiom of agricultural production. Agricultural products, whether plant or animal, remove nutrients from the land on which they are produced. Even well-maintained organic farms that carefully collect and return crop residues and livestock wastes to the soil only replace part of the soil nutrients extracted. The other available nutrient sources internal to the agroecosystem (e.g., rock weathering, soil minerals, soil animals) are unlikely to make up this deficit. Fertilizer costs in most coca producing regions are high (U.S. $ 300 to 400/mt vs. U.S. $ 220/mt on the international market (122)), indicating a need for efficient fertilizer programs and use of alternative nutrient sources (e.g., green manure, nitrogen-fixing plants).

PEST CONTROL

Agricultural losses to pests significantly reduce production each year and costs for pest control place added burdens on producers. It is possible to optimize pest control and reduce pesticide needs using a variety of methods, including crop rotation, crop monitoring, pest-resistant cultivars, timing of planting and harvest, and biological controls.

Pest control may be initiated based on pest scouting—monitoring to determine a pest prob-

lem. Depending on the type of pest identified, the organization of the production system, and the extent of infestation, various control approaches may be used. Crop rotation and manipulation of planting and harvesting dates can break the life cycles of many pest species. Cultural controls such as tillage and water management can render the crop environment less favorable for pest populations.

Integrated Pest Management (IPM) blends the suite of pest control technologies into a single system designed to benefit (economically and environmentally) the user and society. IPM programs attempt to restructure an ecosystem to minimize the likelihood of pest damage. Programs are meant to be adaptive with an objective of improving program efficacy over time. The ultimate goal is to maintain pest populations at near-harmless levels.

SOIL AND WATER MANAGEMENT

Management of the soil and water environment for crop production requires understanding the interaction of these cropping-system components, and the suitability of the chosen crop(s) for the agroecosystem. Production of crops ill-suited to a given region may require more intensive external inputs, such as pesticides and fertilizers, to overcome the associated plant stress responses and to achieve acceptable yield levels (16).

Use of soil- and water-management techniques can adjust or modify the agroecosystem to enhance crop production and thus affect the requirements for external inputs. For example, soil-management practices designed to improve the friability and moisture-holding capacity of soils can facilitate crop root development. This in turn may improve the plants' nutrient extraction capability, thereby reducing the need for external nutrient inputs.

CROP MANAGEMENT

Crop management refers to the numerous decisions that most directly relate to the crop, including cropping pattern (e.g., rotation, intercropping) and crop or cultivar choice. Certain crop-management alternatives and techniques may complement or enhance nutrient and agrichemical management activities. Crop-management decisions may have direct impacts on agrichemical use and on how such compounds will behave and move through the agroecosystem. Crop choice alone has instant implications for the pesticide and fertilization regime a producer will use. Similarly, certain cropping patterns, such as legume-based crop rotations, may supply plant nutrients and break pest cycles for a subsequent crop and thus reduce agrichemical requirements.

▮ Conclusion

Alternative crops must compete with the low-risk economic scenario associated with coca production. Although scattered economic data on potential alternative crops suggest that there are no legitimate economic equivalents to coca[5] (table 4-4), this could change if benefits of legitimate agricultural activities increased. Without improved production techniques, technical assistance, and other associated services, however, the chances are slim that substantial numbers of farmers will voluntarily adopt alternative systems. Despite some encouraging signs that coca profitability is decreasing, alternatives will still need to be economically attractive. Development of systems that allow incremental diversification of coca cropping with a goal of replacement may hold promise.

Constraints to crop diversification fall largely in the areas of support systems. While improved cultivars, cropping combinations, and production technology are available, extension of these to producers is hindered by inadequate extension and technology transfer systems (chapter 5). Primary constraints include:

- Input availability and costs (agricultural chemicals, machinery),
- Labor availability and costs,
- Credit availability and terms,
- Land tenure systems,
- Market availability (domestic and international), and
- Security risks.

Irrespective of the identified difficulties, legitimate agricultural production in the Andean nations could be enhanced. Some crops, production and processing technologies, and markets are available. Although new crops that might improve the economics of agricultural production have been identified, further research is needed to identify appropriate cultivars, production techniques, and market potential. Understanding that crop diversification is as important as interdiction has reached high political levels in the Andean nations and leaders have identified the need for concomitant efforts on these fronts.

FOREST RESOURCES[6]

Bolivia, Peru, and Colombia have substantial areas of remaining natural forests with potential for biodiversity conservation and forest management. These tropical wet forests and tropical pre-montane rainforests contain large numbers of tree species, epiphytic plants, lianas, and vertebrate and invertebrate animals (50). For example, the Palcazu Valley in east-central Peru contains at least 30 species of fish, primarily food fish (10); at least 50 mammalian species, at least 400 bird species, and numerous reptiles and amphibians (17); and between 5,000 and 10,000 vascular plant species. Almost one-half of the nearly 30 mammal species that could be of economic importance are rare or very rare and require protection to ensure their survival (33). Early

---

[5] While coca appears to be more profitable than suggested alternatives, this has not been proven. Classical benefit/cost analyses may not be an appropriate method for such economic analysis because of the illegal nature of the coca economy.

[6] This section was drawn largely from: D. McCaffrey, ''Biodiversity Conservation and Forest Management as Alternatives to Coca Production in Andean Countries,'' contractor report prepared for the Office of Technology Assessment, August 1991.

Table 4-4—Internal Rate of Return (net cash flow/costs) for Some Alternative Crops

Crop	Internal rate of return	Data area	Data year	Year at positive cash flow
Coca	165.4			2
Annatto (Achiote)	20.0	Pucallpa, Peru	January 1992	4
Araza	20.2	Pucallpa, Peru	November 1991	6
Banana (export)	53.8	Colombia		2
Black pepper	22.9	Pucallpa, Peru	January 1991	5
Macadamia	54.0	Colombia		5
Orange	29.0	Pucallpa, Peru	February 1992	5
Passion fruit	41.9	Peru	March 1992	4
Peach Palm	82.2	Ucalyi, Peru	January 1992	2
Pineapple	40.3	Pucallpa, Peru	January 1992	2
Rice	22.3	Tarapoto, Peru	March 1992	1

SOURCES: H. Villachica, Lescano, C., Lazarte, J., Chumbe, V., "Estudio de oportunidades de inversión en desarrollo e industrialización de cultivos tropicales en Pucallpa," Perfil de proyecto para la planta de coloantes naturales y para la planta de conservas de palmito, Convenio FUNDEAGRO, Región Ucayali, Lima Peru, 1992.

Coca—H. Villachica, "Crop Diversification in Bolivia, Colombia, and Peru: Potential to Enhance Agricultural Production," contractor report prepared for the Office of Technology Assessment, April 1992.

Banana—J. Arbelaez, "El Cultivo de Plátano en Zona Cafetera, Federación Nacional de Cafeteros," Bogota, Colombia, p. 40, 1991.

Macadamia—O. Rincon, "El cultivo de Macadamia, Federación Nacional de Cafeteros," Bogota, Colombia, p. 29, 1990.

estimates suggested that between 100 to 1,000 species could become extinct if this forest area was removed (39). Based on ecological similarities, it may be assumed that equivalent levels of biodiversity exist throughout the coca-producing regions in South America.

Deforestation occurs in all parts of each country (table 4-5) and in large part is correlated with coca production. Currently, deforestation affects large areas in the eastern Andean foothills and the Upper Amazonian lowlands of each country. Despite this, promoting protected areas and forest management in these zones could provide conservation benefits and alternative livelihoods for existing populations.

It has been suggested that many areas now supporting subsistence farming, including the production of coca for cocaine manufacture, might best be returned to long-term forestry development as the most ecologically sound land use. Considerable effort and state support would be needed to promote such a program although significant employment and economic benefits could arise from sustainable forest management approaches. However, the intensive subdivision

of the land makes this a very difficult proposal to implement (105).

■ Protected Areas

Protected areas include conventional protected areas (e.g., national parks, forest reserves) and more recently biosphere and extractive reserves. However, some disagree as to how well extractive reserves function as mechanisms of forest/diversity conservation (19). Lands set aside for indigenous peoples also may serve as protected areas. Ownership and management commonly is public although some areas are privately owned. Use restrictions control the level of access and nature of extractive activities in protected areas.

Protected area management typically requires identification of suitable sites based on conservation criteria and formal establishment within the national system of protected areas. Although the size and extent vary among the protected area systems in the Andean countries (table 4-6), the necessary institutional framework exists.

Protected areas also provide indigenous peoples a method to gain or maintain access to culturally important wild resources. For example,

Table 4-5—Forest Areas and Deforestation Rates in Andean Countries, 1980s

Country	Forest area (sq km)	Deforestation rate (sq km/yr)	Deforestation rate annual percentage
Bolivia.....................	668,000	870	0.2
Colombia	517,000	8,900	1.7
Peru	706,000	2,700	0.4

SOURCE: World Resources Institute, *World Resources 1990-1991: A Guide to the Global Environment* (Oxford: Oxford University Press, 1990), table 19.1 In: McCaffrey, 1991.

Table 4-6—Protected Areas in Andean Countries, 1985

Country	Number of protected areas	Total area protected (sq km)	Percent national territory protected
Bolivia.....................	12	47,076	4.3
Colombia	30	39,588	3.5
Peru	11	24,076	1.9

SOURCE: World Resources Institute, International Institute for Environment and Development, *World Resources 1986: An Assessment of the Resource Base that Supports the Global Economy* (Oxford: Oxford University Press, 1990), table 19.1 In: McCaffrey, 1991.

16 Yanesha Native Communities occupy 580 square kilometers of forest and agricultural land in the lower Palcazu Valley (114). The national park and protected forest provide for conservation, research, and tourism, and the communal reserve provides for traditional uses by the Yanesha people. Ultimately, greater economic benefits (in terms of tourism dollars) could arise from the maintenance of these wild areas, as is evidenced through expanding ecotourism markets worldwide (15).

However, national governments do not provide adequate legal backing, sufficient staffing, and financial support for protected areas (18). Thus, protected areas frequently cannot meet desired conservation goals and often exist as ''paper parks'' that do not fulfill their mandate. The Isiboro-Secure National Park in Bolivia possesses many of the qualities that identify a highly appropriate protected area and also provides for the needs of the Yuracare and Mojenio native peoples. However, the park is located in an active area of coca cultivation. Its boundaries are breached increasingly by coca cultivators, log-

gers, and hunters (88,89), and enforcement is inadequate to control poaching.

■ Forest Management

Forest management describes the use of technical practices designed to increase the flow of benefits from forest resources. Management may be strictly for sustainable yield of forest products like timber and wildlife and may provide indirect benefits like erosion control over the long term. Benefits may be harvested or generated continuously or cyclically. Multiple-use management programs seek to provide numerous, often diverse, benefits from forests. Some spatial and temporal separation of benefits may be associated with multiple-use systems since uses may not be compatible (e.g., forest preservation and lumber operations).

Forest management can be applied to primary, secondary, and heavily disturbed natural forest systems. Practices vary depending on the level of disturbance and the desired benefits from management. All of these forest types as well as some

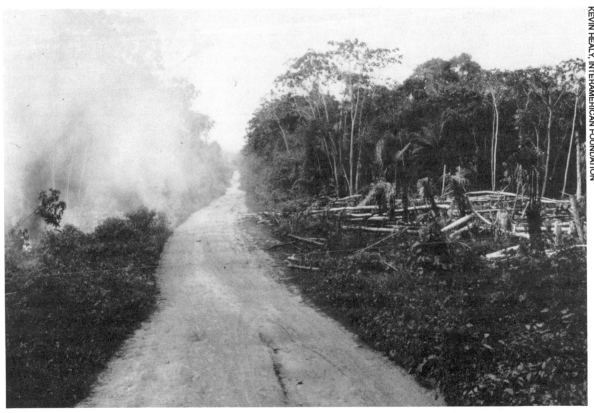

KEVIN HEALY, INTERAMERICAN FOUNDATION

Slash-and-burn forest clearing commonly is used to access agricultural lands, but land productivity tends to be short-lived. Evidence suggests that maintaining forests for sustainable timber operations and extractive reserves may offer longer term economic benefits.

small areas of planted forest are found in the coca-producing regions.

Forest management in the coca-producing regions could offer significant environmental and economic benefits to local populations. Forest systems offer a mechanism to reduce soil erosion, increase soil fertility, sustain biological diversity, and manage water resources. An economic dimension can be added to the environmental benefits by careful and systematic selection of forest trees for economic benefits. Selective removal of undesired species and regeneration of desired species can maintain the basic character of the forest while increasing the flow of economic benefits. Similar principles could be applied to other economically important forest plants and wildlife.

Potential also exists for managing traditional subsistence swidden-fallow agriculture to increase the abundance of economically important plants. Typically, the fallow period of agricultural lands involves allowing regrowth of naturally occurring plants for later removal once soil productivity has been enhanced. Selective removal of plants as opposed to slash-and-burn practices can contribute to maintaining a seed source for desired species. Ultimately the composition of plants can be shifted toward more economic forest species (117).

■ Technical Considerations in Forest Management

Forest characteristics (e.g., species composition, age), site environmental features (e.g., slope, climate), and external factors (e.g., roads, processing facilities) are important considerations in developing forest management and extraction plans (53). There is protocol to manage tropical timber forests based on natural regeneration of harvested tracts (108,110) (box 4-E). Selective cutting, enrichment planting, or plantation establishment regimes may be used to manage and exploit secondary growth and disturbed forests (75).

Incorporating the participation of the local population and providing them with tangible economic benefits can improve the success of forest management efforts (90). Reconciliation of local interests with national policies and identification and quantification of environmental benefits and potential beneficiaries are also necessary for forest management to be effective (80). Ideally, forest management pays for itself by generating high-value products in the short term. Alternatively, external economic incentives may be required to support such management (73).

Pilot forest management activities in undisturbed and secondary growth forests are ongoing in the American tropics. Largely these activities have concentrated on timber production, although some effort has been placed on extractive reserves (90). Funding for these activities has come from private and public sources. The key lesson from these pilot activities is the lack of a single formula for successful forest management in wet tropical environments. Plan development requires careful examination and incorporation of environmental, sociocultural, infrastructural, and political features of a site.

▐ Constraints to Forest Management

Opportunities to manage forests sustainably are constrained by a variety of factors, including:

- High demands placed on forest areas for land and forest products (e.g., conversion of forestland for agricultural purposes and exploitation of existing forest resources),

- Potential for long lag-time between plan implementation and realization of benefits for production systems in disturbed forests,
- Low value placed on forests and the view of forests as an obstacle to development (92), and
- Conventional economic analyses that ignore the value of future forest (76)

Forestry institutions have not grown to meet the additional challenges arising from increasing global concern over tropical deforestation (129). Several features of tropical forests complicate management efforts, including forest complexity, distance from urban centers, and widely varied values placed on forests by various sectors of society (90). The inherent difficulties with forest management are heightened in coca-producing regions that also must cope with economic distortions and environmental difficulties associated with coca production and processing practices (32).

▐ Conclusion

A number of forest management approaches are applicable to the Andean countries. Local commitment and participation are key elements of all of these approaches. Efforts range from largely communal to commercial efforts, yet are based on a fundamental goal of enhancing forest production (table 4-7).

Some private organizations are promoting sustainable logging through negotiations directly with forest communities. This approach allows for gradual exploitation and gives local inhabitants incentive to protect forest to maximize economic benefits over the long term. Selective cutting techniques are used to remove high quality wood for high value markets. Resource sustainability and social equity are criteria for acceptability of potential agreements. Development of such sustainable harvest methods may provide an opportunity to maintain the tropical hardwood market in the face of increasing con-

Box 4-E—Sustainable Forest Exploitation: Case Example in the Palcazu Valley of Peru

Sustainable exploitation of forest resources in tropical areas commonly is viewed as having little potential because of the complexity of managing diverse, old-growth stands. In fact, estimates suggest that less than 1 percent of tropical forests currently are being managed sustainably. However, an innovative forest production system in operation in the Palcazu Valley of Peru is demonstrating that sustainable forest exploitation in tropical humid forests may be possible. The project emerged from an AID-sponsored subproject (the Palcazu Valley Development Project—PVDP) of Peru's Pichis-Palcazu Special Project (Proyecto Especial Pichis-Palcazu— PEPP). PEPP was promulgated by road development (Carretera Marginal de la Selva) along the base of the Peruvian Andes in the early 1980s and was intended to promote agricultural colonization in the region. The AID subproject was to maintain a part of the highway leading to the Palcazu Valley and provide rural development assistance.

The environmental assessment conducted by AID for the PVDP, however, indicated the agricultural potential for the valley was low and the region was environmentally unsuitable for a large-scale colonization scheme. Recommendations for low-impact development were made in the plans for AID's *Central Selva Natural Resources Management Project*, including a widespread production system for primary forest areas. The Tropical Science Center of Costa Rica developed an integrated forest production system based on interspersed, narrow strip clear-cuts in high, primary forest; a 40-year rotation; family or exchanged labor; complete use of all wood in the cut area; and animal traction for removal of products to roadside landings. Trees would not be planted in the clear-cut strips; natural regeneration from bordering high forest trees and stump sprouting would serve to maintain the forest and its species diversity. Production tracts would border primary or secondary roads to facilitate the transport of forest products to nearby processing plants and only processed products would be marketed.

However, PEPP focus remained on agricultural development in the region and land was titled to resident cattlemen for livestock production. The only remaining forested land had been titled to 12 communities of native, forest-dwelling Amuesha (Yanesha) Indians, several of which showed interest in the forestry proposal. Thus, the original forest management scheme was redesigned to fit the Amuesha. Although scaled-down in size and funding, the development of the Yanesha Forestry Cooperative emerged from these efforts in 1985. The techniques envisioned for the larger project (e.g., labor intensive, animal traction, small-sized harvest equipment) were adapted for the Amuesha, including vertical integration, with the forest operators collectively owning the production, processing, and marketing operations.

Despite difficulties encountered by the Cooperative (e.g., an uncompleted processing plant, inadequate transport and road maintenance machinery, lack of working capital, and the threat of violence from insurgents and narcotics traffickers), it has managed to move ahead slowly. Today, the Cooperative product mix includes finished lumber, treated poles and posts, charcoal, and manufactured products. Although some difficulties have arisen in securing national markets for certain products, this may be a result of the existing economic situation in Peru. Nevertheless, shipments have been made to U.S. and European buyers at premium prices and sawn timber has effectively entered local markets. Evidence to date suggests that the Yanesha Forestry Cooperative is a sustainable forest production system.

SOURCES: J.A. Tosi, Jr., "Integrated Sustained Yield Management of Primary Tropical Wet Forest: A Pilot Project in the Peruvian Amazon," Tropical Science Center, Costa Rica, 1991, In: McCaffrey, 1991. M.A. Perl, M.J. Kiernan, D. McCaffrey, R.J. Buschbacher, and G.J. Batmanian, "Views for the Forest: Natural Forest Management Initiatives in Latin America," World Wildlife Fund, Washington, DC, 1991, In: McCaffrey, 1991.

sumer boycotts of tropical wood products for environmental concerns (133).

In addition to sustainable logging opportunities, economic benefits are becoming apparent from extractive reserves. For example, some estimates suggest that while converting forests to pastureland can produce about 220 pounds of meat per acre each year, leaving them standing could produce 2,750 pounds of food. Further, the value of the forest products (nuts, fruits, other) can reach twice the one-time logging revenue. Similarly, review of non-timber forest product value on two sites in Belize suggest that rainforest use as extractive reserves seems economically justifiable based on current market data and currency values (54). Recently, Colombia and Brazil ceded control of certain forests to native Indian populations for extractive reserves. Expanding on this trend will require developing local economies with an interest in conserving and maintaining the forests and demonstration that these activities can be economically attractive. Some current activities that might assist in

highlighting the value of forests include efforts in Costa Rica, where forest samples are being collected and investigated for potential commercial value (104). If such ''prospecting'' assures economic benefits for native communities, it could be incentive for conservation and maintenance of existing forests.

Interest is increasing in forest-related activities (e.g., extractive reserves, logging, nature tourism) in the Andean region. Research in the Chapare region suggests that many of the promising agricultural alternatives to coca are nontraditional tree crops, such as macadamia and peach palm and long-cycle perennials such as passion fruit and black pepper (4). In fact, the Chapare is ideally suited for a land use system based largely on forestry and to a much smaller extent on agriculture (109).

The importance of incorporating forest resource opportunities in substitution programs is clear. For example, according to several estimates, between 66 and 80 percent of coca producers in the Alto Huallaga were settled on

Table 4-7—Forest Management Approaches To Promote Sustainable Resource Exploitation

Project	Type	Location	Activity	Goal
Yanesha Cooperative	Cooperative	Palcazu Valley, Peru	Harvest of undisturbed natural forest using strip clearcutting.	Produce lumber, chemically treated poles and posts, charcoal, and firewood.
Portico	Commercial	Costa Rica	Harvest of single tree species from swamp forests.	Produce high-quality doors for international market.
Boscosa	Public/ private	Costa Rica	Reclamation of cut-over and secondary growth forests, management plans for sustainable use.	
Plan Piloto	Public/ private	Quintana Roo, Mexico	Rehabilitation of degraded forest, increase numbers of economic species through regulated harvest, natural regeneration, and enrichment plantings.	Harvest of economic tree species.
Extractive Reserves	Community	Brazil	Formalizing lands as extractive reserves through petition to national government.	Harvest of forest reserves (e.g., rubber, brazil nuts).
ANAI	Public/ private	Costa Rica	Works with small farmers to protect and manage local forest.	Integrated land use.

SOURCE: D. McCaffrey, "Biodiversity Conservation and Forest Management as Alternatives to Coca Production in Andean Countries," contractor report prepared for the Office of Technology Assessment, August 1991.

steep slopes when the *Proyecto Especial Alto Huallaga* (PEAH) was developed (11,34). Despite this knowledge, the project excluded land in steeply sloping areas—areas classified as suitable only for forestry or protected forest—and focused on areas suitable for agriculture or livestock production. Since the project addressed only the flat areas, the impact on coca producers was limited from the outset. Likewise, a development factor that should have been of major importance, a forestry component, was not even considered. This is a serious shortcoming given circumstances where lands classified as suitable for forestry use constitute a considerable part of the region (12). However, forestry and agroforestry, although promising, should be viewed as components of an overall package of land use practices that could provide stable incomes and improved environmental conditions for populations in the coca-producing regions.

WILDLIFE AND WILDLAND RESOURCES[7]

Wildlife and wildland resources could provide an opportunity to expand renewable resource based development. Andean ecosystems support a broad variety of wildlife species that are, or might be, managed to offer alternative livelihoods for local populations. Potential wildlife markets include hides and fibers, pet, meat, and other animal products (e.g., bone). Techniques exist for managing a variety of amphibians, reptiles, fishes, birds, and mammals to provide these commodities.

Nature-based tourism depends on maintaining certain valued ecosystems to attract foreign exchange. Considerable efforts are being made to incorporate local communities in nature tourism development (e.g., Monte Verde) (7). Wildlife development, and particularly tourism, is likely to be curtailed by social, political, and economic pressures in target areas.

Development of wildlife resources for the national and international markets in wildlife and wildlife products may provide more immediate returns than tourism and may also provide a base for developing tourism industries. Ranching, farming, and collection of wildlife are dependent on maintenance of wild populations and critical habitats. Although farming and ranching may require greater capital investment than hunting, they also offer greater security in terms of supply consistency. Market demand for neotropical wildlife and wildlife products has been increasing steadily and exhibits sufficient profit margins to entice international investors (13,27).

South American wildlife products remain important traditional protein and fiber sources and have been exported for nearly 400 years (70,72). International conservation organizations have focused on sustainable development of wildlife resources, and international wildlife conservation treaties (e.g., CITES, Migratory Bird Treaty) have led to some control over the exploitation and international marketing of wildlife products. Despite these actions, considerable amounts of illegal hides flow from the region.

Wildlife-centered economic development has become more acceptable and research efforts are being undertaken to determine sustainable yields and appropriate husbandry practices. Techniques for raising certain wildlife species with little capital investment have been developed and are easily incorporated in rural communities. For example, experimental programs for ranching of green iguanas have spread from Panama to other neotropical countries (6,127). Licensing and protection policies are being implemented in the region that are making farming and ranching of wildlife more profitable than taking from the wild (97).

---

[7] This section was drawn largely from: R.E. Ashton, Jr., ''Potential Use of Neotropical Wildlife in Sustainable Development,'' contractor report prepared for the Office of Technology Assessment, December 1991.

▮ Wildlife Farming and Ranching

Farming and ranching of reptiles and amphibians have been successful in several countries, including Bolivia. These operations provide hides, meat, and live animals for the international market. Animals tend to be superior to those collected from the wild since they are healthier, accustomed to captivity, and generally parasite and disease-free. A select review of live animal importers showed that 100 percent prefer farmed or ranched animals for these reasons (6).

Wildlife ranching and farming appear to be on the threshold of becoming a major industry in some areas. Only within the last year have South American iguanas and caiman reached the pet markets in the United States. Table 4-8 shows some species that retailers and researchers suggest as having the possibility for sales volumes sufficient to sustain an industry. Underlying research needs include information on sustainable yield levels, life history, and husbandry techniques.

Wildlife farming involves collecting enough stock from the wild to have a viable breeding base to sustain a captive population and produce a marketable commodity. Once the stock is collected, the captive population is sustained through breeding and recruitment from the wild is not required. Although farming may offer an opportunity to propagate rare species without harming wild populations (102), it may also result in little concern for sustaining the wild populations or their habitat since the economic value lies with the farmed populations. Farming may also be used to conceal wildlife harvests, as has been suggested to have occurred in Colombia under some of the recent captive propagation programs (35). Nevertheless, well-organized and managed wildlife farming programs can promote monitoring of exports and provide revenue for enforcement activities and local communities. Constraints to this approach include potentially high startup and operation costs to sustain the captive population.

Wildlife ranching is based on capturing wild stock and raising it to marketable size and quality and requires continuous replenishment from wild populations. While this form of wildlife production is preferred for species with large wild populations, it can affect the viability of those populations if management is inadequate. Indiscriminate collection of wildlife can lead to extinction (102). By necessity, wildlife ranching depends on the maintenance of wild populations and their habitats and thus may yield conservation benefits. Revenues generated through taxes on ranching systems could support enforcement and protection of the resource.

Local communities that may not be able to finance a full-scale ranching system may still participate and receive economic benefits through collection of stock for ranching activities. Cultures that retain strong hunting and gathering systems may then supplement their incomes through supplying ranching needs.

Sustainable harvest from wild populations requires understanding population dynamics. Although such information generally is lacking for many exploitable neotropical wildlife, there are options for developing sustainable harvest programs *in situ*. Harvest levels can be based on empirical evidence during the period that population dynamics data are collected (13) (box 4-F).

EXOTIC SPECIES

The introduction of exotic species for farming or ranching activities is controversial. Concerns center largely on the potential for escape and ensuing displacement of native species and ecosystem disruption, disease transmission to wild populations, and economic consequences resulting from predation of exotic species on native biological resources.

If introduced species are excellent competitors or predators, native species may be displaced and ecosystems disrupted. Displacement may take the form of population decline or range limitations. In either case, if the native species is desirable, or economically important, the adverse impact is

Table 4-8—A Partial List of South American Wildlife Species With Potential for Sustainable Development

Species	Current status	Potential status	Market	Species	Current status	Potential status	Market
Invertebrates				**Lizards**			
Butterflies	G,F	F,R	H	Enyalioides laticeps	G	F,R	P
Beetles	G	G,R	H	Iguana....................	G,F,R	F,R	H,P
Spiders	G	G,F	P	Ctenosaura pectinata	G	F,R	H,P
Tropical fish	F,G	G,F,R	P	Basiliscus sp.	G	F,R	P
Amphibians				Tubinambis sp.	G,R	F,R	H,P
Treefrogs	G	G,R	P	**Snakes**			
Dendrobatids	G	R	P	Boa constrictor	G	F,R	H,P
Bufonids	G	G,R		Corallus sp.	G	F,R	P
Salamanders	G	G	P	Epicrates sp.	G	F,R	P
Crocodilians				Eunectes sp.	G	F,R	H,P
Crocodylus intermedius	G	R	H	Drymarchon corias	G	F,R	P
Crocodylus acutus	G	R	H	Lampropeltis sp............	G	F,R	P
Crocodylus moreleti	G,R	R	H	Spilotes pullatus	G	F,R	P
Caiman crocodilus	G,R	G,R	H	Lachesis muta	G	G	P
Caiman latirostris	G,R	G,R	H	Bothrops sp.	G	F,R	H,P
Melanosuchus niger	G,R	R	H	Crotalus durissus	G	F,R	H,P
Paleochuchus palpebrosus	G	G,R	P	**Birds**			
Paleochuchus trigonatus ...	G	G,R	P	Amazona sp.	G,R	R,F	P
Turtles				Ara sp.	G,R	R,F	H,P
Geochelone denticulata	G	F,R	P	Other Psittacines	G,R	G,R,F	P
Geochelone carbonaria	G	F,R	P	**Mammals**			
Aquatic turtles	G	R	P	Tayassu pecari	G	R	H
				Felis pardalis..............	G	F	H,P
				Panthera onca	G	F	H,P
				Lutra longicaudis	G	F	H,P
				Hydrocherus hydrocherus ..	G,R	R	H,P
				Agouti paca	G,R	F	H,P
				Vicugna vicugna	G,R	R	H

KEY: G = Hunted or collected.
R = Ranched or potential for ranching.
F = Farmed or potential for farming.
H = Animal products industry (e.g., hide, meat, feathers, bone).
P = Live animal trade.

SOURCE: R.E. Ashton, *Handbook on Central American Tourism and Wildlands Protection,* Paseo Pantera Ecotourism Project, Wildlife Conservation International, 1991, In: Ashton, 1991.

quickly apparent. In cases where the species is less obvious or desirable, the impact also may be serious since the ecological balance will have been disrupted. Similarly, when introduced species prey on economic biological resources (e.g., crops, trees, fish), economic disruptions occur in the form of reduced yields, and increasing costs of control measures and management effort.

Nevertheless, species introductions are underway for potential economic gain. Nile crocodiles have been introduced on an Amazonian crocodile farm because of their higher quality hide compared with the native species. Accidental release of this prolific and potentially dangerous species into the Amazon basin could have serious consequences (97).

Asian and African big game have been introduced into some private game hunting ranches in savanna areas in Central and South America. Cattle associations in affected areas have re-

Box 4-F—Information Needs for Developing Sustainable Harvest Practices

- Population size and range.
- Habitat requirements.
- Resilience to human disturbance.
- Mortality and productivity rates.
- Key factors regulating populations and their tendency to increase or decrease.
- Effects of environmental variation (e.g., effects of climatic cycles) on productivity.

SOURCE: S.T. Beissinger and E.H. Bucher, "Can Parrots Be Conserved Through Sustainable Harvesting?" *Bioscience* 42(3):164-172, March 1992.

sponded with demands for strict control of these imports due to the potential for transmission of ungulate diseases to their stock.

INFORMATION NEEDS TO SUPPORT WILDLIFE PRODUCTION

Despite available technologies for wildlife production, species specific information is needed to support a viable wildlife production industry. Some of this type of research currently is underway for caiman and birds in South America. Biological studies are needed that characterize the extent of the resource and identify likely impacts of increased wildlife production and marketing.

Member countries of the Convention on International Trade in Endangered Species of Wild Fauna and Flora (CITES) are required to provide a management plan based on recent surveys and studies on listed[8] species population dynamics and other key aspects affecting their viability. If it is determined that the species can be harvested, limits on the take are set to provide for the population to sustain or increase its numbers.

Allowable take limits must be based on solid scientific information regarding population size, dynamics, reproductive behavior, and current status. Species' feasibility for captive propagation is determined by behavioral, reproductive, and husbandry needs as well as economic value. Most species are not suitable for captive propagation (106) and comprehensive planning is necessary to avoid failure. For example, the United Nations, Man and the Biosphere and the United Nations Education, Science, and Cultural Organization 1970s project with tortoises failed to account for the time required to raise tortoises to market size for food. A component directed to the demand for hatchling tortoises in the pet trade might have been more appropriate.

■ Protection and Enforcement

Enforcement of wildlife protection and management regulations is a primary requirement for developing a sustainable wildlife exploitation program. Game laws typically have been difficult to enforce, and regulations have not been well supported since wildlife is considered part of the public domain (102). Most efforts at protection have been directed by international laws and treaties such as CITES. However, funding for much needed enforcement and education programs typically has been low.

Political will and increased revenues will be necessary to support sustainable development of wildlife resources. Economic pressures from conservation groups and the international market could provide incentive for producing nations to adopt or enforce protection programs. Revenue from legitimate business could help in providing the capital necessary for implementing these programs. The American alligator harvesting program and the International Union for the Conservation of Nature and Natural Resources (IUCN) Crocodile Specialist Group are examples of programs to promote protection, enforcement, and licensing and to facilitate marketing wildlife products.

---

[8] *Listed* refers to the identification of a species as rare or protected under CITES.

■ Economics of Wildlife Opportunities

Economic concerns include startup costs, technology costs, logistics, cost/benefit ratio, and marketing (127). Although there are no data showing that sustainable development of wildlife resources could protect natural ecosystems or become the dominant method for economic development for small rural communities, indications are that well-managed sustainable wildlife industry development can be economically attractive. For example the demand for natural leathers has remained stable and has prompted some to investigate producing leathers from nontraditional sources such as frogs and toads (97). Prices for hides or animal fibers (e.g., vicuna wool) vary and high-quality products may bring significant earnings. For example, high-quality crocodilian hides may bring as much as U.S. $100 for an average caiman or crocodile.

The exotic animal pet trade has grown, mainly over the last decade. Tropical fish exports from several neotropic locations comprise a flourishing multimillion dollar business. Conditions that have led to the popularity increase of exotic pets include:

- Expanding awareness of rainforest biodiversity and intrigue with associated wildlife,
- Affluent populations in urban areas that view exotic pets as status symbols and as being easier to care for (27,51,97),
- Increasing accessibility and availability of exotic pets, and
- Increasing availability of captive care and maintenance techniques and trained exotic pet care experts.

Nearly all species of birds common to the pet trade are being raised in captivity, perhaps as much as 75 to 90 percent of the demand. Farmed or ranched birds could pose an alternative to captive raised animals if accompanied by attractive prices. Costs of transporting live birds and the quarantine requirements may pose major constraints to entrance into this market (6). In addition, competition from illegal imports may hurt the exotic bird market. For example, it has been estimated that nearly 150,000 birds from various countries were imported illegally each year through Mexico, totaling roughly U.S. $1 million in receipts for bird trade (107). As Mexico has become a member of CITES, this situation is expected to change. Considerable research would be required to develop systems appropriate to the raising of mammals for the exotic pet trade. High investment costs and the extensive care requirements are key considerations.

Few areas within Bolivia, Peru, or Colombia have adequate infrastructure to enter the live animal export market. In addition, the current market structure is weighted toward enriching the middleman rather than the supplier. Prices paid to villagers are about 10 percent of the wholesale price. For example, a boa constrictor that might fetch U.S. $250 results in an earning of U.S. $0.50 to $5.00 for the individual capturing the boa. Clearly, market access must be improved to increase economic benefits to the supplier.

Significant concern exists over the importation of disease with live animal trade. Despite mandatory health certificates, quarantine, and other importation restrictions under the Animal Quarantine Regulations administered by the U.S. Department of Agriculture (USDA), illegal imports have spread some diseases.

Quarantine and certification of health requirements will need review if the spectrum of imported wildlife increases. As the agency responsible for quarantine and health certification of imported birds and mammals, USDA must be adequately equipped to handle these tasks at ports of entry. Even today, some importers indicate that the current status of bird and mammal quarantine and staff training for these duties is inadequate and responsible for some wildlife losses.

Regulations regarding importation of wildlife to the United States may need to be reviewed as wildlife production becomes more controlled. Regulations established to curtail overexploitation or illegal takings of wildlife will be inappropriate for farmed or ranched species. For example, under the Public Health Service Act only 4 hatchling to 4-inch carapace turtles or tortoises may enter the United States in a single shipment and they cannot be sold except for scientific or educational use. Clearly, this regulation would pose a considerable obstacle for imports of captive raised turtles or tortoises.

■ Wildlife- and Wildland-Based Tourism

Wildlife-based tourism has grown at least 20 percent annually since 1980 (58,99), and has been described as a reasonable approach for sustainable wildland development. Tourism offers an opportunity to earn foreign exchange and provide employment for local communities. Where tourism is developed properly, it has a greater potential for generating local income than most traditional farming or ranching activities (68).

Nature-based tourism could provide economic opportunities for the Andean countries. However, it should be noted that poorly developed tourism industries all too commonly degrade natural resources and ultimately may reduce development options. There are examples of well-planned, appropriately designed nature tourism attractions that could serve as models for similar development in the Andean countries. Ecotourism is gaining interest globally and expertise in developing these resources is expanding.

Game tourism has not reached the levels of big game hunting in Africa and Southeast Asia, although jaguar, tapir, peccary, white-tailed deer, and birds have been hunted in South America. Fishing in the Amazon has been popular for at least 20 years and has focused on such exotic species as peacock bass and giant catfish. Some game tourism is seasonal in nature due to the migratory behavior of target species (e.g., ducks) and provides only short-term employment for local populations. Sustainable management of game resources will require development and enforcement of optimum harvest limits.

While studies have been conducted on the contributions of nature-based tourism to local cultures, they lack data on the level of economic contribution and volume. In fact, data on nature-based tourism's actual importance to local and national economies are lacking. There are no standard data collection methods by tourism officials or international organizations and researchers' poor knowledge of nature tourism (58,99) has led to ineffective study methods and erroneous conclusions.

Appropriate planning and management of wildland tourism areas must incorporate the needs of the local communities, fair user fees, and equitable distribution and use of revenue to maintain the attractions that sustain the industry. Where nature tourism has been developed, primary criticisms relate to failing to fulfill these needs. Tourism developed around indigenous cultures and wild areas may also offer an opportunity to preserve traditional cultures, skills, and knowledge. Also important is the investment of tourism revenue into the local society in terms of improving quality of life by providing employment, training, and education. Such revenue has been shown to contribute significantly to economic growth (8) and increase support for parks by local communities (62).

Developing successful tourism programs that support local communities should include:

- Written working agreement with communities or local people outlining the use of lands, jobs, interactions with tourists, wildlife protection and associated compensation for undertaking such activities, training, and advancement potential;
- Agreement describing operators efforts to support the local community;
- Agreement to the privacy rights of tourists and local populations; and
- Agreement on marketing goods produced by the local community that assures fair compensation and precludes overharvest of local resources upon which the industry depends.

If nature tourism increases in importance in the Andean countries, mechanisms will be needed to protect wild resources supporting the industry. However, competing demands for resources can pose a constraint to development and implementation of such regulations. For example, the Isiboro-Secure National Park in Bolivia provides a highly diverse forest system that could be of interest to nature tourism, but encroachment on park lands by squatters producing coca has adversely affected its tourism potential.

■ Conclusion

International and domestic markets for wildlife, wildlife products, and nature tourism exist. Developing these resources could contribute to overall economic improvements in the Andean region. Farming and ranching of wildlife species and protecting and preserving of habitats are techniques that could promote development of these sectors.

Revenues from sustainable development and exploitation of wildlife resources can support conservation efforts critical to sustaining the industry. Governments must set appropriate user fees and allocate revenue for habitat protection, monitoring programs, research and education programs, and maintenance of necessary infrastructure. Models of successful efforts (e.g., crocodilian programs) could provide the basis for developing rational revenue allocation schemes.

AQUATIC RESOURCES[9]

Abundant freshwater aquatic systems (e.g., lakes, reservoirs, rivers, and streams) in the Andean nations provide opportunity for sustainable exploitation of endemic and introduced fishes, other vertebrates and invertebrates, and plants. However, little development effort has been placed on improving existing commercial and artisanal fisheries.

Comparisons of estimated productivity and actual harvest suggest that a higher level of sustainable exploitation of Andean aquatic resources is possible. Use of better management, production, and postharvest technologies could increase fishery production. Well-designed management systems that include size, season, and gear restrictions can influence aquatic community composition and sustain high-value fisheries and protect the resource base. Such systems, however, need to be suitable to the local community and local input in developing management plans should be an integral part of such activities.

Use of improved capture technologies can allow more precise exploitation of aquatic communities and greater benefit per fishing trip. Aquaculture technologies offer an opportunity to increase food production through intensive fish farming through stocking to maintain commercial fisheries. Perhaps, the key need for improving the potential contribution of aquatic resources to the Andean countries will be efforts to reduce postharvest losses of aquatic products by improving processing, handling, and storage methods. Infrastructure development could assist in marketing, reduce product cost, and potentially increase economic benefits.

In some regions, coca production and processing have adversely affected aquatic systems and reduced their potential productivity. Aquatic remediation technologies could be applied, although clear definition of the problem will be necessary before undertaking reclamation activities.

■ Existing Fisheries

Commercial and artisanal freshwater fisheries in the Andean countries have not been a focus of development activities. Some commercial fisheries have been developed around introduced high-value species. For example, rainbow trout and pejerry introduced into Bolivian and Peruvian

---

9 This section was drawn largely from: R. Schroeder, ''Fishery/Aquatic Resources in Bolivia, Colombia, and Peru: Production Systems and Potential as Alternative Livelihoods,'' contractor report prepared for the Office of Technology Assessment, October 1991.

lakes supported a commercial trout fishery until severe overfishing caused a significant stock decline (36,119). Pejerry is now the most abundant fish in these lakes and supports a major fishery in Bolivia. Pejerry is also cultured in lagoons and lakes at Cuzco and Apurimac in Peru (31). In addition to lake fisheries, river basins support active fisheries, including the Magdalena, Pilcomayo, Amazon, and Orinoco Basins.

Other aquatic animals and plants may have some potential as food and fiber resources. Amphibians, birds, mollusks, and crustaceans are found in the Titicaca Basin (42,120,121). Economically valuable plants (e.g., bullrush, algae, *Elodea, Myriophyllum,* and *Potamogeton*) are found in lakes and streams and rivers. These plant materials can be used for human and livestock food, construction materials, crop fertilizers, paper production, and medicines (69). Estimates suggest that sustainable totora—*Scirpus tatora* or bullrush—production in Lake Titicaca could feed 265,000 head of livestock. Development of these resources will require strategies to protect against overharvest and to enhance their growth (e.g., cultivation through careful cutting can enhance bed productivity and density).

Aquatic vegetation also provides nursery habitat for economically important fish and invertebrates, feeding areas for birds, and shoreline protection (65). Littoral swamps may extract contaminants from terrestrial runoff. Thus, maintaining or enhancing these resources could provide conservation and economic benefits for local communities.

Fishing communities of the Andean region typically are small and dispersed, with fisheries being largely artisanal and labor intensive. Artisanal fisheries are characterized by low-technology, high effort with seasonal fluctuation, limited fishing range, and landing of small quantities at scattered sites. Fishermen typically are low income, have few opportunities for alternative employment, and wield little political influence (74). Fishing tends to be a part-time occupation due to the seasonal nature of fisheries

and migratory behavior of many economic species; full-time fishermen must migrate along riverine systems to follow stock (124). Fishing trips typically are short (e.g., several hours), and most fishermen are also involved in crop or livestock agriculture. Rapid development of large-scale fisheries could result in resource overexploitation to the detriment of these artisanal fishermen (82). Lack of formal training opportunities in fishing skills also poses a constraint to expansion of fishery development (63).

Fishing craft, gear, and methods vary widely depending on target species, whether the fishery type is artisanal or commercial, and whether the exploited aquatic system is a river, stream, lake, or reservoir. Boats range from paddled dugout canoes to small powerboats. Some traditional fishing gear (e.g., reed rafts, nets of llama wool, traps, and spears) is being replaced by more modern technology.

Marketing typically is dependent on fish traders and some traders may even provide small loans to fishermen (74). Although some products now reach distant markets, difficulties remain for long-distance marketing (81,82). Existing production and market system features reduce the potential for increasing fishery value in domestic markets. In the Lake Titicaca Basin, for example, export of high-value fish is controlled by middlemen and import of frozen marine products has undercut the price of native fish, which make up the greatest part of poor fishermen's catch (9). Thus, annual earnings for fishermen providing for local markets averaged one-half that of export-oriented fishermen (i.e., U.S. $1,200 vs. $2,400) (82).

■ Management of Aquatic Resources

Fishery legislation typically has been difficult to enforce largely due to lack of public acceptability and the remote nature of many of the region's fisheries. A variety of regulatory measures may be needed to promote and sustain fishery development. These can include restrictions on total fishing effort, resource restoration, habitat enhancement, pollution controls, and selective removal of competitive species. Restriction on effort can include catch limits, licensing quotas, gear limitations, closed seasons and areas, and zoning guidelines for waterside development (124).

Ad hoc resource management is accomplished in some areas through community-controlled fishing territories—Territorial Use Rights Fishing (TURFs), whereby aquatic resources are defended from exploitation by outsiders. TURFs may extend from a few hundred meters to several kilometers from shore (64). Although the TURF system is not recognized legally, this informal management system may also function to sustain fisheries by preventing overexploitation. Conflicts between commercial and artisanal fishermen may be promulgated by fishery development since the latter primarily depend on higher yield/lower catch per unit effort fishes while the former depend on larger, high-value species. TURFs may function to defend harvest zones from commercial efforts.

Generally, fishery development focuses on high-value species and seeks to manage the entire system with respect to sustainable yield for these products. Without careful management, overfishing for high-value fish may result in community dominance by short-lived species that support greater sustainable populations. It may be possible to develop a balanced system for producing high- and low-value species, but management requirements are likely to be even greater. Elimination of competitors through a variety of methods (e.g., selective application of electrofishing or ichthyocides) can reduce pressure on desired fishery species. Understanding life history and basic biology of fishes can be used to develop harvest measures specific to certain life stages or species.

Effective management and compliance with fishery regulations also require an understanding of the importance of such measures at the community level. Active fisheries extension serv-

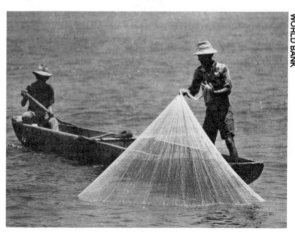

WORLD BANK

Fishing gear vessels typically range from dugout canoes to small motor-powered boats. A dugout canoe allows these two Colombian fishermen to extend the area they can exploit with a castnet.

ices can facilitate understanding of requirements, and community level organizations (e.g., TURFs) might offer opportunities to distribute information. Active local participation in the development of fishery management plans can also promote acceptability and compliance with these efforts. Management planning for the Titicaca Basin, for example, could incorporate the traditional TURF system with more formal management strategies and stress cooperation between the various stakeholders (63)

■ Increasing Fishery Production Potential

Methods to increase or improve fishery production at the commercial and artisanal levels, include use of improved harvest technologies, habitat improvement, and aquaculture. Aquatic systems are subject to numerous and competing demands from other activities (e.g., agriculture, urbanization, recreation). A primary consideration prior to fishery development or enhancement will be the additional surrounding activities that may have an impact on the aquatic system and strategies to integrate such competing needs with fishery development.

HARVEST TECHNOLOGIES

Improved fishing gear and methods could increase production in artisanal and commercial fisheries. Gear/method combinations vary depending on the target species, location, and water system; artisanal fishermen tend to employ a variety of nets, seining, and fishpots. These technologies are simple to implement and provide relatively inexpensive harvest methods. While previously constructed from local materials, nets and lines of more modern materials are now being used. However, boats are used infrequently, restricting the range of exploitation to nearshore environments. Dugout canoes that are handpaddled may be used by some fishermen, but size and storage abilities also create harvest restrictions. Wider use of improved materials in traditional fishing gear and boats with greater capacity for proper catch storage could contribute to improved catch per unit effort in artisanal fisheries. Commercial fishermen also use a variety of nets for capture. Although some commercial efforts on Lake Titicaca focus on nearshore activities (i.e., beach seining for catfish), higher value species are captured from boats by pelagic gillnetting or trawling. Vessels commonly are equipped to store catch on ice to decrease postharvest losses.

HABITAT ENHANCEMENT

Actions that reduce habitat complexity threaten the diversity of fish populations. Variations in stream flow, siltation, and chemical inputs all may result in physical or chemical changes in aquatic ecology. Such effects are common in coca-producing and cocaine-processing areas where erosion from cultivation can contribute large amounts of sediment to nearby riverine systems and periodic dumping of processing chemicals into rivers and streams may change the water's pH balance temporarily.

Resource enhancement can be accomplished through physical (e.g., artificial reefs, fish ladders, current generation) and biological (e.g., stocking, selective exploitation) means. Artificial reefs have been used successfully in temperate lakes to increase abundance of economic fishes and might hold promise for high altitude lakes in the Andean region. Increasing exploitation pressure on competitive species can also improve productivity of desired species. Sufficient natural reproduction and recruitment to maintain a fishery require optimum conditions (e.g., water temperature, flow, clarity, substrate type, complexity) and, most often, regular stocking.

AQUACULTURE

Several organisms have culture potential for high-altitude tropical aquatic systems. Tilapia is the most popular freshwater fish cultured in tropical and subtropical regions. However, early efforts to promote small-pond culture of tilapia in certain regions of the Andes were unsuccessful. The program failed largely because plans lacked a strategy for the local population to produce fish food cheaply and easily (84). An integrated, farming systems approach could have addressed this need.

In Rwanda, small fishponds (0.8 ha) at altitudes of 1,300 to 2,500 meters have been found to be economically viable with production levels averaging 400 kg/ha/yr. Tilapia (*Oreochromis niloticus*) was found to be the most suitable species for this type of culture. Andean river shrimp have commercial aquaculture potential (120,121) and native freshwater prawns in mountain streams and lakes may have similar potential (67). Techniques for shrimp and prawn culture have been used successfully in tropical areas (115).

Aquaculture also can be used to complement capture fisheries by providing fingerlings for stocking. Characterization of the aquatic ecosystem is necessary, since artificial enhancements can alter interspecific competition (41,77). Increasing nutrient and organic content of natural systems and temperature elevations may cause undesirable shifts in natural aquatic communities (28). Algae also may be "stocked" to provide a supplemental food source for fish and be harvested as livestock feed, fertilizer, or for human consumption (135).

Floodplains may provide an area for expanded aquaculture activities by blocking small channels or depressions and constructing drain-in ponds and refuge traps. Annual production can average several hundred to a thousand kilograms of fish per hectare (124). Successful examples of transforming waterlogged soils in tropical floodplains into productive aquaculture/agriculture systems are evident in the Peoples Republic of China. Traditional dike-pond agriculture and aquaculture systems on the Pearl River Delta have been operating for at least 400 years. Fish, livestock, and agricultural crops are produced and material cycling contributes to reduced production costs (box 4-G).

HANDLING, STORAGE, AND TRANSPORT

Infrastructure development has lagged in providing the facilities necessary to promote fisheries in many areas. Indeed, key constraints to greater economic benefits from fishery production in Bolivia seem to center on inadequate infrastructure for processing, handling and storage, and lack of equipment to exploit the resource adequately. These difficulties translate into low prices for the fishermen and high prices for consumers. For example, in 1987 fresh fish prices were nearly three times greater in La Paz (market) than in Trinidad (production center) and only 25 percent of the price was retained by the fisherman (87). Development of roads, ice plants, marketing channels, and credit systems could support increased fishery development (126).

■ Conclusion

Aquatic resource systems of the Andean region harbor significant potential for enhanced production. The numerous lakes and river systems include a variety of harvestable species that could support artisanal and commercial fisheries under good management conditions and application of appropriate technology. Some systems clearly are underexploited and could provide significant increases in domestic food production.

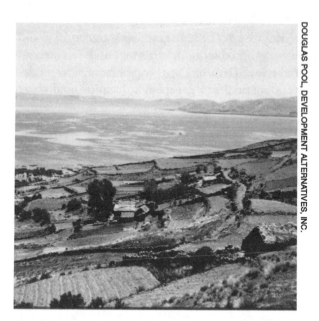

DOUGLAS POOL, DEVELOPMENT ALTERNATIVES, INC.

Productivity estimates for Lake Titicaca, shared by Bolivia and Peru and covering 8,135 square kilometers range from 50,000 to 250,000 metric tons—far above actual yield estimates.

Despite the availability of resource assessment technologies, little information on aquatic resources has been gathered. Fishery research activities that demand the highest priority are stock assessment, aquaculture, fishery expansion, resource administration and management, handling and processing, and technical training to support enhanced fishery production. Assistance of an applied nature designed to address immediate problems could provide rapid results and the basis for demonstration and diffusion of new technologies and approaches to fishery production (14).

Quantitative and qualitative field assessments on the extent of aquatic resources are necessary to develop rational resource management plans. Information on species composition, recruitment, and life history help to establish sustainable harvest parameters. A variety of methods are available for gathering such information, some highly technical and others based on surveys at landing sites and local fish markets (125).

Box 4-G—Dike-Pond Aquaculture Systems

Blending of aquaculture and agriculture systems may hold promise for increasing productivity of floodplains or waterlogged soils. A notable example is the dike-pond system that has been used in the Pearl River Delta for at least 400 years. The system is composed of land and water subsystems linked through agriculture and livestock components. Byproducts from one subsystem become inputs for the other (29).

A diversity of fish are cultured in ponds (bottom, mid-level, and surface dwellers) and sugarcane, fruit trees, mulberry, forage crops, vegetables, and flowers are produced on the dikes. Poultry and livestock are raised near the ponds and silkworms are raised on the mulberry trees. The forage crops produced on the dikes are fed to livestock and fish. The livestock excrement is used to fertilize ponds and pond mud piled on dikes to fertilize crops.

Despite the antiquity of the Chinese system, scientific procedures for quantifying analyzing and experimenting with these farming systems are sparse. The International Center for Living Aquatic Resource Management (ICLARM) is actively researching combined agriculture and aquaculture systems in India and Malawi. These efforts closely resemble those of the Chinese systems. As in agricultural crop substitution approaches, a key need identified through the ICLARM effort is mass farmer participation in the adaptive research and development process (66).

SOURCE: Office of Technology Assessment, 1993.

Models to predict the potential catch productivity of river fisheries can be based on characteristics such as channel length or drainage basin area; correlations with environmental parameters; or habitat variables (124,125). For example, standing stock may show a high correlation with stream width, width-to-depth ratio, extent of riparian vegetation, and dry-season stream flow (59). Primary productivity estimates—requiring examination of morphological, physical, chemical, and biological features of the resource—are also necessary in developing management plans (20).

Some work has been done on quantifying production potential of the riverine systems of the Altiplano (the large, high-altitude inland drainage plateau of Bolivia and Peru) (86) and the Magdalena River Basin of Colombia (52,118). The aquatic systems of the eastern and western cordillera of the Andes have yet unquantified production potential, although these resources could contribute to national protein production (132).

Development of sustainable resource management plans requires information on the current status of a wide variety of parameters, including:

- Resource production and potential,
- Fishing activity,
- Environmental health,
- Historical trends to identify critical variables, and
- Spatial and temporal variations in conditions.

Once this information is available, opportunities for developing sustainable exploitation strategies may improve. Such management strategies should contain at least the following components: resource enhancement/regeneration plans, financial support, regulation and enforcement measures, development of local organizational capacity and coordination, and training and extension.

STRATEGIES TO ENHANCE COCA SUBSTITUTION EFFORTS[10]

Development of the alternative economy being promoted in Andean countries to reduce dependence on cocaine is at a critical stage. Some promising alternative crops have been identified

---

[10] The basis for this section was developed largely from: U.S. Congress, Office of Technology Assessment, Crop Substitution Workshop, September 30-October 1, 1991, Washington, DC.

and efforts continue to improve adoption and productivity of these systems. Largely the focus has been on agricultural crops as opposed to the broad range of renewable resource uses that might offer alternatives to coca production. Indeed, some coca production areas are identified as inappropriate for agriculture, yet suitable for forest management and production. Improving coca substitution programs in the Andean countries might be approached through:

- Diversifying agriculture systems,
- Intensifying agricultural production, and
- Expanding the range of resources exploited.

Some key principles unique to the Andean crop substitution effort create the framework within which improved substitution programs might be developed. First, the degree of economic and traditional dependence of Andean peoples on coca hinder acceptance of coca substitution programs linked to complete eradication of the crop. Coca is a traditional crop in Andean agriculture with a high degree of symbolism; further, it provides the largest share of export earnings for the Andean countries. Programs that approach crop substitution incrementally, therefore, may find greater acceptance than replacement strategies. Transition time from producing coca to producing alternative crops may be lengthy. Programs or projects must consider investment time for producers to make the transition to alternative livelihoods. Programs might focus on creating preconditions necessary to implement crop substitution programs, identifying how these programs fit with existing policies, and assisting in marketing and developing other support structures necessary for success of a substitution program.

Secondly, coca farmers tend to be smallholders, yet national agricultural policies (e.g., land-tenure, agricultural pricing and structure) seem to work against development of smallholder agriculture. Investment in improved agricultural production systems require access to affordable credit—a feature largely lacking for smallholders, particularly in coca production regions. Nevertheless, increasing profitability of national agricultural production is likely to depend on intensifying smallholder production systems. Progress toward the transition to alternative cropping systems in the coca-growing regions will depend on availability of improved technology and techniques, practices and cropping combinations, and a supportive policy environment at the local, regional, national, and international levels.

Finally, the extent of the cocaine economy in Bolivia, Peru, and Colombia highlights the size of the crop substitution task. If substitution programs focus on current coca-producing regions, environmental features will constrain the breadth of alternative crop choices. Coca grows on poor soils with low pH, high aluminum content, and low cation exchange—conditions few other crops will tolerate. Because of coca's value, carrying capacity of coca-producing regions exceeds that allowed through production of legal crops. Substitution efforts that seek to expand the range of resources exploited may be more successful than those that focus solely on a single resource alternative (i.e., regional economic development vs. alternative crops). Sustainable exploitation is key in such goals in order to maintain benefits in the long term. However, sustainable-use systems require development to support such resource use, and economic and sociocultural constraints must be addressed (e.g., market availability, practitioner skill). These features are important considerations and underscore the need for a flexible approach to developing alternative livelihoods for Andeans involved in coca/cocaine production.

■ Strategy: Diversify Agriculture Systems

Diversification of agricultural systems by incorporating high-value crops is the driving force behind current crop substitution efforts in the Andean countries. High-value agricultural exports offer potential to generate foreign exchange

Box 4-H—Estimated Economics of Intercropping Coffee with Annual, Semi-perennial Crops, and Shade Trees

The following table illustrates potential earnings from establishing a coffee, shade tree, semi-perennial, annual cropping system under good soil conditions. During the first 2 to 3 years of the system, annuals and semi-perennials are interplanted with the coffee to provide income (e.g., corn, cassava, bananas). Corn may be planted in October/November followed by bananas in November/December. The coffee seedlings are planted in January/February, and the established corn crop provides shade to promote coffee seedling development. After the corn crop is harvested, legume tree seedlings are transplanted. At this point the banana development is sufficient to provide shade for coffee, and annual crops such as cassava may be interplanted for harvest in 8 to 10 months. Bananas produce 14 months after transplanting and can be harvested for 3 to 4 years. Banana tree density is reduced 30 to 40 percent annually until it reaches 10 percent of its initial planting density. By years 4 to 5 coffee is in full production and legume tree cover is sufficient to provide shade.

Year after planting	Crop	Yield (kg/ha)	Income (U.S.$/ha)
1	Corn	1,500	180
2	Banana	5,000	500
3	Banana	2,000	200
3	Coffee	275	210
4	Banana	1,500	150
4	Coffee	440	335
5	Banana	500	50
5	Coffee	660	503
6	Coffee	990	754
7	Coffee	1,175	880
8	Coffee	1,375	1,048

SOURCE: H. Villachica, "Crop Diversification in Bolivia, Colombia, and Peru: Potential to Enhance Agricultural Production," contractor report prepared for the Office of Technology Assessment, April 1992.

earnings and thereby increase the attractiveness of legitimate agriculture. For example, tropical fruits and nuts, coffee, and spices are impressive in terms of potential income per hectare produced because of their value in European, Asian, and U.S. markets. Although still lower returns than that generated by coca production, these commodities are viewed as having the greatest potential for competing with coca. Yet, at the same time, existing infrastructural constraints to moving these products to market can reduce their value at the producer level and create a disincentive to participate in substitution programs. Integrated systems of high-value and staple crops could

provide a basis for agricultural diversification and increase agricultural profitability (box 4-H).

The Andean countries remain net food importers currently because cheap food imports are more cost effective than internal movement of foodstuff from production site to urban markets. Prices for traditional agricultural products are adversely affected by present agricultural structure and pricing policies. Nonetheless, crop diversification strategies could be approached in an incremental fashion with an initial focus on increasing production of traditional food products for local and regional markets and phasing in of high-value export commodities. Developing systems that integrate legitimate crops with coca offers an

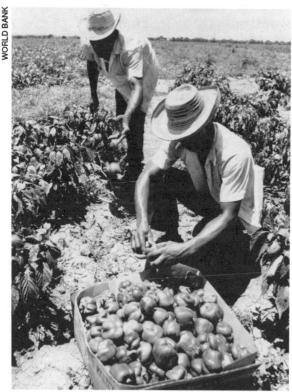

Irrigation networks can increase agricultural production, particularly in areas subject to seasonal rainfall. Here, farmers harvest green peppers on an irrigated cooperative farm.

option to reduce the perceived risk of transition to alternative systems for some coca producers. Coordinated effort could be placed on developing necessary infrastructure to support an agricultural export industry along with value-added processing to increase the economic benefits for local communities.

OPPORTUNITY: INCREASE IMPORT SUBSTITUTION

Diversion of land from legitimate agricultural production to coca production is suggested to have increased the Andean nations' dependence on foreign food imports. Production of typical Andean crops has declined; however, to what degree this may be attributed to expanding coca cultivation or to changes in food consumption patterns is unclear. Although increasing agricul-

tural productivity of the Andean peasant economy through application of selective technological packages is now viewed more optimistically, such approaches may require redesign of certain rural strategies (e.g., Peru's Agrarian Reform) and significant infrastructure development and technical assistance (115).

While the economic conditions of the Andean countries imply that internal markets will not be high-priced, ability to market may be increased if products and markets are in close proximity (e.g., a producer in the Chapare may stand a better chance of getting grain to La Paz than bananas to Chile). Price differentials, however, will constrain this approach and may result in a need for additional economic incentives associated with substitution programs.

Lessons from activities to convert opium cultivators to legal crops in Pakistan could be applicable to the situation in the Andean countries. The Food and Agriculture Organization (FAO) has been assisting the Pakistani Government for the past 10 years to develop alternative employment for opium cultivators with a focus on increasing production of food crops for national markets. Project funds have been provided by the United Nations International Drug Control Programme and the Government of Pakistan. Production of legal crops in the region (wheat, maize, and pulses) has been increased through the application of improved cultural practices and increased inputs. Cash crops (sugar cane, tobacco, horticultural products, and fodder) were introduced as well, largely through development of irrigation technologies, and the livestock sector was strengthened. A major factor in the success of these efforts was the strengthening of supporting infrastructure, including potable water-supply systems, irrigation networks, and gravel and tarmac roads (38) (chapter 3).

OPPORTUNITY: INCREASE THE VALUE OF AGRICULTURE IN DOMESTIC MARKETS

The value of smallholder agricultural production in the Andean countries is low relative to other sectors. To some degree, this is the result of national food policies that maintain low-cost food for urban areas. In addition, international programs may have adversely affected the prices producers can command in local, regional, and national markets. Food assistance under the P.L. 480 program (the Agricultural Trade Development and Assistance Act of 1954 as amended) provides low-cost food imports to the Andean countries, largely staple crops produced in excess in the United States. Competition with these cheap commodities may have contributed to reduced value of Andean agriculture in the domestic market.

OPPORTUNITY: DEVELOP TRANSITIONAL SYSTEMS

Transitional systems that allow coca producers to shift their production systems gradually to legitimate crops may offer an opportunity to ease risk-averse farmers into legitimate agricultural productions systems. While participants in current substitution programs continue to produce some amount of coca, focus remains on coca replacement systems rather than integrated systems. This may have several effects. First, farmers may maintain separate fields for coca and substitution crops, dividing time and effort and potentially reducing yields of the legitimate crops. Secondly, with coca being the ''cash crop,'' farmers are more likely to weight their attention toward the ''sure thing'' as opposed to the alternative, particularly in times of adversity when yields of both may be threatened. Lastly, the replacement approach may discourage participation by risk-averse farmers who are unwilling to eliminate coca or by those who do not have sufficient land or labor to tend separate plots. Alternatively, integrated systems that incorporate alternative crops in coca production could provide source reduction benefits as well as improved agronomic attention to legitimate production by the farmer.

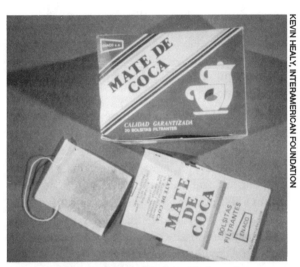

KEVIN HEALY, INTERAMERICAN FOUNDATION

Increasing markets for legal coca products (e.g., coca tea or maté de coca) *may reduce the hardship for producers adopting alternative crop systems.*

OPPORTUNITY: EXPAND MARKETS FOR LEGITIMATE COCA PRODUCTS

Mechanisms to absorb program participants' coca during the transition phase and channel it into legitimate markets offer an opportunity to reduce the coca supply for cocaine production. Options might include expanding the international market for legitimate coca products (e.g., coca tea, pharmaceuticals). However, the large amounts of coca produced are likely to overflow existing legitimate markets.

Alternatively, developing new products from coca may have some merit (61). Potential medicinal and therapeutic applications of coca include: 1) treatment for spasmodic conditions of the gastrointestinal tract, motion sickness, toothache and other mouth sores; 2) caffeine substitute; 3) antidepressant; and 4) adjunct to weight reduction and physical fitness (91). Examination of the other alkaloids found in coca might yield additional industrial possibilities. Although the research and development time required to bring new products to market may reduce the short-term utility of this approach, it could be a useful component in an overall package of efforts to reduce illicit coca production.

■ Strategy: Intensify Agricultural Production

Intensifying agricultural production for domestic and international markets will be necessary for the Andean countries to reduce food imports and produce sufficient quantities of products to interest international markets. This might be done through improving traditional agricultural production systems, facilitating input availability, and reducing disincentives to investment in improved production practices. At least four International Agricultural Research Centers (IARCs) conduct research on crop improvements directly applicable to the Andean region. In fact, many of the advances in staple crop production in the Andean nations have arisen from IARC research efforts (e.g., recent increases in rice and maize yields and production expansion in Peru).

Highly productive forms of agriculture in tropical regions generally focus on some form of polyculture. Improvements in productivity can be generated through carefully planned crop combinations, agroecological suitability, and effective nutrient and energy cycling systems. Integrated systems can be developed that efficiently recycle subsystem by-products through other subsystems, such that the waste from one activity becomes the input to another.

OPPORTUNITY: IMPROVE TRADITIONAL AGRICULTURE SYSTEMS

Traditional production practices developed in the Andean countries could be improved to offer expanded economic benefits for producers. Examination of how these practices promote productivity and sustainability could be used to identify where research and development effort could best be placed. Agroforestry, polyculture, and integrating livestock with agricultural production systems may offer particularly promising opportunities.

Multiple cropping systems have a long history in the Andean region and are ideally suited to the humid tropical zones where crop substitution activities are underway. Agroforestry is of particular interest in substitution programs as many of the alternatives identified are long-cycle tree crops (e.g., tropical fruit trees, nut trees). Currently, only one Consultative Group on International Agricultural Research (CGIAR) institute focuses primarily on agroforestry—the International Council for Research on Agroforestry (ICRAF). ICRAF is located in Kenya, hundreds of kilometers distant from tropical wet forests ecologically similar to those of the eastern Andean foothills and thus these efforts are unlikely to be easily transferred to the Andean countries. Additional agroforestry research was carried out by North Carolina State University at Yurimaguas, Peru. This effort was largely an offshoot of traditional agricultural research, yet it highlighted the importance of perennial tree crops in tropical agriculture. These efforts have ceased, however, largely due to violence in the area.

OPPORTUNITY: DEVELOP SMALLHOLDER AGRICULTURE

Small-scale farms are essentially the rule in coca-producing zones and opportunities to intensify their production are needed. Farming systems could be intensified through the application of modern technology adapted to suit local agroecological conditions. Increasing the availability of agricultural inputs and improving delivery methods may offer an opportunity to intensify agricultural production. Increased productivity at the subsistence level would likely lead to surpluses that could be marketed. Technical assistance exists for many crops and additional work on improved cultivars could increase yields. Assisting smallholders to intensify production may allow them to move gradually to semi-commercial and commercial production. Concomitant with this effort would be strengthening local markets, perhaps to redirect from imports to locally produced commodities.

OPPORTUNITY: ASSIST WOMEN AGRICULTURALISTS

In many regions, women contribute the largest amount of farm work. Yet most efforts to assist farmers have been aimed at men. Traditionally, Latin American women in rural areas have been neglected by development projects (112). Women participate in agriculture in a number of ways, including crop and livestock selection, cultivation, harvest, postharvest handling, and marketing. Significantly, in areas where migration for seasonal labor is common (e.g., High Valleys), women stay at home to care for the crops and livestock. Recently, greater effort has been placed on the role of women in agricultural development, yet, increased efforts could improve the contribution of women farmers in crop substitution programs.

OPPORTUNITY: REMOVE DISINCENTIVES TO INVESTMENT IN IMPROVED SYSTEMS

There are a number of disincentives to investment in agricultural production improvements in the Andean region. These largely stem from national economic and political conditions (e.g., rural poverty, risks to personal security), and most will need to be addressed by national governments. One mechanism open to U.S. and multilateral organizations to improve investment opportunities is to increase the availability and affordability of agricultural credit. Agricultural credit is a key need to improve opportunities for producers to invest in production and land improvements necessary for alternative systems. Coca farmers tend to be small-holders, often without land title, personal capital resources, or access to normal routes of credit. Recent actions on the parts of national governments have improved the outlook for gaining land title, although bureaucratic constraints slow the process.

Within the context of coca substitution programs, opportunities for credit exist. Evidence suggests, however, that insufficient attention has been paid to developing appropriate credit packages for coca farmers. For example, agricultural credit is available to farmers in the Chapare, Bolivia, through an AID grant and is administered through a local private voluntary organization. However, the terms of credit are so high as to make it essentially unavailable for most farmers. Further, in Bolivia credit is conditional on removal of the coca crop, often the sole income-generating activity of the family. Although assistance is provided to develop an alternative production system, income is generally not established until the third year after planting. Yet, repayments for interest are due in year 1 of the loan. Under this scenario it is simple to understand the reluctance to give up coca in exchange for legitimate crops.

Much the same situation exists in Peru where collateral terms are significant (e.g., urban homes) and interest rates vary depending on the credit currency (i.e., 18 percent per year in U.S. dollars and 8 percent per month in Peruvian soles) (122). Although Colombia also lacks agricultural credit for crop diversification for coca, it does provide credit for diversifying coffee. Coffee farmers may receive up to 80 percent of the cost of developing new production sites at 20 percent interest per year. Loan repayment begins with the first harvest and must be completed in 10 years. Delayed payment schedules such as this could likely be appropriate for crop diversification credit.

Issues of credit availability and affordability may increase in importance if substitution becomes more broad-based in order to expand the range of resources exploited. In this case, credit opportunities will be needed for forest, wildlife and wildland, and aquatic resource exploitation—additional activities where producers are likely to be handicapped in meeting existing credit eligibility requirements.

■ Strategy: Increase the Range of Exploited Renewable Resources

The Andean countries have a wide range of renewable resources that could be developed to increase economic opportunities for producers. While much attention has been placed on narrowly defined agricultural opportunities, less emphasis has been directed toward the potential for expanding sustainable exploitation of other resources such as forests, fisheries, wildlife, or wildlands. Indeed, many coca-growing areas are more suitable to some of these options than traditional agriculture. For example, in the Alto Huallaga, where most coca is produced on steep slopes, agriculture is an environmentally, if not economically, unsuitable alternative. In the Chapare, Bolivia, timber operations were the primary economic activity until the mid-1970s when coca expansion eclipsed the industry (85).

OPPORTUNITY: DEVELOP SUSTAINABLE FORESTRY SYSTEMS

Considerable potential exists to manage Andean forests to increase the flow of benefits to smallholders, and even though deforestation affects an increasing area of these forests, substantial areas of natural forest remain. Efforts to promote protected areas and forest management offer alternative livelihoods and environmental benefits. Opportunities include:

- Conserving biological resources,
- Developing extractive reserves, and
- Developing sustainable timber operations.

The importance of sustaining tropical biological resources has been highlighted in the last two decades and recently was underscored by the United Nations Conference on Environment and Development. One mechanism of conservation has been to cede certain forest areas to indigenous populations to sustain their traditional lifestyles while offering conservation benefits. Similarly, extractive reserves offer economic and conservation opportunities. The value of forest products (nuts, fruits, etc.) harvested from an extractive reserve can be longer-term and significantly higher than that offered by one-time logging operations or conversion to agricultural production (104). Opportunities also exist for ''chemical prospecting'' in tropical forests to identify compounds with commercial potential. Sustainable

timber exploitation technologies have been demonstrated in the Palcazu Valley in Peru. Such innovative operations could be tested and adapted to other forest areas in the Andean countries. Despite these potential opportunities, efforts will be needed to increase the understanding of tropical forest management, specifically in the Andean region.

Recently, a cooperative effort between the Nature Conservancy and AID has provided funding (Parks in Peril Project) to ensure protection for threatened national parks in areas of concern. As part of this effort, on-site management will be established in Amboro National Park and Noel Kempff Mercado National Park in Bolivia, La Paya National Park in Colombia, and Pampas del Heath National Sanctuary in Peru. Efforts will include surveying protected area boundaries, recruiting, training, and educating rangers and local communities about park protection, developing park infrastructure, and promoting local community participation (113). The AID Environmental Support Project that supports cooperative efforts between foreign organizations and Latin American countries is active in Bolivian forests in conducting botanical inventories (Amboro and Noel Kempff) and developing sustainable harvest for economic tree species. These and similar efforts can contribute to developing national expertise and highlighting opportunities in forest management in the Andean nations.

OPPORTUNITY: DEVELOP SUSTAINABLE WILDLIFE AND WILDLAND MANAGEMENT SYSTEMS

The Andean region has a diverse range of ecosystems supporting a broad variety of wildlife species that are, or might be, managed to offer alternative livelihoods for local populations. Further, wildland management to sustain wildlife populations may offer an additional opportunity to enhance nature-based tourism industries. Development of wildlife resources for national and international markets in wildlife and wildlife products may provide more immediate returns than tourism but could also provide a base for tourism markets.

Wildlife-centered economic development has become more acceptable, and research efforts are being undertaken to determine sustainable yields and appropriate husbandry practices. Some techniques for raising/producing certain wildlife species have been developed and are easily incorporated in rural communities with little capital investment. For example, experimental programs for ranching of green iguanas have now spread from Panama to other neotropical countries (6,127). Licensing and protection mechanisms implemented in the region are making farming and ranching of wildlife more profitable than taking from the wild (97).

The International Union for the Conservation of Nature and Natural Resources and other international resource organizations are working to create viable legal markets for wildlife and wildlife products in conjunction with protecting habitats and wild populations. Congress could support these efforts by providing funding to these organizations to assist the Andean countries to develop wildlife industries. Coordination with AID, UNDCP, and other donors would be necessary to ensure that an adequate support structure was available to handle transport and marketing opportunities for producers.

OPPORTUNITY: DEVELOP SUSTAINABLE FISHERY PRODUCTION SYSTEMS

The numerous Andean lakes and rivers contain a variety of harvestable organisms and, with application of appropriate technology, their productivity could be enhanced. For example, recent fish production in Colombia's Guajira reservoir was 82/kg/ha/yr, whereas sustainable production has been estimated at 103 to 256 kg/ha/yr (134). Similarly, estimates on the productivity potential for the total fishery of Lake Titicaca range from 50,000 to 250,000 metric tons (maximum sustainable yield)—far above current actual yield estimates. Based on a conservative estimate of U.S. $0.50/kg, the fishery resources of Lake Titicaca

could realize an annual earning potential of U.S. $25 million (56,60,82,94).

Constraints to developing Andean fisheries include a lack of information on the extent and quality of the various resource systems, level of resource extraction, and fishermen themselves; and shortfalls in handling, processing, and storage technologies and transport infrastructure. Current fishery production is characterized by significant postharvest losses that could be reduced through attention to these needs. For example, postharvest losses from the Pilcomayo fishery are relatively low (9.4 percent) compared with those in the Bolivian highlands (30 percent). The primary difference between these examples is the use of ice in transport from the Pilcomayo fishery (87). Poor handling can reduce the value of fishery products and increase losses to spoilage.

Technical assistance to promote enhanced productivity of existing fisheries will be needed. Introduction of efficient gear and harvest technologies and aquaculture practices to support stocking efforts, training in processing techniques for postharvest handlers, and strengthening of administrative and management protocol for fishery offices are a few of the key needs. Training programs similar to those developed for trout hatcheries in rural communities of Maucana, Peru, could improve local economies through fishery enhancement of lakes and streams (96). Currently, AID does not identify fishery production as a priority for resource development in the Andean region and there is only one fisheries specialist (on loan from National Marine Fisheries Service) in AID (103). AID could increase its effort toward fishery development and establish technical assistance as a priority. A development project costing one to several million dollars could produce a 10-fold increase in total local earning for inhabitants of Lake Titicaca (93).

Alternatively, the Andean countries could take advantage of existing international expertise in aquatic resource management and development. International research organizations, such as the International Center for Living Aquatic Resource

Management (ICLARM), Peace Corps, and other institutions (e.g., International Center for Aquaculture at Auburn University) could be tapped to assist in fishery development or enhancement.

CHAPTER 4 REFERENCES

1. Alcorn, J.B., *Huastec Mayan Ethnobotany* (Austin, TX: University of Texas Press, 1984) In: Gliessman, 1992.
2. Allison, J., *An Ecological Analysis of Home Gardens (Huertos Familiares) in Two Mexican Villages*, M.A. Thesis, Biology, University of California, Santa Cruz, CA, 1983, In: Gliessman, 1991.
3. Altieri, M., *Agroecology: The Scientific Basis of Alternative Agriculture* (Boulder, CO: Westview Press, 1987) In: Gliessman, 1991.
4. Alvarez, A., Agricultural Research Scientist, Advisor to Programa de Desarrollo Alternativo Regional, Cochabamba, Bolivia, personal communication, March 1991, In: McCaffrey, 1991.
5. Arbelaez, J., "El Cultivo de Platano en Zona Cafetera, Federacion Nacional de Cafeteros," Bogota, Colombia, 40 p., 1991, In: Villachica, 1992.
6. Ashton, R.E., Jr., "Potential Use of Neotropical Wildlife in Sustainable Development," contractor report prepared for the Office of Technology Assessment, December 1991.
7. Ashton, R.E., Jr., "Land Use Planning and Ecotourism," *Ecotourism and Resources Conservation* 1:91-98, 1991, In: Ashton, 1991.
8. Ashton, R.E., Jr., "Handbook on Central American Tourism and Wildlands Protection," Paseo Pantera Ecotourism Project, Wildlife Conservation International, 1991, In: Ashton, 1991.
9. Avila, L., Charaja, M., and Camapaza, J. (eds.), "Socio-Economic Aspects of Fishing the Bay of Puno," unpublished manuscript, In: Schroeder, 1992.
10. Bayley, P.B., "Fish Resources in the Palcazu Valley: Effects of the Road and Colonization on Conservation and Protein Supply," Report to USAID/Peru, JRB Associates, McLean, VA, 1981, In: McCaffrey, 1991.
11. Bedoya, E., "Las Causes de Deforestacion en la Amazonia Pruana: Un Problema Estructural,"

Working Paper No. 46 (Binghamton, NY: Institute for Development Anthropology, 1990) In: Painter and Bedoya, 1991.
12. Bedoya, E., Intensification and Degradation in the Agricultural Systems of the Peruvian Upper Jungle," *Lands at Risk in the Third World*, P.D. Little and M.M. Horowitz (eds.) (Boulder, CO: Westview Press, 1987) In: Painter and Bedoya, 1991.
13. Beissinger, S.T., and Bucher, E.H., "Can Parrots Be Conserved Through Sustainable Harvesting?" *Bioscience* 42(3):164-172, March 1992.
14. Bonetto, A, "Report on the Limnological Studies To Be Carried out in the Amazon of Peru," FAO Project PNUD/FAO-PER/76/022, Part 4, *Informacion de Instituto del Mar de Peru* 81:173-205, 1981, In: Schroeder, 1992.
15. Boo, E., "Ecotourism: The Potentials and the Pitfalls," World Wildlife Fund, Washington, DC, 1990, In: McCaffrey, 1991.
16. Boyer, J.S., "Plant Productivity and Environment," *Science* 218:443-448, Oct. 29, 1982.
17. Brack, A., "Ecological Evaluation of the Palcazu River Valley (Pasco, Peru) and Guidelines for Environmental Conservation Program, Report to USAID/Peru, JRB Associates, McLean, VA, 1981, In: McCaffrey, 1991.
18. Brockman, C.E. (ed.), "Perfil Ambiental de Bolivia," USAID, La Paz, Bolivia, International Institute for Environment and Development, Washington, DC, 1986, In: McCaffrey, 1991.
19. Browder, J.O., "The Limits of Extractivism," *BioScience* 42(3):174-182, March 1992.
20. Brylinsky, M., and Mann, K., "An Analysis of Factors Governing Productivity in Lakes and Reservoirs," *Limnology and Oceanography* 18:1-13, 1973, In: Schroeder, 1992.
21. Budowski, G., "Home Gardens in Tropical America: A Review," paper presented at the First International Workshop on Tropical Homegardens, Bandung, Indonesia, Dec. 2-9, 1985, In: Gliessman, 1991.
22. Chavez, A., "Andean Agricultural Research and Extension Systems and Technology Transfer Activities: Potential Mechanisms To Enhance Crop Substitution Efforts in Bolivia, Colombia, and Peru," contractor report prepared for the

Office of Technology Assessment, December 1991.

23. Christanty, L., *An Ecosystem Analysis of West Javanese Homegardens*, East-West Center, Honolulu, HA, working paper, 1981, In: Gliessman, 1991.

24. Christanty, L., Abdoellah, O., Marten, G., and Iskander, J., "Traditional Agroforestry in West Java: The Pekarangan (Homegarden) and Kebuntalun (Annual-Perennial Rotation) Cropping System," In: Marten, G. (ed.), *Traditional Agriculture in Southeast Asia* (Boulder CO: Westview Press, 1986) In: Gliessman, 1992.

25. Conway, P., "Silk for Life—Project Proposal," Silk for Life, Madison, WI, January 1991.

26. Coutts, R., and Zuna, F., "Present State of Fishery Technology in Bolivia," Departamento Nacional Desarrollo Pescadero, La Paz, Bolivia, 1981, In: Schroeder, 1991.

27. Crutchfield, T., Owner, Reptile Enterprises, Bushnell, FL, personal communication, 1991, In: Ashton, 1991.

28. Darschnik, S., and Shuhmacher, H., "Trout Farms Causing Disturbance in the Natural Stream Continuum," *Archeological Hydrobiology* 110:409-439, 1987, In: Schroeder, 1992.

29. DENG, Hanseng (Guangzhou Institute of Geography), "Application of Dike-Pond Systems to the Degraded Lands in South China," Paper Submitted at the China Tropical Lands Workshop, 9-13 September, 1991, University of Hong Kong, Kadoorie Agricultural Centre, Shek Kong, New Territories, 1991.

30. Development Alternatives, Inc., "Environmental Assessment of the Chapare Regional Development Project, Bolivia," DAI, Bethesda, MD, 1990, In: Stevenson, 1992.

31. Deza, A., "Incubation of Eggs of Kingfish *Basilichthus bonariensis* in Cuzco," *Hydrobios* 9(1-2):24-28, 1985, In: Schroeder, 1992.

32. Dourojeanni, M., "Amazonia Que Hacer?" Centro de Estudios Tecnologicos de la Amazonia, Iquitos, Peru, 1990, In: McCaffrey, 1991.

33. Dourojeanni, M., "Fauna and Wild Area Management in the Palcazu Valley," Report to USAID/Peru, JRB Associates, McLean, VA., 1981, In: McCaffrey, 1991.

34. ECONSULT, "Informe Final de la Evaluacion del Proyecto USAID No. 572-0244 Desarrollo Rural del Alto Huallaga," Lima, Peru, 1986, In: Painter and Bedoya, 1991.

35. Edwards, S.R., Coordinator, IUCN Sustainable Use of Wildlife Initiative, Washington, DC, personal communication, 1991, In: Ashton, 1991.

36. Everett, G., "The Rainbow Trout *Salmo fairdneri* (Rich.) Fishery of Lake Titicaca, *Journal of Fishery Biology* 5:429-440, 1973, In: Schroeder, 1991.

37. Everett, G., "The Rainbow Trout of Lake Titicaca and the Fisheries of Lake Titicaca," Report to the Government of Peru, 1971, In: Schroeder, 1992.

38. Food and Agriculture Organization, *FAO In Action* vol. 43, Jan./Feb. 1987.

39. Foster, R.B., "Brief Inventory of Plant Communities and Plant Resources in the Palcazu Valley, Peru," Report to USAID/Peru, JRB Associates, McLean, VA., 1981, In: McCaffrey, 1991.

40. Francis, C.A., *Multiple Cropping Systems* (New York, NY: McMillan, 1986).

41. Franzin, W., and Harbicht, S., "An Evaluation of the Relative Success of Naturalized Brook Charr, Salvelinus fontinalis, populations in South Duck River and Cowan Creek, Duck Mountain Region" *Manitoba Canada Technical Report on Fisheries and Aquatic Science* 1370, 25 p., 1985, In: Schroeder, 1992.

42. Gibson, H., "Lake Titicaca," *Verh. International Vercin. Limnological* 15:112-127, 1964, In: Schroeder, 1992.

43. Gliessman, S., "Diversification and Multiple Cropping as a Basis for Agricultural Alternatives in Coca Producing Regions," contractor report prepared for the Office of Technology Assessment, February 1992.

44. Gliessman, S.R., "Integrating Trees Into Agriculture: The Home Garden Agroecosystems as an Example of Agroforestry in the Tropics," Gliessman, S.E. (ed.), *Agroecology: Researching the Ecological Basis for Sustainable Agriculture* (New York, NY: Springer Verlag Ecological Studies Series, 1990) pp. 160-168.

45. Gliessman, S.R., "Plant Interactions in Multiple Cropping Systems," In: Francis, C.A. (ed.)

Multiple Cropping Systems (New York, NY: McMillan, 1986) In: Gliessman, 1992.

46. Gliessman, S.R., Garcia, R., and Amador, M., "The Ecological Basis for the Application of Traditional Agricultural Technology in the Management of Tropical Agroecosystems," *Agro-Ecosystems* 7:173-185, 1981, In: Gliessman, 1992.

47. Gomez-Pompa, A., "On Maya Silviculture," *Mexican Studies* 3:1-17, 1987, In: Gliessman, 1992.

48. Gonzalez Jacome, "Homes Gardens in Central Mexico," I.S. Farrington (ed.) *Prehistoric Intensive Agriculture in the Tropics*, BAR International Series 232, Oxford England, 1985, In: Gliessman, 1992.

49. Goodland, R.J.A., Watson, C., and Ledec, G., *Environmental Management in Tropical Agriculture* (Boulder, CO: Westview Press, 1984) In: Gliessman, 1992.

50. Gow, D., Clark, K., Earhart, J., Fujita, M., Laarman, J., and Miller, G., "Peru An Assessment of Biological Diversity," USAID, DESFIL, Washington, DC, 1988, In: McCaffrey, 1991.

51. Henson, T., Owner, Tropical Wildlife, Ltd., Suriname, personal communication, 1991, In: Ashton, 1991.

52. Hoffman, M.S., *The World Almanac and Book of Facts 1991* (New York, NY: Pharos Books, 1990), In: Schroeder, 1992.

53. INADE-APODESA, "Manejo de Bosques Naturales de la Selva Alta del Peru: Un Estudio de Caso del Valle del Palcazu," Instituto Nacional Desarrollo—Asistencia a la Politica de la Selva Alta, USAID Conco Consulting Corporation, Tropical Science Center, Lima, Peru, 1990, In: McCaffrey, 1991.

54. *International Ag-Sieve*, "Tropical Rainforest Plants: The Bottom Line," 5(1):3, 1992.

55. Janzen, D.H., "Tropical Agroecosystems," *Science* 182:1212-1219, 1973, In: Gliessman, 1992.

56. Johanesson, K., Vilchez, R., and Bertone, D., "Acoustic Estimation of Icthyomass and its Distribution in Lake Titicaca," FAO Report FAO/GCP/RLA/025 (NOR), 1981, In: Schroeder, 1991.

57. Kass, D.C.L., "Polyculture Cropping Systems: Review and Analysis," *Cornell International Agriculture Bulletin* 32:1-69, 1978.

58. Kaye, M., President, Costa Rica Expeditions, San Jose, Costa Rica, personal communication, 1991, In: Ashton, 1991.

59. Kozel, S. and Hubert, W., "Testing of Habitat Assessment Models for Small Trout Streams in the Medicine Bow National Forest, Wyoming," *North American Journal of Fishery Management* 9:458-464, 1989, In: Schroeder, 1992.

60. Laba, R., "Fish, Peasants, and State Bureacracies: The Development of Lake Titicaca," *Comparative Political Studies* 12:335-361, 1979, In: Schroeder, 1991.

61. Latin America and Caribbean Commission on Development and Environment, *Our Own Agenda*, Inter-American Development Bank, United Nations Development Programme, p. 38-39, 1989

62. Leaky, R., Director, Kenya Wildlife Protection, Nairobi, Kenya, personal communication, 1991, In: Ashton, 1991.

63. LeVieil, D., "Territorial Use-Rights in Fishing (TURFs) and the Mansgement of Small-Scale Fisheries: The Case of Lake Titicaca (Peru), PhD Dissertation University of British Columbia, Canada, 1987, In: Schroeder, 1992.

64. LeVieil, D., and Orlove, B., "Local Control of Aquatic Resources: Community and Ecology in Lake Titicaca, Peru," *American Anthropology* 92, 1990, In: Schroeder, 1992.

65. LeVieil, D., and Orlove, B., "Socio-Economic Importance of Lake Titicaca Macrophytes," unpublished manuscript, In: Schroeder, 1992.

66. Lightfoot, C., Integration of Aquaculture and Agriculture: A Route to Systainable Farming Systems," *International Ag-Sieve* 4(5):4-5, 1992.

67. Lin, S., Shy, J., Yu, H., "Morphological Observation on the Development of Larval Machrobracium asperulum (Crustacea, Decapoda, Palaemonidae) Reared in the Laboratory," *Journal of Fisheries Society* Taiwan. 15:8-20, 1988, In: Schroeder, 1992.

68. Lindbergh, K., "Policies for Maximizing Nature Tourism's Ecological and Economic Benefits," World Resources Institute, Washington, DC, 1991, In: Ashton, 1991.

69. Little, E., ''Handbook of Utilization of Aquatic Plants,'' FAO Fishery Technical Paper (187):176 p., 1979, In: Schroeder, 1992.

70. Mares, M. and Ojeda, R., ''Faunal Commercialization and Conservation in South America,'' *Bioscience* 34:580-584, 1984, In: Ashton, 1991.

71. McCaffrey, D., ''Biodiversity Conservation and Forest Management as Alternatives to Coca Production in Andean Countries,'' contractor report prepared for the Office of Technology Assessment, August 1991.

72. McGrath, D.G., *The Animals Products Trade in the Brazilian Amazon* (Washington, DC: National Wildlife Federation, 1986), In: Ashton, 1991.

73. McNeely, J.A., ''Economics and Biological Diversity: Developing and Using Economic Incentives To Conserve Biological Resources,'' International Union for the Conservation of Nature and Natural Resources, Gland Switzerland, 1988, In: McCaffrey, 1991.

74. Medina-Pizzali, A., ''Small-scale Fish Landing and Marketing Facilities,'' FAO Fishery Technical Paper, 291:68, 1988, In: Schroeder, 1992.

75. Ministerio de Agricultura, ''Plan Nacional de Accion Forestal 1988-2000,'' Lima Peru, 1987, In: McCaffrey, 1991.

76. Myers, N., ''Discounting Depletion: The Case of Tropical Forests,'' *Futures* December 1977, In: McCaffrey, 1991.

77. Nagoshi, M. and Kurita, H., ''Relationship Between Population Density and Production of the Redspot Masu-Trout Oncorhynchus rhodurus in Japanese Mountain Stream,'' *Bulletin of the Japanese Society of Fisheries* 52:1875-1879, 1986, In: Schroeder, 1991.

78. Ninez, V. ''Introducton: Household Gardens and Small Scale Food Production,'' *Food and Nutrition Bulletin* 7(3):1-5, 1985 In: Gliessman, 1991.

79. Norton, G., and Ganoza, V., ''The Benefits of Agricultural Research and Extension in Peru,'' NCSU/AID, Lima, Peru, 1985, In: Chavez, 1991.

80. Organization of American States, ''Minimum Conflict: Guidelines for Planning the Use of American Humid Tropical Environments,'' Washington, DC, 1987, In: McCaffrey, 1991.

81. Orlove, B., ''Barter and Cash Sale on Lake Titicaca: A Test of Competing Approaches,'' *Current Anthropology* 27:85-98, 1986, In: Schroeder, 1992.

82. Orlove, B., LeVieil, D., and Trevino, H., ''Social and Economic Aspects of the Lake Titicaca Fisheries,'' unpublished manuscript, 1990, In: Schroeder, 1992.

83. Orlove, B., and LeVieil, D., ''Some Doubts About Trout: Fisheries Development Projects in Lake Titicaca,'' In: B. Orlove, M. Foley, and T. Love (eds.) *State, Capital, and Rural Society: Anthropological Perspectives on Political Economy in Mexico and the Andes* (Boulder CO: Westview Press) 1989, In: Schroeder, 1991.

84. Painter, M., Institute for Development Anthropology, Binghamton, New York, personal communication, October 1991.

85. Painter, M., and Bedoya-Garland, E., ''Institutional Analysis of the Chapare Regional Development Project (CRDP) and the Upper Huallaga Special Project (PEAH),'' contractor report prepared for the Office of Technology Assessment, July 1991.

86. Parenti, L., ''A Taxonomic Revisionof the Andean Killifish Genus *Orestias* (Cyprinodontiformes, Cyprinodontidae),'' *Bulletin of the American Museum of Natural History* 178:107-214, 1984, In: Schroeder, 1992.

87. Pattie, P.S., Arledge, J., Asmon, I., Avram, P., Castilla, O., Gertsch, M., Kraljevic, I., Riordan, J., and Smith, J., *Agriculture Sector Assessment for Bolivia*, prepared for Agriculture and Rural Development Office USAID/Bolivia Mission, IQC Contract Number PDC-1406-1-00-7007 (Washington, DC: Chemonics International Consulting Division, January 1988).

88. Paz, S., Sociology Student, Universidad May San Simon, Cochabamba, Bolivia, personal communication, March 1991, In: McCaffrey, 1991.

89. Perez, C., Advisor to Programa Desarrollo Alternativo Regional, Cochabamba, Bolivia, personal communication, March 1991, In: McCaffrey, 1991.

90. Perl, M.A., Kiernan, M.J., McCaffrey, D., Buschbacher, R.J., and Batmanian, G.J., ''Views for the Forest: Natural Forest Management Initia-

tives in Latin America,'' World Wildlife Fund, Washington, DC, 1991, In: McCaffrey, 1991.

91. Plowman, T., ''Coca Chewing and the Botanical Origins of Coca (*Erythroxylum* ssp.) in South America,'' D. Pacini and C. Franquemont (eds.), *Coca and Cocaine: Effects on People and Policy in Latin America*, Cultural Survival Report #23 (Peterborough, NH: Transcript Printing Company, 1986), pp. 5-33.

92. Repetto, R. ''The Forest for the Trees? Government Policies and the Misuse of Forest Resources,'' World Resources Institute, Washington, DC, 1988, In: McCaffrey, 1991.

93. Richerson, P., Professor, Aquatic Ecologist, Institute of Ecology, University of California—Davis, personal communication, 1991, In: Schroeder, 1991.

94. Richerson, P., Widmer, C., and Kittel, T., ''The Limnology of Lake Titicaca (Peru-Bolivia), a Large, High Altitude Lake,'' University of California Davis Institute of Ecology Publication, 14:78, 1977, In: Schroeder, 1991.

95. Rincon, O., ''El cultivo de Macadamia, Federacion Nacional de Cafeteros,'' Bogota, Colombia, 29 p, 1990, In: Villachica, 1992.

96. Rodriguez, A., ''Pisciculture program in the 'Central de Capacitacion' for work in San Juan Bautista, Matucana, Peru,'' Documenta 10:8-13, 1982, In: Schroeder, 1991.

97. Ross, P.R., Executive Officer, Crocodile Specialist Group, personal communication, 1991, In: Ashton, 1991.

98. Ruthenberg, H., *Farming Systems in the Tropics*, revised edition (Oxford: Clarendon, 1980) In: Gliessman, 1992.

99. Ryel, R., ''Ecotourism: An Economic Alternative for Natural Resource Destruction,'' *Ecotourism and Resource Conservation* 1:31-44, 1991 Miami FL, In: Ashton, 1991.

100. Sanchez, P., and Benites, J., ''Opciones Tecnologicas para el Manejo Racional de Suelos en la Selva Peruana,'' 1st Symposium on the Humid Tropics, Belem do Para, 1986, In: Chavez, 1991.

101. Schroeder, R., ''Fishery/Aquatic Resources in Bolivia, Colombia, and Peru: Production Systems and Potential as Alternative Livelihoods,'' contractor report prepared for the Office of Technology Assessment, October 1991.

102. Shaw, J.H., ''The Outlook for Sustainable Harvests of Wildlife in Latin America,'' *Neotropical Wildlife Use and Conservation* (Chicago, IL: Chicago University Press, 1991) In: Ashton, 1991.

103. Simmons, K.E., Executive Vice President, RDA International, Inc., personal communication 1991, In: Schroder, 1991.

104. Smith, E., ''Growth vs. Environment,'' *Business Week* May 11, 1992, pp.66-75.

105. Stevenson, B.McD., ''Post-Harvest Technologies to Improve Agricultural Profitability,'' contractor report prepared for the Office of Technology Assessment, March 1992.

106. Terborgh, J., Emmons, L.H., and Freese, C., ''La Fauna Silvestre de la Amazona: El Despilfarro de un Rescurso Renovable,'' V. de Lima 46:77-85, 1986, In: Ashton, 1991.

107. Thomsen J.B., and Brautigam, A., ''Sustainable Use of Neotropical Parrots,'' *Neotropical Wildlife Use and Conservation* (Chicago, IL: Chicago University Press, 1991) In: Ashton, 1991.

108. Tosi, J.A., Jr., ''Integrated Sustained Yield Management of Primary Tropical Wet Forest: A Pilot Project in the Peruvian Amazon,'' Tropical Science Center, Costa Rica, 1991, In: McCaffrey, 1991.

109. Tosi, J.A., Jr., ''Ecological Analysis and Land Use Capacity in the Area of the Chapare Project,'' Report to USAID/Bolivia, Cochabamba, Bolivia, 1983 In: McCaffrey, 1991.

110. Tosi, J.A., Jr., ''Sustained Yield Management of Natural Forests,'' Forestry Sub-Project, Central Selva Resources Management Project, Palcazu Valley, Peru, Tropical Science Center, San Jose, Costa Rica, 1982, In: McCaffrey, 1991.

111. Trenbath, B.C., ''Biomass Productivity of Mixtures,'' *Advances in Agronomy* 26:177-210, 1974, In: Gliessman, 1992.

112. United Nations, UNIFEM, ''Action for Agenda 21,'' United Nations, New York, New York, 1991.

113. U.S. Agency for International Development, ''Tropical Forests and Biological Diversity—USAID Report to Congress 1990-1991,'' USAID, Washington, DC, May 1992.

114. U.S. Agency for International Development, ''The Palcazu Valley (Oxapampa - Peru), Land

Use Planning for Sustained Development, An Experience Applicable to the Amazon Region,'' Ronco Consulting Corporation, Washington, DC., 1989, In: McCaffrey, 1991.

115. U.S. Congress, Office of Technology Assessment, Crop Substitution Workshop, Sept. 30-Oct.1, 1991, Washington, DC.

116. U.S. Congress, Office of Technology Assessment, *Integrated Renewable Resource Management for U.S. Insular Areas*, OTA-F-325 (Washington, DC: U.S. Government Printing Office, June 1987).

117. Unruh, J.D, ''Iterative Increase of Economic Tree Species in Managed Swidden-Fallows of the Amazon,'' *Agroforestry Systems* 11(2):175-197, 1990.

118. Valderrama, M., and Zarate, M., ''Some Ecological Aspects and Present State of the Fishery of the Magdalena River Basin, Colombia, South America,'' *Proceedings of the International Large River Symposium* 106:409-421, 1989, In: Schroeder, 1992.

119. Vaux, P., Wurtsbaugh, W., Trevino, H., Marino, L., Bustamente, E., Torres, J., Richerson, R., and Alfaro, R., ''Ecology of the Pelagic Fishes of Lake Titicaca, Peru-Bolivia,'' *Biotropica* 20:220-229, 1988, In: Schroeder, 1992.

120. Vegas-Valez, M., Ruiz, L., Vega, A., and Sanchez, S., ''The Shrimp *Chryphiops caementarius* (Palaemonidae): Embryonic Development, Stomach Content, and Controlled Reproduction: Preliminary Results,'' *Review of LatinoAmerican Aquaculture* 9:11-28, 1981, In: Schroeder, 1992.

121. Vegas-Valez M., Ruiz, L., Vega, A., and Sanchez, S., ''The River Prawn Chryphiops caementarius (Palaemonidae): Embryonic Development, Stomach Content and Reproduction Under Laboratory Conditions,'' Preliminary Note, Summaries Workshop of Natural Sciences, 1980, In: Schroeder, 1992.

122. Villachica, H., ''Crop Diversification in Bolivia, Colombia, and Peru: Potential to Enhance Agricultural Production,'' contractor report prepared for the Office of Technology Assessment, April 1992.

123. Villachica, J., Lescano, C., Lazarte, J., Chumbe, V., Estudio de oportunidades de inversion en desarrollo e industrializacion de cultivos tropi-cales en Pucallpa. Perfil de proyecto para la planta de coloantes naturales yu para la planta de conservas de palmito, Convenio FUNDEAGRO, Region Ucayali, Lima Peru, 1992.

124. Welcomme, R., ''River Fisheries,'' FAO Fishery Technical Paper, (262):330 p., 1985, In: Schroeder, 1992

125. Welcomme, R., ''River Basins,'' FAO Fishery Technical Paper, (202):60 p., 1983, In: Schroeder, 1992.

126. Welcomme, R., and Henderson, H., ''Aspects of the Management of Inland Waters for Fisheries,'' FAO Fisheries Technical Paper (161):36 p., 1976, In: Schroeder, 1992.

127. Werner, D.I., ''The Rational Use of Green Iguanas,'' *Neotropical Wildlife Use and Conservation* (Chicago, IL: Chicago University Press, 1991) In: Ashton, 1991.

128. Willey, R.W., ''Intercropping—Its Importance and Research Needs. Part 1. Competition and Yield Advantages,'' *Field Crops Abstracts* 32:1-10, 1979, In: Gliessman, 1992.

129. Winterbottom, R., ''Taking Stock: the Tropical Forestry Action Plan After Five Years,'' World Resources Institute, Washington, DC, 1990, In: McCaffrey, 1991.

130. World Resources Institute, *World Resources 1990-1991: A Guide to the Global Environment* (Oxford: Oxford University Press, 1990), In: McCaffrey, 1991.

131. World Resources Institute, International Institute for Environment and Development, *World Resources 1986: An Assessment of the Resource Base that Supports the Global Economy* (New York: Basic Books, Inc., 1986) In: McCaffrey, 1991.

132. Wurtzbaugh, W., Associate Professor, Fisheries Biologist, Department of Fisheries and Wildlife/Ecology Center, Utah State University, personal communication, September 1991.

133. Wright, M., ''Selling Timber without Selling Out,'' *Tomorrow: The Global Environment Magazine* 1(2):87, 1991.

134. Zarate, V. Valderrama, B., Sanchez, M., and Martinez, R., ''Evaluation of the Fisheries of the Guajiro Reservoir and Some Management Criteria,'' *Trianea* 3:215-226, 1989, In: Schroeder, 1991.

135. Zhou, W., ''A Preliminary Report on the Introduction and Utilization of Blue Algal Bloom in Some Lakes of Our Country (China),'' *Transatlantic Oceanoligical Limnology* 4:54-57, 1987, In: Schroeder, 1991.

Technologies To Support Alternative Crop Production | 5

Whatever the product, supporting technologies are needed to enable producers to compete in global markets. Key needs in the Andean region, include:

- Research, extension, and access to technologies that can improve production of commodities;
- Processing, transport, handling, storage, and communication infrastructure; and
- Improvements in product quantity and quality and trade programs to increase competitiveness of Andean products.

Meeting these needs is the ultimate challenge facing national and international development organizations.

INTRODUCTION

Research and extension plays an enormous role in providing alternative livelihoods for coca producers and promoting their adoption. Development of suitable technology packages for coca farmers will depend in large part on the ability of research and extension specialists to conduct interdisciplinary and adaptive work. Existing research and extension systems are not well-equipped to fulfill this role and economic disparities and political conditions restrict the level of national funding for these efforts. Technology transfer can provide assistance in this arena, but improvements are needed.

Adequate infrastructure (including processing and storage facilities, transportation pathways and vehicles, and communication pathways) is critical in supporting production and marketing of Andean products. Ability to move necessary inputs into producing regions and raw or processed materials out to wider

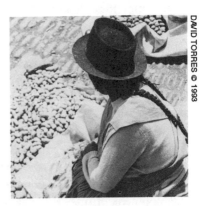

markets depends on effective, affordable transportation. Information on markets and prices is necessary for practitioners to make production decisions. Currently, agricultural marketing is hindered by the lack of: specialized packing facilities; cooling facilities; airport-based cool storage; ability to load refrigerated shipping containers at product source; and specialized processing installations nearby production areas. Private-sector investment in supporting production and marketing is hindered by the lack of affordable credit, and government inability to service international loans hinders national investment in comprehensive roads and other services or in sizable construction projects.

Infrastructure development—particularly transportation systems—is controversial. Some argue such development will assist narcotics traffickers and others cite the disastrous environmental consequences of some early road-building projects in the Amazon region. Nevertheless, while it is *possible* that improved infrastructure would benefit narcotics traffickers, it is *certain* that producers of legitimate products are handicapped by its absence.

Production of alternative crops is not yet at a level where Andean producers can enter international markets effectively—small production units make product quantity a key constraint to effective competition. There is a need for importers willing to accept small shipments with a vision towards expansion as producer capability and production area increase. Marketing agricultural products also can be complicated by the strict product quality and safety requirements of importing nations. Such restrictions can be difficult for developing countries to meet without proper training and assistance programs. Trade programs that stimulate Andean exports to the United States and other countries can complement alternative development efforts. For example, the Andean

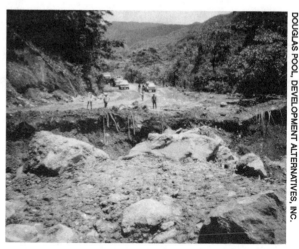

DOUGLAS POOL, DEVELOPMENT ALTERNATIVES, INC.

Reliable roads are essential for profitable agriculture in the Andean region. Here, heavy rains have washed out a road in the Chapare, Bolivia, disrupting farmer access to agricultural inputs, markets, and agricultural extension.

Trade Initiative (ATI) offers specialized trade arrangements for the Andean nations with the United States. This action addresses the need in part, but greater effort is likely to be necessary.

ANDEAN AGRICULTURAL RESEARCH AND EXTENSION SYSTEMS[1]

Bolivia, Peru, and Colombia possess the essential institutional foundations to develop effective national research and extension systems. However, each country has a unique situation and must overcome certain problems evident in existing systems. Proper action to improve the functioning of research and extension is a basic condition for future agricultural success. All three countries require foreign financial aid and/or specialized technical assistance. Peru requires financial aid urgently to rebuild its system. In Bolivia, the need for technical assistance probably is more acute.

Whatever the amount and quality of technical and financial assistance granted to the affected

---

[1] The information contained in this section was drawn largely from A. Chavez, ''Andean Agricultural Research and Extension Systems and Technology Transfer Activities: Potential Mechanisms To Enhance Crop Substitution Efforts in Bolivia, Colombia, and Peru,'' contractor report prepared for the Office of Technology Assessment, December 1991.

countries, its usefulness will depend on actual measures taken by governments to secure permanency and progress for research and extension agencies and their programs. A real and effective political commitment to technical innovation and modernization of agriculture must be made, particularly in Bolivia and Peru, including adequate funding for research and extension activities, respectable salaries for personnel, and appropriate regard for the entities in charge of these activities.

Agricultural research and extension systems vary significantly among Bolivia, Peru, and Colombia. Funding levels, staff size and capability, and institutional arrangements comprise key differences. Government instability has constrained agricultural modernization in Bolivia and Peru where the research and extension systems are under central government control. Colombia's system has been participatory and stable, with an obvious direction toward modern agriculture.

Agricultural research and extension systems typically are based on national research organizations, agricultural colleges, and private nongovernmental organizations. Regional political pressures in Bolivia and a strong private sector in Colombia influenced diversification of their respective research systems, while the Peruvian system has remained unchanged. A review of institutional frameworks and resources highlights the importance of foreign assistance and international cooperation in promoting Andean research and extension systems.

▌ Bolivia

INSTITUTIONAL FRAMEWORK

Bolivia's agricultural research system has four main components established in the 1970s that conduct basic and applied research and provide extension services to most agricultural producers:

- Bolivian Institute of Agriculture and Livestock Technology (*Instituto Boliviano de Tecnología Agropecuaria* (IBTA))—IBTA

is the leading national research institute, and its subcomponent the IBTA–Chapare, is the main research and extension agency for Bolivia's coca substitution program.
- Tropical Agriculture Research Center (*Centro de Investigación Agrícola Tropical* (CIAT))—CIAT is a regional research agency for Santa Cruz, the country's most dynamic agricultural sector.
- Pairumani Plant Genetics Research Center (*Centro de Investigaciones Fitogenéticas de Pairumani (Santa Cruz)* (CIFP))—CIFP is a technical branch of the Patino foundations.
- Bolivian Institute of Science and Nuclear Technology (*Instituto Boliviano de Ciencia y Tecnología Nuclear* (IBTN))—IBTN focuses on chemical analysis and tissue culture.

In addition to these organizations, several Department development corporations (*Corporaciones Departmentales de Desarrollo*), universities, and nongovernmental organizations (NGOs) perform agricultural research on short-term, specific problems for local clientele. However, little coordination exists among the formal research and extension system and these groups.

IBTA direction is determined by the Ministry of Agriculture (MACA)—an organizational structure that has created substantial difficulties for IBTA. Politically-oriented changes in Directors and research priorities have fragmented IBTA's meager financial resources. The Government of Bolivia's investment in agricultural research through IBTA has declined, resulting in manpower reduction policies and complete reliance on foreign assistance.

IBTA research is commodity-oriented and geographically restricted to the Altiplano and Valley areas. IBTA operates three experiment stations, three substations, and two germplasm centers, all poorly equipped and staffed. Research conducted by IBTA will continue to focus on genetic improvement and field management of commodities in the Altiplano and Valley regions.

IBTA was responsible for Bolivia's extension service, operating seven regional offices with a total of 80 extension posts. The national extension system failed, however, due to poor coordination with other research agencies, poorly paid and inadequately trained staff, and lack of well-established extension methodologies and monitoring and evaluation methods.

IBTA-Chapare operates under the Regional Alternative Development Project (*Proyecto de Desarrollo Alternativo Regional* (PDAR)), and carries out research and extension activities for Bolivia's coca substitution program. IBTA-Chapare operates two experiment stations: La Jota—for research on crops, soils, and pest control; and Chipiriri—for research on livestock and poultry. In addition, IBTA-Chapare undertakes many studies, and extension[2] and promotional activities through NGOs and other regional entities. It also maintains close technical relationships with several national and international research entities.

Centro de Investigación Agrícola Tropical has a regional research focus on production systems in Santa Cruz emphasizing grains, tree crops, and livestock. CIAT also performs research in rhizobiology, fertilizer management, and postharvest problems. Research programs of the *Universidad Autónoma "Gabriel Rene Moreno,"* which concentrate on beans, corn, and cassava, complement CIAT activities. Additional activities include horticulture research at the Okinawa Experiment Station and sugarcane research at the Sugarcane Producers Association Experiment Station.

CIAT receives national and international funding to carry out its research and extension activities. Domestic funding ($1.6 million annually) primarily comes from regional public entities and local producer associations. External financial assistance comes from seven international donors. CIAT is managed by a Board of Directors under an Executive Director appointed by the Minister of Agriculture for a 5-year term.

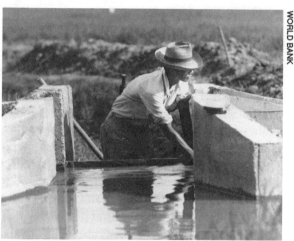

Irrigation networks can be important supporting infrastructure for regions experiencing a dry season. IBTA–Chapare research on improving agricultural production in the High Valleys includes an irrigation component.

A Regional Research Council meets twice a year to coordinate research activities in Santa Cruz.

The *Centro de Investigaciones Fitogenéticas de Pairumani* focuses its research efforts on developing new varieties of grain legumes, maize, and wheat. Most of its research is done in Cochabamba. Although CIFP has a significantly smaller annual budget than some of the other institutions, it has been successful in genetic improvement of maize for silage, and development of some new maize varieties for human consumption.

The *Instituto Boliviano de Ciencia y Tecnología Nuclear* recently began to address agricultural matters in its chemical analysis and tissue culture work. These areas of expertise allow IBTN to complement IBTA research in soil-water relationships, soil fertility, and high-altitude cropping systems.

RESEARCH AND EXTENSION PRIORITIES

Bolivian near-term agricultural policy goals include: 1) improving rural economies, 2) increasing food production, 3) integrating the

---

[2] Extension activities include 87 demonstration production units reaching more than 7,000 producers.

agricultural economy with international markets, 4) promoting agricultural exports with competitive advantages, 5) developing and implementing sustainable agricultural systems, and 6) improving crop substitution activities (18). A national council (*Consejo Nacional de Investigación y Extensión Agropecuaria*—CNIEA) directs Bolivian research and extension activities to achieve national agricultural goals. CNIEA is headed by the Deputy Secretary of Agricultural Production and includes representatives from major public and private entities that conduct research and extension. Although all agencies involved in research and extension continue to pursue individual agendas, CNIEA can play a critical coordination role in Bolivian agriculture.

A major priority is to rebuild a national extension service. This has been accomplished partially through regional and local systems and international donors through their agricultural development projects (e.g., Cochabamba Regional Development Project). An estimated 130 NGOs are active in extension and reach between 100,000 and 150,000 small farmers—roughly one-third of the national farm population (37). Some Department development corporations also provide extension services through regional or local agricultural projects. Finally, a growing number of farmer cooperatives and commercial firms provide extension assistance and information to farmers.

Ideally, research priorities are set according to local or regional conditions and actual production problems and patterns. Involving farmers and producer organizations can be key in setting realistic research and extension priorities. These groups can assist in identifying primary production problems. For example, CIAT research priorities closely reflect local agricultural problems in Santa Cruz. The close relationship between CIAT and local farmer associations and extension specialists fosters such applied priority setting. Conversely, lack of farmer representation in IBTA-Chapare and lack of transitional production systems may have constrained priority setting in connection with coca substitution activities.

IMPROVING EXISTING RESEARCH AND EXTENSION SYSTEMS

Agriculture is beginning to be revitalized to supply domestic markets at reasonable prices and expand and diversify exports. Accordingly, much attention is focused on Bolivia's agricultural research and extension system. International financial and technical support, and specific commodity projects by different research and extension agencies represent important contributions to Bolivian agricultural development.

A need exists for enhanced coordination among institutions within the system such that national and regional research priorities can be established and institutional research plans harmonized. An improved relationship between research and extension is also needed to enhance technical assistance to farmers and to keep research relevant to their needs. Also necessary are attention to agricultural regions that lack research and extension services and comprehensive training in the skills and expertise needed to modernize Bolivian agriculture.

■ Peru

INSTITUTIONAL FRAMEWORK

Agricultural research and extension activities in Peru have been provided almost exclusively by central government institutions. Accordingly, these institutions have been characterized by instability. Over the last two decades, institutional structures and responsibilities for research and extension have changed frequently due largely to political changes. The current political flux of Peru may result in further alterations of the existing research and extension systems.

National crop, forestry, livestock, and agroindustry research are the responsibility of the National Institute for Agrarian and Agroindustry Research (*Instituto Nacional de Investigación Agraria y Agroindustrial* (INIAA)) established in

1987, while extension activities have been placed under regional governments. Most of these units are ill-equipped for extension activities and currently the system barely operates. Another reorganization is planned to give extension responsibilities to the INIAA.

Peruvian universities rarely are involved in providing research for government or private institutions; most university research activity is confined to student thesis work. Exceptions to this situation are the National University of San Marcos Graduate School (*Universidad Nacional Mayor de San Marcos* (UNMSM)) and the National Agrarian University (*Universidad Nacional Agraria* (UNA)) at Lima. UNMSM has made major contributions related to animal health and livestock production systems. UNA, the most important academic center for agricultural and biological sciences in Peru, has managed to develop and maintain a highly qualified cadre of agricultural professionals since the 1960s. Foreign investment and institution-building efforts have fostered UNA's position as a key contributor to agricultural development.

General financial and political crises that have ravaged the university system since the 1970s have adversely affected UNA, however, and its academic quality and research potential have declined. Tropical forestry research on species inventory and on tropical woods characterization for industrial uses is one of the few research fields that UNA has pursued continuously. Four universities at Tingo Maria, Tarapoto, Iquitos, and Pucallpa, cover Amazonian ecosystems, but their research capabilities are very limited.

The Peruvian Amazon Research Institute (*Instituto de Investigaciones de la Amazonía Peruana* (IIAP)) was created to promote and coordinate research in the Amazon region. IIAP has few technical and financial resources, however, and thus its activity and power fall far short of its chartered mandate. Currently, the only vehicle for research coordination in Peru is the Peruvian Amazon Research Network (*Red de Investigación de la Amazonía Peruana* (REPAP)), an Interna-

tional Research Center for Development (*Centro Internacional de Investigaciones para el Desarrollo* (CIID))-funded research network established in 1989 to develop sustainable production systems for the Amazon region.

Research and extension funding has diminished significantly over the last 5 years and recent budgets have provided only for payroll and not operating expenses. Thus, most technical personnel sit idle; the few ongoing research activities are totally dependent on foreign interests and funding. The public extension system has declined in importance as nonpublic organizations (e.g., national and local commodity organizations, universities and technical institutes, and the commercial sector) began to provide extension services. However, these services tend to address specific needs in the most favored agricultural areas rather than possessing a broader national agricultural agenda. The government has not made any systematic effort to organize or extend these alternative extension services nationally. Thus, most Peruvian farmers lack systematic and permanent technical support.

Institutional instability, unrealistic salary policies, and political maneuvering have constrained attempts to establish permanent professional research and extension teams in Peru. In fact, government actions have reduced the number of public research and extension personnel. INIAA's professional staff has been reduced already by 40 percent (around 200 positions).

PRIORITIES FOR AGRICULTURAL RESEARCH AND EXTENSION

Research and extension were neglected during the late 1960s and throughout the 1970's (16) as resources were directed to irrigation projects and land reform. During the 1980s, government interest and investment in research and extension improved substantially with financing from the World Bank, U.S. Agency for International Development (AID), and the InterAmerican Development Bank (IDB). Even then, total public investment in agricultural technical change remained small. Today, Peru's agricultural structure is based on *minifundia*—small landholdings—with 72 percent of units smaller than 5 hectares (approximately 12.5 acres). Undoubtedly, this will present great challenges to research and extension.

Economic policies promoting low-priced basic food imports since the 1960s have adversely affected domestic food production. A widening gap between domestic supply of and demand for basic foods led to prioritization of research programs on rice, maize, potatoes, grain legumes, and wheat. During the second half of the 1980's, the number of research programs expanded as demand for work on other products grew. Research in oilseeds, horticulture, fruits, soil and water management, forestry, and agroindustry were added to the agenda. However, increases in funding did not accompany the expanded agenda of research and extension institutions. In recent years, agricultural priorities have shifted from domestic to export markets.

Extension priority was given to the northern coast and the most important Andean valleys. In the Amazon region, only the big valleys of the northeast received some support. The Andean highlands, with the largest and poorest peasant population, and new agricultural areas in the Amazonian region, remained almost unattended.

IMPROVING RESEARCH AND EXTENSION SYSTEMS

The key constraints to improving the agricultural research system in Peru revolve around the lack of a functional national extension service, poor coordination of activities, and low funding levels. The impulse given to agricultural research and extension during the first half of the 1980s lost steam as economic and political difficulties increased. The number of international donors decreased, which in turn has resulted in redistribution of existing outside funding. The sectoral project supported by IDB came to an end in 1986 and the World Bank stopped disbursing in 1987. AID's financial support continued, but had to be

redistributed among a growing number of research programs and to all experiment stations. The situation continues to decline with most experiment stations being transferred to regional governments or the private sector. The majority of these organizations do not have the financial means or the technical expertise to manage research.

∎ Colombia

INSTITUTIONAL FRAMEWORK

International assistance has been very important to the Colombian research and extension systems. During the 1960s, most foreign assistance was from the United States, and focused on institution building. In 1963, the Ford, Rockefeller, and Kellogg Foundations played critical roles in the organization and implementation of research and extension programs. By the end of the 1960s, 18 international agencies were cooperating with the Colombian Agricultural Institute (*Instituto Colombiano Agropecuario* (ICA))—the most important agricultural research institution in Colombia. ICA was created in 1962 as part of the government restructuring of the public agricultural sector and has been the most important source of technical and financial assistance to agricultural producers. The Institute maintains a large, highly trained staff to provide a broad and diverse human-resource base for agricultural research and extension. This may be the most important single factor contributing to modernization of Colombian agriculture. Key factors in ICA's success were government financial and political commitment to research and extension, and the involvement of the private sector and key public agencies (13).

ICA has been instrumental in promoting the use of modern agricultural techniques in Colombia. Improved cultivars and practices are now used on nearly 40 percent of Colombian cropland. The Institute supplies most of the basic seed used for agricultural production and is active in developing improved varieties. For example, ICA released 236 new varieties and cultivars of the country's most important crops, 34 of them between 1986 and 1990.

ICA's institutional framework for research and extension includes 4 national research centers, 12 regional research centers, 7 experiment stations, 29 diagnostic centers for animal health, and a network of 66 regional centers for extension, training, and technology dissemination. Training is a high priority for ICA. Between 1986 and 1990, ICA spent $7.7 million, or 6 percent of its total budget, for training. About 35 percent of ICA's budget supports direct research and extension activities (15 and 20 percent, respectively) (14).

Government support for research and extension has accounted for 55 to 75 percent of ICA's budget. Government contributions grew steadily between 1964 and 1990, but currently are decreasing. With fewer financial resources and numerous loan repayment obligations, ICA is looking for avenues to increase income. Possibilities include increasing competition with the private sector.

Colombia also has a complex network of private institutions in the agricultural sector. The private sector has expanded its role in genetic and agronomic research as well as in certified seed production. In the 1980s, significant private research effort was placed on sugar cane and coffee. Oil-palm producers recently have organized a research center (CENIPALMA), and flower and banana producers are planning their own research centers. Benefits for producers could be achieved through a vigorous coordination effort among the numerous private and public research and extension institutions.

Private-sector support of university research has improved capabilities of the Agronomy Department and the Graduate School of Colombia's National University. However, the majority of Colombia's universities do not play important roles in agricultural research or extension. Despite Colombia's strong institutional framework for agricultural research and extension, productivity improvements are hampered by financial instability for exports (due to an overvalued Colombian peso), lack of security in many agricultural regions, institutional confusion, and lack of coordination.

Colombia is now in the process of decentralizing public functions and responsibilities. Agricultural extension will become the responsibility of Municipal Units of Technical Assistance (*Unidades Municipales de Asistencia Técnica Agropecuaria* (UMATAs)). Tax revenues will be transferred to the UMATAs for rural development. The Integrated Rural Development Fund (*Fondo de Desarrollo Rural Integrado* (DRI)) is implementing a strategy for local agricultural development working through the UMATAs. At the same time, a compromise between centralized and decentralized approaches to extension is emerging in the National System of Technical Assistance for Small Producers (*Sistema Nacional de Transferencia de Technología Agropecuaria* (SINTAP)). SINTAP will focus on small producers and development of local production options. Local extension priorities will be set by the UMATAs. Finally, ICA is preparing a set of local, regional and national agricultural projects.

PRIORITIES FOR AGRICULTURAL RESEARCH AND EXTENSION

The Alta and the Media Guajira (1.7 million hectares), and parts of the Orinoquia region (2.1 million hectares farmland and 13 million hectares grassland) have been identified as high productivity zones, which should be prioritized for research. Research priorities by topic include:

- Agricultural production in acid soils,
- Low-cost production systems for Andean valleys, and
- Biotechnology.

Production option priorities are not clear and, in general, insufficient attention is given to prioritizing the research use of public resources. ICA, perhaps due to its large size, is finding it difficult to focus on research subjects consistent with the

Box 5-A—Necessary Conditions for Successful Technology Transfer

1. Technology should fit the local biophysical and socioeconomic environment of the adopters and should have proven successful elsewhere under similar conditions, at least on a pilot scale.
2. Technology is transferred most effectively by direct people-to-people actions involving individuals with experience in applying the technology. Media presentations (e.g., pamphlets, books, radio) may assist, but personal interactions are necessary.
3. Technology transfer agents must be well-qualified and experienced in applying the technology and able to communicate effectively to potential adopters. Development of expertise in local organizations is necessary to continue technology transfer beyond the bounds of development assistance projects and time frames.
4. Facilitators or middlemen are needed in addition to transfer agents and capable adopters to help new technologies compete with established resource use methods.
5. Adopters and transfer agents should be involved in choosing, planning, and implementing technology transfer so that it will meet actual needs and is appropriate to the setting in which it will be implemented.
6. Interests of all parties involved in technology transfer should be identified and addressed in the technology transfer effort; all must see how the technology will benefit them.
7. Early definition of participant roles is needed so that all are aware of the subsequent steps in the transfer process and the relationship between their actions and those steps.
8. Demonstrations of the technology should take place under environmental, economic, and sociocultural conditions similar to those where it will ultimately be implemented.
9. Commitment of financial resources should be sufficient to carry out the technology transfer until it is self-supporting.
10. The transfer process must include mechanisms through which all participants can contribute effectively to interim evaluations and adaptations.

SOURCE: Derived from a Technology Transfer Workshop held for the Office of Technology Assessment study of *Technologies to Sustain Tropical Forest Resources*, OTA-F-214 (Washington, DC: U.S. Government Printing Office, March 1984).

regionalization process. Demands from the local extension systems and the growing involvement of the private sector in research further complicate this task. Several observers and public officials propose focusing ICA research on basic crops, small-farming production systems, and natural resource management.

IMPROVING RESEARCH AND EXTENSION SYSTEMS

Colombia's political and economic system is in flux. The new constitutional rules and the macroeconomic policies of the Colombian *aperatura* may create opportunities for social and economic development. However, institutional adjustment to these new conditions could be difficult. The size and role of national research and extension institutions are likely to change as fiscal support

funds dwindle and local, regional, and private-sector entities begin to replace them. ICA in particular has had difficulties prioritizing effectively in light of expanding responsibilities. Reduced government financial contributions and debt repayment obligations may exacerbate these difficulties. Conversely, extension funding does not seem to be a problem. The SINTAP project alone is likely to provide a significant amount to extension (nearly $130 million). The central government is providing value-added tax revenues for extension activities through the UMATAs. Private-sector institutions can and are willing to play an important role in promoting technical innovation in agriculture, in some cases through research contracts with universities. The government then could concentrate its efforts on small producers and improving rural economies.

Box 5-B—Horizontal Cooperation for Agricultural Research and Extension

Technology transfer among Latin American countries can link regions with similar environmental conditions and promote research and development of suitable technologies. For example, PROCITROPICOS, a cooperative agreement recently signed by a number of national agencies for agricultural research (NAARs) of Latin American countries, is focusing on cooperative or joint research programs, scientific and technical information exchange, and technology transfer. Efforts will be devoted to three main tropical ecosystems (i.e., humid-tropic, tropical savanna, and Amazon highlands) common to Bolivia, Brazil, Colombia, Guyana, Peru, Suriname, and Venezuela. The PROCITROPICOS will be supported by the Inter-American Institution for Cooperation on Agriculture (IICA) of the Organization of American States. Programs and activities of PROCITROPICOS should contribute to policy formulation and determination of production options conducive to sustainable development in the tropics. Sustainability criteria for the Latin American tropics and practical measures and actions for achieving sustainable production systems will be a main research focus (PROCITROPICOS Agreement, 1990).

Another cooperative program for research and technology transfer among Andean countries, PRO-CIANDINO, was initiated in 1985 by IICA and the InterAmerican Development Bank. The participant NAARs are from Bolivia, Colombia, Ecuador, Peru, and Venezuela and the program is governed by a council of NAAR directors. The program includes two major activities: joint research by two or more participants on specific problems that affect production of selected commodities; and horizontal technology transfer through a training program and experts consultation. PROCIANDINO initially focused on potatoes, maize, grain-legumes, and extension methods, and recently has expanded to include crop and livestock production problems in the Andean region. PROCIANDINO generally is praised as an effective mechanism for horizontal cooperation although delays in financing operating expenses and equipment purchases have hampered the research component. Through this project, scores of technicians and professionals from the NAARs have been able to experience and observe different ways of solving common problems.

SOURCE: A. Chavez, "Andean Agricultural Research and Extension Systems and Technology Transfer Activities: Potential Mechanisms to Enhance Crop Substitution Efforts in Bolivia, Colombia, and Peru," contractor report prepared for the Office of Technology Assessment, December 1991.

■ Agricultural Technology Transfer

Technology transfer is a temporary activity and provides a mechanism to build local expertise throughout the technology development and diffusion process (box 5-A). Activities that are conceptualized and implemented such that a long-term professional partnership is established between native and foreign experts may be most successful. Project cycles of at least 10 years probably are necessary to produce relevant results spanning technology generation to technology adoption by the average producer. Examples include the joint programs established by International Agricultural Research Centers (IARCs) and specific financing sources (e.g., the Trop-Soils and the Small-Ruminants programs in Peru) or bilateral assistance groups (e.g., AID Seed Program in Bolivia). Development of local abili-

ties in this way increases the potential for continuation of efforts after foreign assistance has ended. Regional technology transfer activities also have proven to be very useful. Collaborative research programs among Latin American countries (box 5-B) could be enhanced organizationally and financially and used more intensively.

In the early 1970s, key Bolivian national research groups (e.g., IBTA and CIAT) were created under U.S. technology transfer programs. Today, a number of bilateral and multilateral assistance organizations provide a wide array of technical expertise. CIAT in Santa Cruz is working with British, Japanese, and Dutch donors, and foreign consultants comprise a large part of CIAT's technicians (box 5-C). While some difficulties exist with donor coordination, this may be addressed with the establishment of CNIEA to facilitate and coordinate national planning for development. World Bank projects to integrate public and private-sector development efforts could increase professional and economic security in the research system. These stabilization measures are likely to improve the effectiveness of technology transfer activities and increase their long-term contribution to Bolivian agriculture.

In Peru, technology transfer activities contributed heavily to establishing the research and extension programs and helping to train Peruvian researchers that became the technical core of INIAA's research programs. Responsibility for technology transfer currently is being shifted from central government institutions to regional governments. Privatization of public functions and activities is gaining momentum, but where this trend will take Peru's technology transfer system is unclear. Peru has developed a relatively extended and well-qualified human-resource base through cooperation with international donors (box 5-D). However, institutional instability and erratic salary policies have eroded this base considerably and security problems reduce Peru's ability to receive and handle technology transfer projects effectively. These difficulties must be addressed to improve training efforts, consolidate key institutions, and maximize technology transfer benefits.

Technology transfer and financial assistance have been integral parts of the Colombian research system. Technology transfer contributed significantly to improved product quality control when the Colombian private sector initiated a strong drive to increase agricultural exports in the 1970s (primarily coffee, cut flowers, and bananas). Financial assistance in connection with technology transfer activities similarly has been important for national institutions. From 1979 to 1984, technology transfer projects brought approximately $5 million in grant money to the ICA and in 1986, ICA held nearly 200 technology transfer agreements with 30 different foreign entities (14) (box 5-E). Technology transfer has greatly diversified ICA's research agenda, al-

---

Box 5-C—Bolivian Seeds Project

One of the most fruitful technology transfer experiences in Bolivia, and one that carried important lessons for other developing countries, was the Seeds Project (Project T-059), initiated at the end of the 1970s with AID funding. The underlying concept was that properly organized and trained producers could succeed. Thus, the main project strategies of technical assistance and financial support for seed production infrastructure were revised to focus more on producer organizations and training. Technical support was given to a public office (MACA—Departmento de Semillas) and financial support was given to upgrade public-sector seed plants that were operating at very low capacities. The project advisor was based in Santa Cruz instead of La Paz where the project benefited from liberal ideas of local agricultural leaders and restricted national government ability to dominate the project. From Santa Cruz, the project expanded to El Chaco, Chuquisaca, to part of Tarija.

Producer participation was significant, particularly in the training activities and several small- to medium-sized seed enterprises were organized. Increasing numbers of institutions and producers became involved in the new production and marketing activities. For instance, the experiment stations became specialized producers of foundation seed. The project triggered a qualitative change in the local farmers' technical environment and promoted the institutional structure needed by a modern seed industry. Commercial demand for certified seed experienced tremendous growth, from 200 metric tons in 1970 to more than 10,000 metric tons in 1988 with a continuing growth trend.

SOURCE: A. Chavez, "Andean Agricultural Research and Extension Systems and Technology Transfer Activities: Potential Mechanisms to Enhance Crop Substitution Efforts in Bolivia, Colombia, and Peru," contractor report prepared for the Office of Technology Assessment, December 1991.

---

though there is some indication that this may have operated to the detriment of the institution (e.g., by increasing responsibility beyond institutional capacity).

Increasing agricultural productivity and profitability will be critical to support crop substitution approaches as part of a long-term strategy to

---

Box 5-D—Collaborative Technology Transfer Efforts in Peru

The Trop-Soils and Small-Ruminants collaborative programs are examples of long-term technology transfer activities. The Trop-Soils program, focusing on problems of tropical soils of the Amazon region, involved a team of Peruvian professionals and technicians working full-time with foreign scientists. The effort has resulted in a number of important contributions in productive, economically efficient, and ecologically sustainable soil management technologies. The program also has a successful training component; helping young Peruvian scientists in graduate studies and providing hands-on training in specialized tasks for laboratory and field technicians. The Trop-Soils program has been in operation for nearly 12 years, although security concerns have had an adverse impact on the level of activities at the Yurimaguas experiment station.

The Small-Ruminants program, focusing on native cameloid stock, is now in its 11th year. This effort also has been an important and useful experience for Peruvian research. In addition to National Institute for Agrarian and Agroindustry Research (INIAA) and Institute for Tropical and High Altitude Veterinary Research (IVITA), the leading Peruvian partners, the program involved several regional universities, cameloid production units, and an array of Peruvian professionals and scientists. The program trained 90 Peruvian professionals seeking advanced degrees, and generated about 700 publications. These two results are probably the program's most useful contributions to research in this field and to the diffusion of technical knowledge to producers.

SOURCE: A. Chavez, "Andean Agricultural Research and Extension Systems and Technology Transfer Activities: Potential Mechanisms to Enhance Crop Substitution Efforts in Bolivia, Colombia, and Peru," contractor report prepared for the Office of Technology Assessment, December 1991.

---

reduce coca cultivation. Most coca production occurs in areas characterized by low land-productivity and poverty. Research, extension, and technology transfer efforts can work to develop packages of practices suitable to these regions. A comprehensive crop-substitution strategy is likely to require:

- Enhanced research and extension activities,
- Financial assistance for research and extension,
- Foreign expertise to share professional research and extension responsibilities on a long-term basis, and
- Enhanced cooperation among Latin American countries.

Several issues that should be addressed jointly by research and extension specialists to improve technology transfer include: improved communication among researchers, extension agents, and producers; prioritization of technology dissemination efforts; and adaptation of extension methods to local conditions. External reviews and evaluations have identified research areas deserving of future attention, and point to new opportu-

nities to improve technology transfer activities. In general, greater attention toward natural resource management is needed as well as refocusing crop research to include cultivation practices, integrated management of pests and diseases, and postharvest problems. A multidisciplinary approach and close cooperation with specialized international programs and research centers will be needed to achieve these goals.

INFRASTRUCTURE TO SUPPORT AGRICULTURAL PRODUCTION AND MARKETING

Processing, handling, and storage facilities and transportation and communication networks are critical needs for successful alternative development. Alternative crops must compete with an easily produced, processed, and transported commodity—coca—with a known and largely stable market. Producers need information on legitimate crop markets for production decisions, easily available and affordable inputs, and scheduled and reliable transport services. Lack of attention to transport and communication development

---

Box 5-E—The Panela Project

The Dutch-supported Panela project, initiated in 1983 in Colombia, is an excellent example of successful technology transfer. Panela-cane, a small farmer's crop, is a popular sugar substitute in many villages and rural areas, as well as an important ingredient in traditional Latin American dishes. The panela industry provides employment and a year-round income to many peasant families throughout the Colombian valleys and Piedmonte area.

Project goals were to improve panela-cane varieties and cultivation methods and to improve traditional panela processing plants and methods. The Instituto Colombiano Agropecuario (ICA) established a pilot center in Santander (Barbosa) to promote adoption of the new technologies and results have been very promising. A new panela-cane variety has generated yield increases by as much as 30 percent.

The project also has produced technical recommendations for improving harvest efficiency and transport to mills. At the mills, new mechanical and chemical methods for cleaning juices were introduced, bringing extraction efficiency to 70 percent—a significant rise for a small-scale industry. Purity of juices also has improved. Finally, the project increased the efficiency of cookers and established the use of milled cane residual as fuel.

There are several important aspects of the Panela-project that made it a successful technology transfer experience. It addressed an important social and economic sector; changes and innovations in techniques and equipment were progressive and locally developed; and finally, the project had a long-term planning perspective—basic diagnosis and prioritization of problems led to application and extension of solutions. At present, ICA is extending the achievements of the Panela project with the involvement of nine Centros Regionales de Capacitación, Extensión, y Difusión de Tecnología (CRECEDs) and several nongovernmental organizations.

SOURCE: A. Chavez, "Andean Agricultural Research and Extension Systems and Technology Transfer Activities: Potential Mechanisms to Enhance Crop Substitution Efforts in Bolivia, Colombia, and Peru," contractor report prepared for the Office of Technology Assessment, December 1991.

---

compounds the comparative disadvantage for producers of legitimate crops in remote areas by increasing costs above competitive levels (box 5-F).

Despite the clear need for infrastructural support for alternative crops, constraints to development include:

- Insufficient financing and credit mechanisms,
- Difficult environments for building physical infrastructure,
- Small and dispersed production units complicating facility siting, and
- Tenuous security in some production areas.

In addition, the potential for efforts to benefit coca production and cocaine trafficking reduces interest in infrastructure development. Nevertheless, adequate infrastructure will be necessary to improve opportunities for coca farmers to undertake alternative crop production.

■ Value-Added Processing Opportunities[3]

Preservation and processing techniques can increase storage life and quality, minimize wastage and spoilage, and facilitate shipping and marketing of agricultural products. Processing also may increase value for producers and market demand. Efforts to develop value-added processing in the Andean region are ongoing, although they have met with some difficulties. In most cases appropriate technologies exist, but the facilities are lacking. In addition, inadequate or lack of electrical distribution networks in producing areas is another significant problem.

---

[3] The information contained in this section was drawn largely from B. McD. Stevenson, "Post-Harvest Technologies to Improve Agricultural Profitability," contractor report prepared for the Office of Technology Assessment, May 1992.

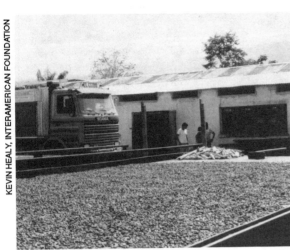

KEVIN HEALY, INTERAMERICAN FOUNDATION

Simple techniques can be used for primary processing of some tropical food products. Here, cocoa is being sundried; the intermediate product will be packed and shipped to another cooperative facility.

An essential part of the analysis of any value-added proposal is quantifying raw material availability, processing costs, and current market prices for the transformed product. The latter information is more readily available than the former. International commodity markets are transparent in the sense that there are many information systems, including the commodities exchange reports from major trading countries. It is important that the Andean countries have access to this information. Subscription to information services on a regular basis could be a part of alternative development projects to address this need.

A variety of Andean tropical food products are suitable for processing for domestic and international markets. Tropical fruits can be juiced, aseptically packed, frozen, canned or dried. While none of these options currently are available in the Chapare in Bolivia, canning facilities are available in Cochabamba and Santa Cruz, and conventional juice extraction plants are also available in Cochabamba. Investment in processing opportunities in the production zone could reduce transport costs and improve product competitiveness.

Box 5-F—From Production to Market: Development Dilemma

Although difficult, identifying potential alternative crops is simpler than developing the industrial base to make the crop economically sustainable. The problem can be illustrated using a real example from the Chapare region. Maracuya (passion fruit) has demonstrated good production characteristics under small farm conditions. The fruit has been processed locally and international buyers have expressed enthusiasm for the single strength juice extract, such that an order was placed for approximately 18 tons of product, to be shipped in 55 gallon drums, frozen. At present total production in the Chapare is unlikely to exceed this quantity per year. However, freezing facilities are not in place, and due in part to high transport, processing, and handling costs, the product is costing approximately 50 percent more than that from competitive sources.

Each of these factors can be addressed within the context of Cochabamba Regional Development Project (CORDEP), but making the transition from supplying local market to that of exporting will require investment in plant material, extension effort to expand the production base, increased efficiency in processing, establishment of frozen goods transport systems, and reduction of transport costs that currently reflect the distance of the production area from the nearest seaport in Arica, northern Chile. Thus, the problem becomes less one of marketing and more one of production and infrastructure. This is typical of a number of products with which alternative development programs are working. There is insufficient raw material to begin an agroindustrial operation, except with multilevel investment starting with the expansion of the production base.

SOURCE: B. McD. Stevenson, "Post-Harvest Technologies to Improve Agricultural Profitability," contractor report prepared for the Office of Technology Assessment, May 1992.

Similarly, nut crops can be harvested, shelled, and packed for transport with a minimum of infrastructure and can provide good returns despite a somewhat lengthy waiting time before trees are productive. In addition, many other value-added products can be derived from the raw material. Macadamia production is still developing in the Chapare and private-sector interest in nut processing is increasing.

Tea and coffee are being produced and achieving quality acceptable to international buyers. Primary processing is done in the production area and the resulting product is readily transported and offers good possibilities for export income. The small quantity of local production remains in all cases the biggest deterrent to international traders who generally require quantities much in excess of the local production capability. Table 5-1 identifies some specific possibilities for value-added processing in Bolivia and many of these crops are also produced in Peru and Colombia.

INVESTMENT IN AGROINDUSTRY

Investment in processing and storage facilities is a key need to promote alternative development in the Andean region. Although international donors have provided assistance in plant development (table 5-2), the private sector is reluctant to invest similarly. Nevertheless, there are examples of successful private sector investment, including the fruit-juice extraction plant in Cochabamba and rehabilitation of the Montero canning plant, which has expanded to process pineapples and palm hearts from the Chapare and Santa Cruz regions. In these cases, investors identified sufficient production of raw material to provide a base from which processing could expand. The citrus-juice processing plant may have a beneficial impact in import substitution and the pineapple canning operation may have export potential if costs can be contained to competitive levels.

The United Nations program has several agro-industrial plants now entering production and is providing infrastructure complementary to production increases. However, several of these plants are encountering problems in terms of their production economics, largely a reflection of the scale of plants built as pilot operations. For example, essential oils plants now entering operation in the Chapare highlight the problems. The

Table 5-1—Andean Tropical Fruits and Nuts With Market Potential

Fruit	Processed form
Banana	Pulped for industry; dried for snack food; processed for stock food.
Papaya	Processed for pectin extract; dried.
Passion fruit (Maracuya)	Juice concentrate (frozen or aseptically packed); pulp (full-strength or concentrate; with or without seeds.
Pineapple	Canned as slices, dices, pulp or puree; juice concentrate (frozen or aseptically packed).

Nut	Processed form
Castana (Brazils)	Shelled, whole and pieces; confectionery (chocolate-coated); ground as marzipan.
Macadamia Nuts	In shell; shelled, whole and pieces; confectionery (chocolate-coated).

SOURCE: B. McD. Stevenson, "Post-Harvest Technologies to Improve Agricultural Profitability," contractor report prepared for the Office of Technology Assessment, May 1992.

lemon-grass oil and mint oil projects are small-scale, and have a design capacity to process raw material from 120 and 75 hectares, respectively. Processing costs are high and production is unlikely to service capital and operating costs. Additional effort is needed to assist the small industries and organize growers to support the activity.

Credit for investment in agriculture typically has been deficient in the Andean countries. Largely a result of unfavorable credit terms and eligibility requirements, this situation has contributed to sluggish adoption of alternative agricultural livelihoods. For example, in Bolivia loans are being made to small producers at commercial terms. One concern is that loans are pegged to the value of the U.S. dollar, and also are at a commercial interest rate—currently 13 percent per annum. The combined inflation rate of perhaps 15 percent and the interest rate produce a real interest rate approaching 30 percent per

Table 5-2—Value-Added Processing Investment in the Chapare Region

Industry	Source of finance	Dollar value capital	Comment
Coffee pre-processing	AID Project 412	$ 73,835	Started in 1980; Project 412 in 1990.
Latex pre-processing	INC - AID	$ 32,900	Started in 1970; Project 412 in 1990.
Tea processing	China - 1984 AID Project 412	$ 108,000 $ 166,728	In production.
Glucose plant	Universidad Mayor de San Simon/UNDCP	$ 307,174	Installation now underway.
Vinegar plant	Universidad Mayor de San Simon/UNDCP	$ 175,298	Installation now underway.
Yuca and banana drying	AID Project 412	$ 73,897	Not yet in operation.
Banana and kudzu drying	Universidad Mayor de San Simon	$ 105,572	Starting production.
Mint oil extraction	AID Project 412		Starting production.
Lemon balm plant	AID Project 412	$ 103,200	Working; low oil return per hectare.
Milk plant	P.L. 480 United Nations	$3,200,000	Project incorporates health aspects.

KEY: UNDCP—United Nations International Drug Control Programme.
P.L. 480—Public Law 480, the Agricultural Trade Development and Assistance Act of 1954, as amended.
SOURCE: B. McD. Stevenson, "Post-Harvest Technologies to Improve Agricultural Profitability," contractor report prepared for the Office of Technology Assessment, May 1992.

annum. This is not sustainable on many agricultural programs. The loan situation is further complicated by significant failure rates, in part due to some borrowers withholding payments in the expectation that they may be forgiven the loans, the seasonal nature of cash flow, and the difficulty in achieving product sales at profitable levels. The lack of profitability, in turn, is a function of product quality and lack of infrastructure to reach major markets (28).

Any product-processing will require training local people to assume responsibility for the technical standards of the processing phase. This can be done either through training gained in a second country already experienced in the particular process, or through technology transfer and training in the host country. Both systems have merit, but the failure most commonly seen in sending people for second country training and experience is that the training is of a general nature and is too brief for technical competence to be achieved. Often the trainee returns and is diverted to an unrelated activity, or denied the resources necessary to implement new technology.

Building national capacity to take full and ongoing responsibility for implementation of new production systems is a primary goal of development efforts. The economics of bringing a single expert from overseas to teach groups of local people are obvious in terms of the multiplier effect achieved. Training programs could emphasize the use of overseas expertise within the developing country, rather than the general tour approach which frequently is seen as an excursion rather than a learning exercise. It is also important that invited expertise is of a technical level sufficient to achieve the desired level of competence in trainees. Frequently, the needed expertise is at a field practitioner level and not at the level of the professional consultant. Preparation of instruction manuals in the language of the recipient country is fundamental, and should form a part of the brief of any overseas expert engaged.

PRODUCT QUANTITY TO SUPPORT PROCESSING OPPORTUNITIES AND MARKET PENETRATION

There is a lack of product quantity to maintain some processing equipment at even pilot levels. Defining local production costs requires close liaison with the extension arm of the local development organization. This can be achieved through careful analysis of "real costs" incurred in the field which frequently differ greatly from the cost structure implied by an experimental or model evaluation. The theoretical cost of inputs may be much greater than the costs actually being incurred by low technology producers. Crop yields will usually reflect the reduced inputs and so the real production function must be known to make realistic crop recommendations. A responsible and adequately equipped field evaluation group should be an integral part of an extension effort, and should have input into the marketing process.

In some cases, the costs of production and processing can create a disincentive for producers to expand activities (e.g., Chapare lemon balm and mint oil plants). An example is the milk production plant nearing completion in the Chapare. Efforts are now commencing to increase the milk production capacity but may be complicated by high dairying costs in the region. Further, the zone is not a traditional milk-consuming area and lacks the infrastructure for refrigerated collection facilities and sales points. If the plant is to succeed, development in all these phases will be vital.

In areas where production units are small, contract farming could be developed whereby a processor contracts with producers to supply a certain quantity and quality product for processing. Thus, processors are assured of sufficient product quantity and quality and producers are assured of a market. However, a highly sophisticated level of agronomic research is required to support contract farming. Technology packages are needed that can assure a certain product quality from set production practices—information not currently available for most of the alternative crops being promoted in the Andean region.

Emphasis on product quantity and expanding production areas will be needed to reach volumes that will allow greater market penetration. Meanwhile, the short-term need is for buyers to accept small product lines with a view to developing a relationship with Andean exporters. Tariff incentives within major consumer nations and the formation of commercial links with developing countries would complement the donor government investment in regional development.

Producer Organizations

Producer organizations offer an opportunity to organize and mobilize capital and people in developing communities where conventional corporations are unable or unwilling to invest because of inadequate return, high risk, or lack of capital. These organizations provide an avenue for bulk purchase of supplies (e.g., seeds, agrichemicals, equipment); processing and marketing of products; financing; and even in some cases research and development of new crops or farming practices.

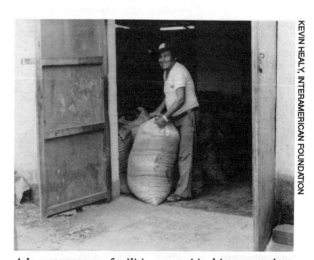

KEVIN HEALY, INTERAMERICAN FOUNDATION

Adequate storage facilities are critical in supporting production and marketing of alternative crops. Here, cocoa is being stored in the El Ceibo cooperative storage facility in the Alto Beni, Bolivia.

Producers organized into cohesive common interest groups could pool individual production to meet market product quantity requirements. The present marketing system relies heavily on intermediaries who buy products directly from individual farmers at the farm gate. Development of producer organizations could offer opportunities for smallholders to increase their bargaining power and disseminate market information (box 5-G).

In some instances, producer organizations may collectively purchase and work land, either by subdividing the land or sharing in the production of the entire tract. The more highly organized food producer organizations provide fully integrated programs for their members. Vertical integration also can offer expanded benefits by linking production, processing, and marketing. Although some efforts have been made to accomplish this in Bolivia, local politics have intervened to limit the efficiency and overburden organizations with administrative costs. Retaining an independent manager could help to avoid these problems. Involvement by the financing institution to assure internal factions do not adversely affect overall operations could be continued until the unit has attained economic independence and has demonstrated viability.

A major advantage of producer organizations is the built-in incentive for members to use services offered, increasing organization revenue. However, members generally lack incentive to purchase more than one share, limiting organization capital. There also is a danger of shortsighted decisions by members with diverse interests or limited knowledge of market economies. Some argue that not enough profit motivation exists in a producer organization to assure sufficient earnings for future growth. Nonetheless, the organization structure and similar constructs seem, in some cases, to be encouraging successful agricul-

tural production and marketing in some areas of the Andean region.

Alternative Trade Organizations

Alternative trade organizations (ATOs) seek to establish an equitable system of trade between developed and less developed countries (LDCs). Their mission is to trade with small-scale, democratically organized LDC producers and help them obtain higher prices and increased control over the market (9).

The ATOs of the 1990s emerged out of three different trends in marketing strategies: 1) church related, 2) development focused, and 3) politically motivated. The groups with a religious base were formed primarily in the United States, while the development and politically focused organizations are rooted in Europe. Today, ATOs are most developed in Europe where they have significant government and union support. Sales of the international ATO movement totaled approximately $75 million in 1987, $8 million of which came from sales in the United States (4).

ATOs focus on returning control and profit to the peasant producers. However, they have tended to remain in marginal markets where, although they may influence conventional business, they are unlikely to pose a great threat (9). Yet, ATOs and their products are finding greater acceptance in the national and international marketplace. As ''green consumerism'' has flourished and the awareness of global interdependence has increased, ATOs have created a niche for themselves in the world economy (box 5-H). Thus, ATOs may have a unique and potentially important role to play in marketing Andean alternative crops or products.

■ Transportation[4]

Profitable agricultural production in part depends on access to affordable necessary inputs and markets. A general lack of transportation

---

[4] The information for this section was drawn largely from J. DeVincenti, ''Infrastructural Needs to Support Agricultural Alternatives to Coca in Bolivia,'' contractor report for the Office of Technology Assessment, December 1991.

Box 5-G—Some Successful Andean Cooperatives

El Ceibo is a federation of 37 producer cooperatives of cocoa beans in the Alto Beni region of Bolivia. Representing some 900 peasant families, the organization offers its members multifaceted services that include agroprocessing, transport, marketing, agricultural extension, and diverse training programs in bookkeeping, accounting, agriculture, and rural development. The federation owns and manages its own industry, producing cocoa powder, baker's chocolate, cocoa butter, and chocolate candy. It sells these products nationally and internationally in Western Europe and Chile. In 1991, El Ceibo exported $600,000 worth of its products to alternative trade organizations and networks of health food stores for organic products.

The key to **El Ceibo's** success is a dynamic system of self-management that allows members to run their own business and services and acquire important rural development skills through intensive job training and experience. The participatory structure fosters a broad distribution of developmental benefits to peasant members and even non-members in the Alto Beni and high levels of motivation throughout the organization. By processing and marketing their products themselves, they are able to add value to their cocoa beans and attain the highest prices available to peasant producers. The positive economic incentives have permitted a continuous growth in member cooperatives and cocoa bean production over the past 14 years.

Asociación Central de Comunidades Productoras de Café (ACCOPCA) is an "association" of coffee farmers located in the La Paz department of Bolivia within the Yungas area. The group was originally created by the Centro de Investigación y Promoción del Campesinado, as an alternative to cooperatives, the traditional method of organizing small farmers in Bolivia. It was hoped that ACCOPCA would be more agile, representative, dynamic, and functional than a cooperative. Originally, the group reached out to *campesinos* through a radio program that provided farmers with information about local organizations and marketing power and a bulletin in the publication KUNATSA. ACCOPCA achieved legal status in 1980 and today there are 732 campesinos members who live in 23 small communities around the town of Coripata. The association offers a wide variety of services for its members in an attempt to develop a system based on self-management. They have established programs that address issues such as crop disease, pest control, crop diversification, and coffee marketing and export.

ACCOPCA is highly organized and its leadership structure is intact and essential to the successful management of the group. The traditional cultural framework for conducting group activities is a fundamental part of ACCOPCA philosophy. ACCOPCA markets coffee through the European Alternative Marketing Organization OS-3, which also works with El Ciebo. In 1987, ACCOPCA was recognized for the quality of its coffee at the international trade fair in West Germany and received the "Premio Internacional de Alimentación" in 1988 in Barcelona, Spain.

SOURCE: K. Healy, "From Field to Factory: Vertical Integration in Bolivia," *Grassroots Development*, vol. 11, No. 2, 1987, pp. 2-11.

---

infrastructure is apparent in the Andean region and may be the most limiting factor to improving agricultural production potential. Scheduled air service is available to numerous locations, but the transport hubs where bulk cargo shipments are possible are far fewer. Airport capacity ranges from modern international airports with adequate storage and handling capabilities to those less able or entirely lacking cargo services. Transport by water to distant markets can be an important export/import mechanism for the Andean region.

Some extensive riverine systems in the Andean region are important cargo navigation systems. For example, Bolivian riverine systems provide for cargo transport from the Chapare to northern points and also to the Atlantic Ocean through Paraguay and Brazil. Rail transport provides another link for certain areas, but rail networks are not extensive. For example, systems in Bolivia serve the east and west of the country and are linked to other national systems but are not linked to one another. Further, they can be expensive and

---

Box 5-H—Profiles of Two Alternative Trade Organizations

The *Max Havelaar Foundation*, founded by two Dutch alternative trade organizations (ATOs) along with churches and several consumer organizations, is the largest alternative trade effort in the world. The Foundation's goal was to move alternative trade coffee into the mainstream by creating a trademark open to all roasters meeting certain purchasing criteria: direct purchase from democratic farmers' organizations, a minimum purchase price, a long-term contract with the farmers, and generous credit terms for the farmers. Over a dozen small and medium-sized Dutch coffee roasters joined the initiative.

The Havelaar Foundation began its effort in 1988. Within the first year the goal was to capture 2 percent of the Dutch market. As of December 1990, Havelaar reached 2.25 percent of overall coffee consumption in the Netherlands. Havelaar now is available in most Dutch supermarkets and has ten times the market penetration than either of the founding ATOs alone.

Every year the Foundation purchases approximately 6 million pounds of coffee from peasant farmers. Its mandated purchase price is nearly 50 percent higher than the world market price. Because the Havelaar program demands direct payment to the growers' associations as well as favorable financing, the economic benefits to farmers may be two or three times those of the conventional coffee system.

Pueblo to People, a Texas based ATO is one of the largest in the United States. The non-profit organization was founded in 1979 to promote marketing outlets and economic support to democratically based grassroots organizations in Central America. The ATO returns $0.40 to $0.45 of each sales dollar to the producer, while the difference pays for the organization's operational expenses. Since the organization was founded in 1979, Pueblo to People has paid over $4 million to peasant producers in Latin America. It reported that in 1990, $1.3 million was returned to its Latin American producers and projected that $1.5 million would be returned in 1991 (29).

Today, Pueblo to People works with eighty groups from seven different Latin American countries (29). Pueblo only works with groups that meet its social criteria, which are often the least profitable and economically risky producers. Furthermore, Pueblo looks to work with groups organized for social as well as economic reasons. Its influence allows peasants to learn organizational skills and democratic methods as well as earn income. Pueblo to People sells its products in a retail store located in Houston, Texas, and through a mail-order catalogue.

A major focus of ATOs is educating consumers about the culture and lifestyle of producers and returning a fair price to producers. For example, Pueblo to People achieves its education goal through its catalogue that contains a blend of information about products, producers, and the mission of the organization.

SOURCE: Dickinson, R., "Alternative Trade Organizations, Peasant Farmers and Coca," contractor report prepared for the Office of Technology Assessment, January 1992.

---

do not provide a modern or efficient mode of transport (23). Currently, Bolivia is investing in railway expansion in some areas (e.g., northeast of the Chapare to Trinidad).

ROAD SYSTEMS

Road access in many coca-producing areas is a function of weather conditions, thus restricting access for extension workers and producers. The lack of a comprehensive network of feeder roads and adequate road maintenance make transport costs a significant barrier to increased agricultural production and contribute to high production and market costs for Andean products. For example,

fertilizer costs in remote areas are nearly twice that of the cost on the international market (34). Adverse road conditions take a heavy toll on vehicles adding further costs that are ultimately reflected in market prices (27).

The existing Peruvian and Bolivian road systems are largely the result of national government efforts in the 1950s and 1960s. These roads were constructed to promote colonization of remote areas of the country and increase production and availability of agricultural products (e.g., Belaunde Highway, Peru; and LaPaz-Santa Cruz, Bolivia). Although efforts to improve Bolivian roads have been made, the situation has not improved appreciably. For example, while the network of Bolivian roads has increased by at least 100 percent in the last 20 years, only 3.7 percent of the network is paved, 22.6 percent is gravel, and nearly 74 percent is dirt (22). Poor drainage conditions of the dirt roads continue to cause transport interruptions in rainy seasons. The current condition of Bolivian and Peruvian road systems is poor and, for a variety of environmental and security reasons, little ability exists to maintain or improve conditions.

Colombia placed considerable effort on developing its transportation network; however, transport costs remain high reflecting the difficult nature of the country, lack of modern transfer and transport facilities, and the generally low efficiency of operators. Infrastructure for farm-to-market access and intraregional connections received lower priority than interregional connections and today remain the weak link in the domestic transport system. Rural road construction and improvement and maintenance of the existing national highway network have been started recently to address this situation (38).

The virtual absence of refrigerated transport vehicles in the Chapare region is a primary constraint to improving marketing of agricultural products. Of the handful of refrigerated trucks in the Chapare, perhaps three are dedicated to the fresh produce business. Little incentive exists for private investment in such transport due to the unreliability of specialized vehicles, high maintenance costs, and low returns in the fresh product market. The Bolivian bananas arriving by road to Arica in Chile must compete with the sophisticated Ecuadorean production and transport systems, which achieve a quality product at a lower price.

Loading and transportation time in addition to difficult road conditions further affect marketing potential. At a minimum, the trip from Chimore in the Chapare, to Arica in northern Chile is a total of 700 kilometers, taking 3-1/2 days of constant driving. Although much further, the trip to the major Argentinian market of Buenos Aires benefits from excellent roads across the frontier. However, it is still 4 days minimum and involves transfer of the cargo at the border.

Despite these difficulties, small shipments have been made to both destinations and products sold in both markets. In order to assure buyers of a specific quantity and quality of desired produce it will be necessary to address infrastructure problems. For example, although Bolivian exports to northern Chile and Argentina have been described as success stories, recurring problems with product quality have created consumer resistance to the Bolivian product. These problems arose from lack of a well-established cold chain and transport infrastructure in advance of opening new markets and further highlight the danger of entering a new market before the basic export infrastructure is in place. To date, buyers have shown perseverance in helping Bolivian products become established in their markets, although it is questionable how much longer buyers will assume abnormal losses as a normal business hazard (28).

STORAGE, PACKING, HANDLING FACILITIES

Storage infrastructure from production point to market is insufficient. This situation contributes to seasonal price fluctuations resulting in low producer prices during harvest season and high consumer prices in off seasons with the greatest benefits accruing to the intermediaries. There are two cold storage units now approved for construction by AID in the Chapare and the first may be operational in 1992. Similarly, grain storage capacity is limited and silo capacity is needed.

In the Chapare, nearly all local market produce is transported by open truck, without any attempt at primary processing or packing. Size and dispersal of production units in the coca-producing regions complicate efforts to design packinghouses for fresh products. At present packing technology in the Chapare region is a field operation using small, rain-protected packing sheds where fruit is washed and treated with fungicide dips to extend storage life. The availa-

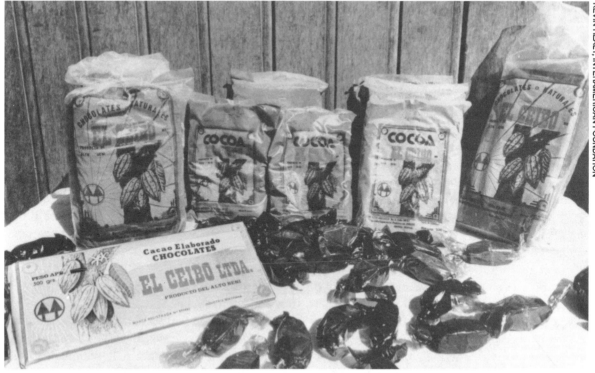

El Ceibo, a federation of 37 cocoa producer organizations in the Alto Beni, Bolivia produces cocoa powder, baker's chocolate, cocoa butter, and chocolate candy for national and international markets. Exports totaled U.S. $600,000 in 1991.

bility of a clean water source at the packing site is paramount to a successful operation. Despite the region's high rainfall, this need can be limiting, often requiring shallow wells adjacent to packing facilities. In addition, lack of rural electricity sources requires manual pumping to fill washing tanks. It is anticipated that electricity will be available in the next 2 years to much of the Chapare, facilitating mechanization of crop processing and handling and is a high priority for improving postharvest handling in the region.

■ Communications

Effective communications systems are critical to producer decisionmaking on crop, market, processing, and transport opportunities. Currently, communication networks in coca-producing areas are inadequate. For example, in the Chapare communications are provided by Institutional radio and two or three public telephones. The system is inefficient and is a further deterrent to private-sector involvement. Establishment of communications systems in remote areas, however, is likely to be subject to the same constraints as road development. While wireless communication technologies can reduce the need for physical structures (e.g., telephone poles, underground cables), they are costly.

Information availability does not pose a key constraint in itself since many information systems exist. Moving the information to producers, however, is a primary need. Development efforts could include mechanisms to develop local information collection and dissemination for producers of legitimate crops through cooperatives or other joint activities. Subscriptions to international information services would be needed to support this activity (27). Producer organizations

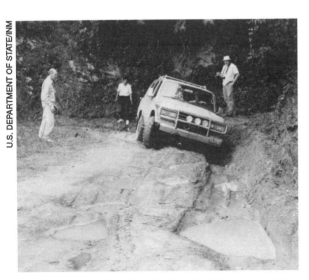

U.S. DEPARTMENT OF STATE/INM

Poorly developed and maintained road systems take a heavy toll on vehicles, particularly in areas with heavy rains. Little incentive exists for private investment in transport due to the unreliability of specialized vehicles and high maintenance costs.

may provide a mechanism to pool producer resources to invest in communications and disseminate information to members.

Improved communications are nececessary to assist in promoting export opportunities and coordinating complex transport interlinking. The remote nature of producing regions and producer inability to purchase or maintain communications systems are areas to be addressed to support alternative crop production. In large part these constraints could be addressed through development efforts in coordination with national governments.

Engineering activities in tropical regions frequently are difficult and some past activities have been linked to significant environmental problems making such development unpopular with the public at large as well as potential donors. Financial resources are the limiting factor in

every phase of infrastructure development, followed closely by construction capability. Funding resources alone likely are insufficient to solve the problem.

Thus, the broad-based infrastructure needs for improving production and marketing of legitimate crops include: 1) road development and maintenance; 2) additional and improved vehicles; 3) processing, handling, and storage facilities; 4) reliable energy sources; and 5) information systems via communications networks. Addressing all of these needs is likely to require significant investment on the parts of national governments and donor organizations. Without such investment, however, efforts to develop alternative crops and livelihoods will continue to be disadvantaged.

AGRICULTURAL TRADE POLICIES[5]

The United States is a key trading partner with many South American countries; U.S. exports comprise nearly 43 percent of the market share in Colombia and 20 percent in Bolivia (19,11). U.S. investment in Latin American and Caribbean agribusiness has grown significantly since 1987. Primary targets have been Mexico, Brazil, and, to a lesser extent, Argentina, Venezuela, and Colombia (36). This trend is expected to continue under new trade initiatives designed to promote opportunities for U.S. producers and exporters in conjunction with increasing trade flexibility for the Andean countries.

The United States enforces a broad range of trade policies, ranging from import quotas and tariffs to complex food safety, sanitary, and phytosanitary requirements to protect domestic industries and human, plant, and animal health. While some protectionist policies have been waived temporarily,[6] meeting food safety and

---

[5] The information for this section was drawn largely from L. Turner, "Primer on U.S. Agricultural and Trade Policies: Opportunities and Constraints to Crop Substitution in the Andean Nations," contractor report for the Office of Technology Assessment, February 1992.

[6] The debate over this came to a head in the late 1980s in a dispute between the U.S. Department of Agriculture and AID/Bolivia over U.S. technical support for Andean soybean producers. Domestic concerns focused on the potential for Bolivian production to adversely affect the U.S. industry. Development groups argued that the Bolivian production was unlikely to even reach 1 percent of the global soybean market.

quality requirements remains a significant challenge for potential importers. Training and technical assistance can help improve compliance with regulations and also help build local expertise to address similar problems in domestic food systems.

■ Trade Policy Initiatives

A number of agreements and initiatives are intended to promote extra- and intra-Andean trade. U.S. administrative initiatives include the Uruguay Round (under the General Agreement on Trade and Tariffs (GATT)), the Andean Trade Preference Act (ATPA), and the recently proposed Enterprise for the Americas Initiative (EAI) (box 5-I). The result of these actions on Andean economies is not yet clear.

Agriculture emerged as the most contentious issue in the Uruguay Round of GATT negotiations. Developing nations abandoned negotiations contending that an agricultural commitment was essential to their continued participation in GATT. Efforts to increase trade of Andean products will need to examine potential trade strategies with respect to GATT rules to avoid challenge and possible retaliatory action from other GATT nations.

Emphasis on trade assistance for the Andean countries has included several commitments: to expedite Generalized System of Preferences (GSP) review under GATT, to provide technical assistance for the agricultural sector, to explore opportunities for expanded textile trade, and to reestablish an International Coffee Agreement (ICA). Although some of these areas have been pursued, restoration of ICA remains elusive although it is considered critical in the Andean region. International trade in coffee largely has been controlled by export quotas established under the ICA. The latest ICA collapsed after contentious debate leading to a sharp reduction in world coffee prices. Coffee exports, nevertheless, are substan-

tial for Colombia, and comprise part of Bolivian, Peruvian, and Ecuadorian income. Colombian coffee exports accounted for 51 percent of the country's 1985 legal export earnings, 7 percent for Ecuador, 5 percent for Peru, and 1 percent for Bolivia (34). Current interest in negotiating an ICA likely will focus on modifying quotas to reflect demand for different varieties of coffees and prohibitions on sales to nonmember nations.

■ Trade Preference Programs

Providing preferential trade arrangements with developing countries is one approach to stimulate their economic growth and has been included in GATT in a variety of forms. This approach is reflected in U.S. trade policy in the GSP, the Caribbean Basin Initiative (CBI), and most recently the Andean Trade Initiative (ATI). The latter two are specialized forms of the GSP and reflect U.S. efforts to provide greater trade advantages to specific beneficiary countries (table 5-3).

The GSP program promotes economic development by opening trade opportunities for lesser developed countries by offering zero- or reduced-duty on certain imports. The Andean nations are beneficiary nations individually, and as part of the Andean Group—an association allowed to be treated as a single country for purposes of GSP eligibility. Products that exceed a certain level of competitiveness may be removed from the U.S. GSP program, although the President may waive these limitations. Similarly, countries may be removed from the GSP program as level of development increases, market penetration increases, or as a sanction protesting other practices of the participating country (e.g., trade practices, worker rights violations).

The GSP program covers raw and processed products; however, value-added products must comply with the rules of origin.[7] If the raw material originates from a non-GSP country, the

---

[7] At least 35 percent of the cost or value of the article must be attributable to direct costs of processing in the beneficiary country.

Box 5-I—Selected Trade Policies Affecting Andean Trade

A number of trade agreements, economic policy reforms, and legislation affect Andean trade. Many have occurred in the past several years and how they will affect national economies is not yet clear. The following briefly summarizes some initiatives likely to play a role in the international trade activities of the Andean region.

Andean Pact

The Pact was a result of a trade framework established in the 1969 Cartagena Agreement. Members include Venezuela, Colombia, Bolivia, Peru, and Ecuador. The goal was to harmonize member trade and investment regimes through preferential tariff structure for member countries, develop a common external tariff, and develop agreements on investment and intellectual property rights. Recent activities under the Pact include:

- Subsidy program elimination for intra-Andean trade and agreement to create a common Andean market by 1996,
- Establishment of free trade between Venezuela, Colombia, and Bolivia in January 1992 with expected additions of Peru and Ecuador in July 1992,
- Tentative agreement on common external tariffs for most goods, although the treatment of the agricultural sector remains unclear,
- Initiation of national treatment of foreign investors, and
- Establishment of minimum standards on patent and trademark protection, allowing individual members to implement stricter laws (19,20).

Andean Trade Initiative

Authorized through the Andean Trade Preference Act of 1991, the Andean Trade Initiative (ATI) establishes preferential trade arrangements for Bolivia, Colombia, Peru, and Ecuador with the United States. ATI provides duty-free access for certain Andean exports for a 10-year period pending country-specific determination by the President. Products excluded from duty-fee status include textiles, footwear, canned tuna, petroleum, rum, and leather goods. As a result of the ATI a number of Andean exports are expected to increase as well as Andean demand for U.S. goods and services to support economic expansion (6). Trade has yet to be visibly affected by the ATI, making projections difficult.

Enterprise for the Americas

This initiative offers market access, financial and technical resources, and debt reduction to countries that liberalize trade and investment regimes, maintain sound economic policies that promote investment and competition, and responsibly manage international debt obligations. The intent is to stimulate economic growth in the entire Western Hemisphere through increased trade and investment and reduction of official debt. Key components include:

- *Trade*—hemispheric free trade, an incremental approach beginning with smaller free-trade associations such as the North American Free Trade Agreement (among the U.S., Canada, and Mexico) and the Andean Pact;
- *Investment*—stimulate investment reform and privatization through the Inter-American Development Bank programs, Investment Sector Loan Program (ISLP), and Multilateral Investment Fund (MIF); and
- *Debt*—reducing debt obligation to the United States through a variety of mechanisms including congressional reduction of food aid debt and debt-for-nature swaps (26).

Some benefits associated with this initiative have been visible in Bolivia:

- Development of a bilateral framework agreement establishing the U.S.-Bolivia Trade and Investment Council,
- Elimination of $371 million in debt to the United States, and
- Grant of an Investment Sector Loan in 1991 (11).

SOURCE: Office of Technology Assessment, 1993.

Table 5-3—Exports Expected to Increase Under the Andean Trade Initiative

Country	Product
Bolivia	Cereals (including rice), cut flowers, wood products, and spices.
Colombia	Cut flowers (particularly roses and chrysanthemums), fresh tuna and skipjack, glazed ceramic products, raspberries, grapes, tropical fruits, and melons.
Peru	Rope, zinc, copper wire, lead, precious metals, asparagus, seafood (including yellowtail, mackerel, and sardines), tomatoes, and dried potatoes.
Ecuador	Cut flowers, fresh tuna and skipjack, pineapple and grape juice, iron and steel wire, limes, tropical fruits, and melons.

SOURCE: E. Turner, "Primer on U.S. Agricultural Trade Policies: Opportunities and Constraints to Crop Substitution in the Andean Nations," contractor report prepared for the Office of Technology Assessment, February 1992.

final product must be "substantially transformed" in the beneficiary country. Changes in product and country coverage are made through general and annual reviews, and any interested party may petition for such a change.

■ Tariff and Quota Policies

A variety of restrictions control imports to levels that will not adversely affect U.S. producers. Largely, these controls take the form of tariffs and quotas on specific commodities. Tariffs are the preferred means for restricting imports under GATT. Although member countries have been encouraged to maintain tariffs at existing levels, or not to increase them beyond a specified level, such a proposal has not been agreed upon.

Tariffs imposed by the United States and other major importing nations tend to escalate as products move through the processing chain. This approach is suggested to have inhibited growth of processing industries in some developing countries (5). Review and possible revision of tariff schedules for processed Andean products could complement crop substitution efforts and contribute to growth of the value-added industries.

Import restrictions may be placed on certain products that may undermine any USDA domestic commodity program (1).[8] These section 22 fees and quotas are designed to keep product prices above the government price support level and to protect U.S. producers by stabilizing domestic prices, particularly during times when world prices are low. Such import restrictions apply to all nations, irrespective of other trading arrangements with the United States (e.g., CBI, ATI).

The Sugar Tariff Rate Quota system is designed to protect the domestic price-support program for sugarcane and sugar beets. Sugar imports are restricted by a country-by-country tariff rate quota system in effect since late 1990.[9] Imports up to the quota amount are subject to a small duty and levels above that are dutiable at a significantly higher rate. This system helps support a U.S. market stabilization price much higher than the world price (21.5 cents vs. 9.2 cents) (17). Bolivia recently requested an expansion of its sugar quota from 16,000 to 100,000 metric tons to help provide alternatives for some farm laborers involved in coca production (10). The request was denied, however, and critics suggested the benefits would accrue to plantation owners and processors rather than the target population (24).

Tariffs are also imposed on sugar-derived products such as alcohol fuels. A schedule of

---

[8] An investigation on the effect of imports on U.S. commodity programs is conducted by the U.S. International Trade Commission; however, ITC's report is merely advisory and the President may set fees or quotas irrespective of its content.

[9] Revised based on a GATT ruling that the 1981 absolute quota system was not in conformity with GATT rules. Yet, the effect of the new program, in terms of restricting sugar imports, was identical to the old quota program.

tariffs was developed to curb imports of alcohol fuels in 1980 and protect U.S. corn and ethanol producers, although ethanol auto fuels remain a small part of the overall gasoline pool (i.e., less than 1 percent). Tariffs for ethanol imports currently run $0.54 cents per gallon (21). Proponents of ethanol fuel suggest the market will expand in response to environmental concern over fossil fuel use and carbon dioxide reduction policies. While ethanol largely is produced from sugarcane and corn, many plants may be used as feedstocks. Technology exists to use a variety of grasses in an ammonium freeze explosion process to produce ethanol. Tariff reductions for ethanol could provide incentive for industry development in the Andean nations. In addition to U.S. imports, several South American countries are large users of ethanol auto fuels (e.g., Argentina, Brazil).

Countervailing duty and anti-dumping laws seek to preclude unfair competitive advantage importing countries might have over U.S. producers as a result of foreign subsidies or by marketing products at less than their fair market value. Imports suspected of violating these conditions are investigated by the U.S. Department of Commerce and International Trade Commission.[10] Additional duties may be imposed on products determined to violate these laws. Subsidies and other assistance promoting agricultural development in the Andean nations potentially could be challenged under U.S. countervailing and anti-dumping laws (15).

▌ Food Safety and Quality Requirements

Imports to the United States are subject to quality and grade standards and requirements deemed necessary to protect human, animal, and plant health. The USDA's Animal and Plant Health Inspection Service (APHIS) and Agricultural Marketing Service (AMS) are responsible for phytosanitary and produce quality programs, respectively. The U.S. Department of Health and Human Services' Food and Drug Administration (FDA), the USDA Food Safety Inspection Service (FSIS), and the U.S. Environmental Protection Agency (EPA) are responsible for regulating health and safety programs. Phytosanitary regulations can pose unique challenges for developing countries. They can restrict trade if applied in an arbitrary manner or if compliance assistance is difficult to obtain. Provision of technical assistance and training could offer benefits for industry development domestically and internationally.

PHYTOSANITARY REQUIREMENTS

Plant, live animal, and meat product imports are subject to APHIS inspection and quarantine requirements. Inspections may be conducted at port-of-entry or in producing countries. APHIS personnel are authorized to enter cooperative programs with counterparts in foreign countries to control or eradicate pest problems. Such programs may minimize potential infestations in the United States as well as provide valuable training for importing countries that can contribute to improvements in national food systems (2, 3). Currently, APHIS personnel are stationed in Peru and Colombia to assist in complying with U.S. phytosanitary requirments; this may expand as a result of Andean Trade Preference Act.

SANITARY AND FOOD SAFETY REGULATIONS

Imported goods (except meat and poultry products) are subject to FDA inspection for compliance with health, safety, packaging, and labeling requirements. Food products that are unsafe, produced under unsanitary conditions, or that contain illegal additives or pesticide residues are prohibited from entry. Imports are subject to inspection and testing at time of entry, although it is estimated that no more than 1 percent of FDA-regulated food imports are actually tested.

---

10 U.S. Department of Commerce investigations examine whether or not subsidies are being supplied directly or indirectly, or if the product is being sold in the United States at less than fair value. The International Trade Commission investigations focus on the potential injury to U.S. producers.

Inspection programs have been criticized for failing to provide adequate protection.

All domestic and importing commercial processors of heat-processed, low-acid canned foods and acidified foods and shellfish are required to register and file processing information with FDA. Requirements for sanitary food production facilities are explained in the FDA's Current Good Manufacturing Practice Regulations (available only in English). While the FDA does not have authority to conduct foreign plant inspections, personnel may travel to help solve public health threats at the request of foreign governments.

Food importers must have access to current U.S. food and safety labeling regulations to export effectively. Further, facilities to monitor compliance with import regulations could assist in improving the domestic food system and international marketing of food products. If food processing is to take a greater role in providing alternative livelihoods in the Andean countries, assistance in the form of compliance training is a key need.

MEAT AND POULTRY INSPECTION

FSIS is responsible for assuring the safety, quality, and accurate labeling of meat and poultry products. Importing countries inspection systems must be equivalent to the U.S. system and be evaluated and approved by FSIS. Currently, no South American countries are authorized to ship meat and poultry products to the United States (33). Development of meat or poultry product industries for export to the United States will require development of Andean inspection facilities, technical assistance, and training.

MARKETING ORDER REGULATIONS

AMS is responsible for regulating produce quality standards. Inspections are conducted only at point-of-entry and costs for this service are charged to importers. There are 15 marketing orders that regulate minimum grade, size, and quality requirements for imports. Although marketing orders apply only to quality of imports, meeting these requirements may also pose challenges for poorly developed export systems. Available infrastructure, handling, and shipping technologies in the Andean nations currently are inadequate to handle increased export opportunities.

Trade incentives form a principal thrust of the U.S. strategy for promoting agricultural production in the Andean countries. Recent trade initiatives indicate a U.S. commitment to improving the ability of these countries to compete in the international marketplace. Yet, the value of these trade concessions may be overshadowed by future agreements with other countries (e.g., North American Free Trade Agreement). Nevertheless, complementary efforts are needed to assist the Andean countries to comply with the numerous phytosanitary, sanitary, safety, and quality requirements for imports.

It may be useful to evaluate trade incentives with respect to their contributions to the overall Andean economy. This could include promoting development of related economic sectors rather than the narrow agricultural focus of current substitution efforts. It may also be useful to evaluate the impact of trade incentives in terms of the global trade environment, recognizing that development of trade agreements with other nations could adversely affect U.S. demand for certain Andean products.

The need for restrictions on agricultural assistance activities should be re-evaluated in relation to the actual "threat" to U.S. agricultural production. Previous reports suggest the potential effect of certain increased Andean agricultural imports on U.S. producers was negligible. Further, in light of the emphasis on trade liberalization and reducing subsidies and barriers to trade, these may become key issues in future GATT negotiations.

STRATEGIES TO SUPPORT RENEWABLE RESOURCE-BASED ALTERNATIVES TO COCA

One way of summing up is to insist that advising "shock treatment" for countries with weak or missing market institutions or limited technical capacity—that they go "cold turkey on policy reform—must be rejected as little more than self-indulgent intellectual sloth. It reflects a lack of willingness to invest the intellectual energy necessary to understanding the economies and the societies for which reform prescriptions are being written (25).

Strategies to enhance coca substitution efforts must address a wide variety of constraints from production to marketing. Producers are unlikely to cease coca production in favor of alternative crops or activities if they cannot be assured that a market exists and that the mechanisms are in place for production, harvest, processing, and transport. A shift from a production- to market-driven approach is evident currently in Cochabamba Regional Development Project. Nevertheless, the support structure necessary to sustain alternative livelihoods is lacking or inadequate.

Recent U.S. policies have been designed to increase comparative advantage for certain Andean products (e.g., ATI) in U.S. markets. Revision of credit programs could improve the opportunities for smallholders to obtain financing for entering legitimate production systems. Credit revisions could mimic current U.S. subsidy programs, providing loans to farmers at lower rates than presently exist in the Andean countries. Such an effort with planned obsolescence as a goal, could be relatively short-term, provide appropriate grace periods prior to repayment (i.e., allow for real production to occur), and perhaps augment or replace eradication payments as a method of inducing change. Further, supporting national governments in encouraging greater domestic food production could increase the viability of Andean agriculture. Such an effort could incorpo-rate financial incentives and loan programs, and improved export and import policies.

Strategies to improve support for alternatives to coca in the Andean region will likely require attention to:

- National research and extension systems,
- Opportunities for value-added processing and increased product competiveness,
- Infrastructure to exploit and export the product, and
- Increased trade opportunities (31)

▌Strategy: Support National Research and Extension Systems

Enhancing agricultural profitability in the Andean nations will require continuing and significant investment in research and extension to develop alternatives and demonstrate techniques and technologies to potential adopters. However, national funding for research and extension activities may be difficult to secure and U.S. international academic research and extension activities are declining.

While research and extension activities were large components of early AID crop substitution efforts in Bolivia, the level of effort has dropped. Continued devotion of funding and effort to long-term research and extension activities is hampered by pressure to produce immediate results. Research on developing alternatives and demonstration and extension of this information to potential adopters are long-term propositions—conservatively running 10 to 15 years while standard project lengths are only 5 years (31).

To overcome this situation, emphasis could be placed on local and national research centers to promote institution building and skill development, thereby improving the potential for activities to continue after direct assistance is withdrawn. Agronomic management research could be oriented to on-farm, farmer participation production trials, involving the local farm population in direct participatory research. Extension activities could emphasize on-farm demonstration and farming systems to maximize the diffusion of new technologies and practices to rural adopting populations. On-farm trials should be maintained for sufficient time to demonstrate effectiveness and promote technology/practice diffusion (7,27,31).

■ Strategy: Improve Opportunities for Value-Added Processing

Increased agricultural productivity is likely to do little for producers' economic well-being if producers cannot effectively and efficiently apply improved postharvest technologies. Such applications will be necessary for alternative crops to become significant in terms of total agricultural exports. Current formal exports of some alternative crops (e.g., turmeric, ginger) are at no more than trial levels. Success will be dependent on the establishment of cost-effective, postharvest processing, as well as the enhancement of producer efficiency through reduced production costs and increased yields (27,31).

For the Andean countries to increase their agricultural export earnings and reduce agricultural imports, major public and private-sector investment will be necessary. AID is a major contributor to Andean country development of legitimate economies. The channeling of that contribution is a joint effort between the offices of the recipient government and the AID coordinating office in the benefiting country. The effectiveness of the AID investment can be enhanced in a number of ways:

Implement Training Programs—Emphasis could be placed on specific technical training at the production technique and processing level, involving the import of short-term expert assistance with a group training responsibility. Programs with specific training objectives, directed to practical-level personnel who can be integrated into production or processing units such as they are expected to manage in their home country, could recieve priority. The need for language training as part of a training proposal should be reviewed and adjusted to promote participation in educational exchanges. Professional training cannot be neglected, but this too must be monitored carefully to ensure trained people remain in positions justifying their preparation and benefiting the AID program (27).

Prioritize AID Investment—Where investigation results have demonstrated agronomic potential of a crop, the processing and marketing infrastructure should be developed along with the expansion of production, so that market outlets for production will be in place when production goals are realized (27).

Promote Producer Organizations—The development of strong producer organizations that can aggregate products for sale to processors, intermediaries, or consumers could overcome the problem small individual producers have in negotiating just prices for their product (27). A grassroots development strategy may be the most appropriate mechanism for assisting rural communities in processing, storage, marketing, and transport of a diversity of agricultural commodities. Grassroots organizations typically have strong support from local populations and understand local cultures, aspirations, and priorities. Abundant organizational skills exist within Bolivian grassroots organizations, *sindicatos*. These groups have a long tradition of solving development problems and promoting rural reform in the Chapare and elsewhere in Bolivia. Bolivian crop substitution programs might work cooperatively with *sindicatos* to promote peaceful crop substitution and alternative development efforts (31). (See chapter 2.)

Promote Private Investment in Processing—Loans to the private sector at realistic interest rates could promote entrepreneurial activity, and ultimately replace the need for AID and other contributing institutions to maintain the present high level of investment in infrastructure and agroindustry. Careful investment evaluations should be conducted, and full market histories and the long-term strategy should be a part of the Project Evaluation (27).

▌ Strategy: Promote Infrastructure Development

Infrastructure is inadequate to support alternative development (e.g., paved roads, bulking and storage facilities, agroprocessing plants). The high cost associated with infrastructure development in remote areas is prohibitive in terms of normal financial assistance. Economic studies must explore fully the infrastructure and integrated development of alternatives, and environmental impacts should be identified and mechanisms to mitigate them included in project design and planning (27).

Infrastructure development is approached slowly, however, because of the potential benefits that might accrue to coca transporters (e.g., road developments are seen as potential landing strips for narcotics traffickers). Although infrastructure development might initially contribute to the coca economy, alternative development and production cannot occur without adequate transportation and marketing routes. Interdiction, monitoring, and enforcement of illegal activities also could be simplified with improved transportation networks (8).

Investment in transportation infrastructure, accompanied by expanded credit programs in production systems can help coca-dominated economies move to more profitable, exportable alternatives (8,27,31). Long-term involvement with this development, and greater emphasis on expanding legal production rather than eliminating coca, could ultimately achieve coca reduction goals. Resources must be channeled in an ordered, well-planned basis with the knowledge that the political requirements for short-term, demonstrable achievements will precede the overall success of the program (27).

▌ Strategy: Increase Trade Opportunities for Andean Products

An increased share in the international market can contribute to improving the economies of the Andean countries. Current crop substitution ap-

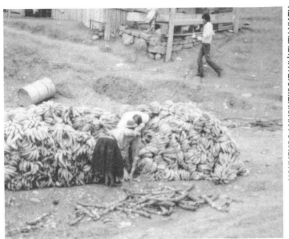

KEVIN HEALY, INTERAMERICAN FOUNDATION

Locally produced bananas are being prepared for transport. However, these producers are at a disadvantage compared with other highly sophisticated production and marketing systems.

proaches have focused on this approach, largely through promoting production of high-value crops, to generate foreign exchange for national governments. However, meeting complex food safety, sanitary, and phytosanitary requirements is often difficult for developing nations. There are some avenues for assistance in developing capacity for meeting these standards. Additionally, developing national abilities to ensure quality and safety standards for produce could help in meeting U.S. import requirements as well as those of other countries. Compliance with these standards could contribute to increased competitiveness of Andean products in international markets and could yield additional benefits by increasing the range of trading partners, encouraging foreign investment, and improving national food systems (27,30,31).

Improve Ability to Meet Quality and Safety Standards for International Markets—Increased exchange among U.S. agencies and potential Andean exporters could assist in identifying key needs to facilitate trade. Such exchange would allow greater insight into the difficulties faced by foreign producers/exporters and familiarize them with U.S. requirements for importing products.

Again, technical assistance will be a critical component (27,30).

Reduce Import Tariffs for Andean Products to Complement Crop Substitution Programs— Although the ATI and certain waivers have reduced import barriers for some Andean products, this effort could be expanded to provide reduced tariffs for all products linked to alternative development projects. While this may run counter to some U.S. commodity support regulations, import levels would likely be low, creating little competition with U.S. producers. Further, the program could contain a clearly identified time frame after which review and possible revision could be undertaken (30,31).

Provide Incentives for Value-Added Processing— Typically, tariffs increase as products move through the processing chain, i.e., raw materials generally are subject to lower tariffs while processed items have higher tariffs. This aspect of U.S. trade policy has been suggested to reduce incentive for development of value-added industry in exporting nations. U.S. tariff policies on value-added products could be reviewed and modified if they are determined to affect development of processing industries in the Andean region adversely (27,30).

CHAPTER 5 REFERENCES

1. 7 U.S.C. 624, In: Turner, 1992.
2. 7 U.S.C. 147(b), In: Turner, 1992.
3. 21 U.S.C. 114(b), In: Turner, 1992.
4. Benjamin, M., and Freedman, A., *Bridging the Global Gap: A Handbook to Linking Citizens of the First and Third Worlds* (Washington, DC: Seven Locks Press, 1989) pp.117-139.
5. Buckley, K., "The World Market in Fresh Fruit and Vegetables, Wine, and Tropical Beverages— Government Intervention and Multilateral Policy Reform," September 1990, In: Turner, 1992.
6. *Business America*, Caribbean Basin and Andean Trade Initiatives, March 23, 1992, pp. 6-7.
7. Chavez, A., "Andean Agricultural Research and Extension Systems and Technology Transfer Activities: Potential Mechanisms to Enhance Crop Substitution Efforts in Bolivia, Colombia, and Peru," contractor report prepared for the Office of Technology Assessment, December 1991.
8. DeVincenti, J., "Infrastructure Needs to Support Agricultural Alternatives to Coca in Bolivia," contractor report prepared for the Office of Technology Assessment, December 1991.
9. Dickinson, R., "Alternative Trade Organizations, Peasant Farmers and Coca." contractor report prepared for the Office of Technology Assessment, January 1992.
10. Embassy of Bolivia, "Proposal for Bolivian Sugar Quota Increase," paper submitted by the Embassy of Bolivia to U.S.Trade Representative, March 16, 1990, In: Turner, 1992.
11. Hatfield, L.Z., "Bolivia's New Legislation Attracts Foreign Investment," *Business America*, March 23, 1992, pp. 19-20.
12. Healy, K., "From Field to Factory: Vertical Integration in Bolivia," *Grassroots Development* 11(2):2-11, 1987.
13. ICA, Instituto Colombiano Agropecuario, "25 Años de Tecnología Agropecuaria al Servicio de Colombia," Bogota, Colombia, 1987, In: Chavez, 1991.
14. ICA, Instituto Colombiano Agropecuario, "La Tecnología al Servicio del Cambio, Memorias de Gerencia 1986-1990," Gabriel Montes Llamas, Gerente General, Bogota, Colombia, 1990, In: Chavez, 1991.
15. Ingersoll, D., Chief, Agriculture Division, U.S. International Trade Commission, personal communication, October 1991, In: Turner, 1992.
16. ISNAR, "El Modelo de Investigación, Extensión, y Educación en el Perú, Estudio de un Case," ISNAR R30s, The Hague, 1987, In: Chavez, 1991.
17. Lord, R., and Barry, R., "The World Sugar Market—Government Intervention and Multilateral Policy Reform," Economic Research Service, September 1990, In: Turner, 1992.
18. MACA, Ministerio de Asuntos Campesinos y Agropecurarios, "Republica de Bolivia, Política Agropecuaria 1991-1993," Mayo, La Paz, Bolivia, 1991, In: Chavez, 1991.
19. MacNamara, L. "Andean Regions Makes Integration Effort," *Business America*, March 23, 1992, p. 5

20. MacNamara, L., "Colombia, Vanguard of Economic Reform," *Business America*, March 23, 1992, p. 17-18.
21. Migdon, R.S., "Alcohol Fuels," Congressional Research Service, Library of Congress, Issue Brief, January 8, 1991, In: Turner, 1992.
22. Ministerio de Industria y Turismo and UN Industrial Development Organization PNUD/UNIDO, *Investment Promotion Programme*, La Paz, Bolivia, 1990, In: De Vincenti, 1991.
23. Morowetz, D., "Bolivia's Exports and Medium-Term Economic Strategy: Prospects, Problems, and Policy Options—Beyond Tin and Natural Gas, What?" working paper, U.S. AID, Bureau on Latin America and the Caribbean, Regional Office, November 6, 1986.
24. Paarlberg, R., Professor, Wellesley College, personal communication, August 20, 1991, In: Turner, 1992.
25. Ruttan, V.W., "Solving the Foreign Aid Vision Thing," *Challenge*, May-June 1991, pp. 43-46.
26. Schaeffer, W., "Enterprise for the Americas Initiative Offers New Trade, Investment Opportunities," *Business America*, March 23, 1992, pp. 2-4.
27. Stevenson, B.McD., "Post-Harvest Technologies to Improve Agricultural Profitability," contractor report prepared for the Office of Technology Assessment, 1992.
28. Stevenson, B.McD., "Final Report Consultancy to the PDAR; Marketing and Post-Harvest Requirements," December 1990, In: Stevenson, 1992.
29. Stewart, J., Product Development and Producer Relations, Pueblo to People, Houston, TX, May 1992, In: Dickinson, 1992.
30. Turner, E.H., "Primer on U.S. Agricultural Trade Policies: Opportunities and Constraints to Crop Substitution in the Andean Nations," contractor report prepared for the Office of Technology Assessment, February 1992.
31. U.S. Congress, Office of Technology Assessment, Crop Substitution Workshop, Sept. 30-Oct. 1, 1991, Washington, DC.
32. U.S. Congress, Office of Technology Assessment, *Technologies to Sustain Tropical Forest Resources*, OTA-F-214 (Washington, DC: U.S. Government Printing Office, March 1984).
33. U.S. Department of Agriculture, FSIS, "Meat and Poultry Inspection: Report to the U.S. Congress," March 1, 1991, In: Turner, 1992.
34. Villachica, H., "Crop Diversification in Bolivia, Colombia, and Peru: Potential to Enhance Agricultural Production," contractor report prepared for the Office of Technology Assessment, April 1992.
35. Vogt, D., "International Coffee Agreement: A Status Report," U.S. Congress, Library of Congress, Congressional Research Service, March 22, 1990, In: Turner, 1991.
36. Wilde, Jr. T.E., "U.S. Agribusiness Trade and Investment Rise in Latin America and the Caribbean," *Business America*, March 23, 1992, p. 4.
37. World Bank, Bolivia, "Agricultural Technology Development, Research Program Development," Working Paper, Washington, DC, 1990, In: Chavez, 1991.
38. World Bank, *Colombia: Second Rural Roads Project*, Washington, DC, 1990, In: DeVincenti, 1991.

Coca
Biological
Control
Issues | 6

Biocontrol is something akin to gambling—
it works, sometimes (13).

E radication[1] has been a component of U.S. supply reduction efforts for illegal narcotic crops (e.g., opium poppies, marijuana, and coca) for nearly two decades. Some experts believe that eradication must precede alternative development in the Andean nations. Others view coca eradication as futile and a threat to the culture and traditions of native Andean populations. Although key requirements, host country consent and cooperation are unlikely to be easily obtained (27,28).

INTRODUCTION

The level of coca reduction necessary to have a clear and measurable impact on cocaine availability is an unknown. Further, new processing technologies have changed the relationship between coca leaf production levels and cocaine availability. For example, an intermediate product of cocaine processing, "agua rica," appears to have excellent storage properties allowing processors to stockpile supplies. Thus, even with a reduction in cultivated area, a reduction in cocaine availability may not occur for years, if at all. Further, current cocaine extraction techniques are only about 50-percent efficient; improved extraction could yield the same amount of cocaine from a much reduced leaf production base (28).

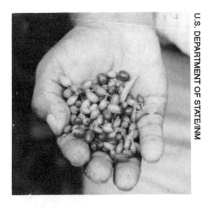

U.S. DEPARTMENT OF STATE/INM

---

[1] For the purposes of this discussion, *eradication* will refer to complete erasure of all traces of coca within a defined area. The area could be defined as small as a single plot or as large as a country.

331–054 – 93 – 8

Eradication efforts have included voluntary and involuntary removal of the target crop. Although coca eradication programs have relied solely on manual techniques, possible application of chemical methods have attracted attention. Renewed interest in application of biological control methodology to coca reduction also is evident. The U.S. Department of Agriculture has responsibility for research and development of coca control methods, including research on chemical control methods and classified research on biological control.

MANUAL COCA CONTROL

Manual eradication of coca can be dangerous and inefficient. The Special Project for Control and Eradication of Coca in the Alto Huallaga, *Projecto de Control y Reducción de los Cultivos de Coca en el Alto Huallaga* (CORAH), in the mid-1980s attempted manual coca eradication in Peru. CORAH workers destroyed 5,000 hectares of coca in 1985 with ''weed whackers'' and machetes (15). Although the manual eradication program had some success, the problems were extensive. Between 1986 and 1988, 34 CORAH workers were killed by insurgent groups (31). CORAH's association with the Mobil Patrol Unit of Peru's Civil Guard, *Unidad Móvil de Patrullaje de la Guardia Civil del Peru* (UMOPAR), an organization accused of using repressive and abusive tactics on local growers, led to great public resistance to eradication. Manual methods also can be ineffective. For example, some fields eradicated manually by coppicing coca shrubs showed invigorated growth later (10).

CHEMICAL COCA CONTROL

Chemical coca eradication thus became of greater interest as it was expected to reduce risk, achieve more uniform results, and increase the potential treatment area. Nonetheless, proposals met with some resistance. Largely driven by political, social, and economic realities in coca-producing countries (see chapter 2), resistance

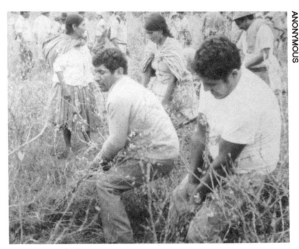

ANONYMOUS

Uprooting coca shrubs is one method of manual eradication, but it can be a difficult and slow process. Here, workers are uprooting coca in an eradication program in Bolivia.

has been bolstered by public concern over the release of chemicals in the environment. Herbicide formulation, chemical properties, and application methods most affect their environmental fate and thus the potential for creating environmental or human health hazards.

▮ Formulation

Herbicides are formulated as liquids (aqueous, oil, emulsifiable concentrates), solids (dust, wettable powders, granules, encapsulated products), and gases (fumigants). The type of formulation depends on the chemical nature of the pesticide, target pest, and other pesticidal properties (29). Granular and pelletized herbicide formulations are preferred because the drift and volatilization concerns are reduced relative to sprays. However, the density of granular products can affect performance and deposition. Because moisture is needed to release the active ingredient, release rates can be highly variable depending on precipitation patterns. Controlled-release formulations (e.g., starch-encapsulated herbicides, ethylene vinyl acetate copolymers incorporated with active ingredients) could contribute to regulated release (29), particularly under high moisture conditions

Table 6-1—Overview of Some Coca Control Herbicides

• Hexazinone	Effective brush control through basal or injection application. Low toxicity, particularly to fish and birds, but potential for groundwater contamination. This herbicide is a persistent compound that will render the soil inhospitable to recropping for approximately one year.
• Imazapyr	Label restricts aerial application to helicopter use and may only be applied to noncrops. Low toxicity to fish and birds. Herbicide is slow-acting and may take up to several months to destroy the target completely.
• Picloram	Restricted use herbicide that can be used on rangeland, pastures, grains, and noncrop areas to control broadleaf and woody plants. Low acute toxicity although it is water soluble and persistant. It can move offsite in surface water and has been detected in surface and groundwater.
• Tebuthiuron	Registered in the United States for control of brush and woody plants in noncrop areas and, at reduced rates, in pastures and rangeland. Has low acute toxicity based on available data. Virtually non-toxic to fish and birds although concern exists about the potential for groundwater contamination. Product labeling bears numerous restrictions about risk to desirable vegetation as well as for livestock grazing and hay production.
• Triclopyr	Registered in the United States for noncrop, pasture, and rangeland uses. Label restricts aerial application to helicopters. Low to moderate acute toxicity and toxic to fish. For 1 year after application lactating animals cannot be grazed on affected soil, and grass may not be harvested.

SOURCE: T. Adamczyk, "Chemical Eradication of Coca," contractor paper prepared for the Office of Technology Assessment, 1991.

common in many coca-producing areas. Several herbicides have been identified as prospective eradication agents for coca. Public information about the toxicity and environmental fate of these herbicides has been derived mainly from tests conducted in the United States, although the U.S. Department of State conducted field tests in Peru in the late 1980s (1).

■ Application

Technologically, herbicide application is challenging. Irrespective of formulation, ground-based and aerial methods are the basic mechanisms for delivering an herbicide to its intended target. Ground-based application offers precision; however, the inaccessibility of most coca plots, steep terrain, and bulky, heavy equipment can make this type of application inefficient. Security for applicators further constrains potential for ground-based application.

Aerial application of herbicides may use rotary- or fixed-wing aircraft. Helicopters can treat small areas surrounded by obstructions, like many coca plots, and also lower special equipment to avoid major off-site dispersal problems for liquid formulations (1). Several herbicides screened for coca eradication (e.g., Imazapyr and Triclopyr) have restrictive labeling limiting aerial application to helicopters (table 6-1).

Disadvantages of using helicopters include the complexity and expense of maintenance, low fuel/distance efficiency, and susceptibility to hostile ground fire. Thus, helicopter application is unlikely to fulfill the needs of a broad-range chemical eradication effort (1). Fixed-wing aircraft are cheaper to maintain than helicopters, can cover large application areas, and have good fuel-to-distance efficiency. The faster application speed of a fixed-wing aircraft also may reduce the security risks associated with involuntary eradication programs. However, for accurate application, the optimum altitude is 5 to 20 feet above the target. Higher altitudes result in a wider dispersal swath and increased likelihood of herbicide loss due to wind drift, propeller and wing-tip vortices, and volatilization. Low-altitude application, however, requires clear, unobstructed approaches with ample space to allow a safe climb at the end of the run (1), conditions largely lacking in many coca production zones.

Liquid herbicide application also depends on mixing and loading sites within a reasonable distance of the treatment area. Sites require a water source, containment equipment, equipment for cleaning and decontaminating aircraft, mixing and pumping gear, and protective clothing for pilots and ground support personnel. While security concerns would be significant for such operations near coca production zones, long ferrying times between loading sites and target zones reduce application efficiency.

■ Herbicide Testing

Testing is a critical step in herbicide evaluation. Thorough testing investigates herbicide efficacy, environmental fate (e.g., mobility and persistence), effects on non-target species, and potential for adverse human health effects. Although a number of candidate herbicides have been tested, the most extensive testing has been performed on tebuthiuron (table 6-2). In addition to tests in the United States, field tests of tebuthiuron were conducted in Peru in 1987.

Executive Order 12114 requires an analysis of potential environmental impacts for certain extraterritorial activities that:

- May significantly affect the environment of the global commons outside the jurisdiction of any nation,
- May significantly affect the environment of an innocent bystander nation, or
- Provide a foreign nation with a product which is prohibited or strictly regulated by Federal law in the United States (e.g., herbicides).

Only actions falling in the first category require the preparation of an Environmental Impact Statement (EIS) under the National Environment Policy Act (NEPA). Second category actions require preparation of bilateral or multilateral studies or a Concise Environmental Review (CER). Final category actions, which would include coca eradication, require preparation of a CER. However, Executive Order 12114 also contains exemptions that might be applicable to a coca eradication effort. Exempted, for example, are actions determined not to have a significant environmental effect, actions taken by the President of the United States, and actions taken at the direction of the President or Cabinet in matters of national interest. Procedures may also be modified to account for unique foreign policy needs, confidentiality, and national security.

Although similar to an EIS, a CER is less rigorous and provides little guidance as to the content of the documents or the procedures by which those documents should be drafted. For example, Order 12114 states without elaboration that a CER may be composed of environmental assessments, summary environmental analyses, or other appropriate documents (9). The Department of State guidelines for implementing Order 12114 require the responsible officer of a proposed program to determine whether the action is likely to have a significant extraterritorial environmental impact. If so, the officer may prepare either an EIS, CER, or cooperative study to evaluate the effects subject to the requirements of Order 12114. Of these choices, only the EIS has specific requirements for document contents and public and Federal agency involvement (33).

Prior to testing tebuthiuron in Peru, the Department of State conducted a CER. However, the document was criticized for several reasons:

- Lack of Andean public and expert involvement in the review process,
- Reliance on existing data on the effects of tebuthiuron in temperate rather than tropical environments,
- Lack of discussion of the need for or alternatives to the proposed action, and
- Lack of review of measures for mitigating the effects of the herbicide.

The latter omission is especially important because of the assumption that applicators would use proper safety equipment and protective clothing, an assumption frequently not borne out in the developing world (6).

The Peruvian Government's agreement to the testing of tebuthiuron in April 1988 provoked

Table 6-2—Coca Herbicide Screening Summary

Chemical	Application rate (lb active ingredient/acre)	Success against target[a]	
		E. Coca	E. Novogranatense
Tebuthiuron[b]	2,4,6	S	S
Tebuthiuron[c]	1,2,4,8,16	S	S
Hexazinone[b]	2,4,6	S	S
Hexazinone[c]	1,3,6	S	S
Triclopyr[b]	3,6,9	M	M
Triclopyr[c]	4.5,9,13.5	S (13.5)	S (13.5)
Cacodylic Acid[c]	12	—	U
Cacodylic Acid[c] + Krenite	6	U	U
2,4-D[c]	1,2,4,8	M	M
Glyphosate[c]	4,8,16	M	S
Thidiazuron[c]	2	S	M
Picloram[c]	2,4,8	S	S
Ethyl metribuzin[c]	2,4,8	S	U
Imazapyr[c]	4	S	S

[a] Control Experiments were conducted in the field and greenhouse. Control codes are: U=Unsuccessful; S=Successful; M=Marginal, in need of further study.
[b] Testing in Kauai, Hawaii
[c] Testing in Frederick, Maryland

SOURCE: U.S. Department of Agriculture, Agricultural Research Service, Beltsville Agricultural Research Center, 1992.

public outcry from those concerned over such a large-scale use of an herbicide and the lack of data on its use in tropical areas. In response, the CER was redrafted and the State Department consulted with the U.S. Environmental Protection Agency, the U.S. Department of Agriculture, and outside experts. However, environmental advocates and residents of the Alto Huallaga still were not incorporated into the process (6,31). Testing resumed in January 1989, but was quickly halted when the Peruvian Government withdrew its support for the project.

Although the new CER described plant recolonization and herbicide residue in the soil it did not include specific data on colonizing plant species and their value (e.g., economic, environmental). Also neglected was examination of the potential impacts on associated water resources even though tebuthiuron is known to leach through the soil profile (table 6-1) (34). The adequacy of the new CER became academic when the producer of tebuthiuron refused to sell any more of the product to the Department of State.

Analysts suggest a process more open to public participation might have resulted in better execution of the proposed program. Early involvement of interested parties would have made public the deep opposition of many Peruvians to herbicide use and the environmental concerns associated with large-scale herbicide use in tropical areas, and, thus, allowed the State Department to develop strategies to address these concerns and defuse opposition (6).

Rigorous analysis of the potential environmental and health impacts of the application of tebuthiuron and other herbicides has yet to be completed. Some proponents of herbicide-based coca eradication suggest the candidate herbicides pose no greater environmental risk than coca cultivation and processing in the long term. Critics maintain use of an herbicide designed to control brush and woody plants in the Andean region could generate numerous unanticipated adverse effects. However, such arguments remain anecdotal at this juncture, with little hard data to support either side.

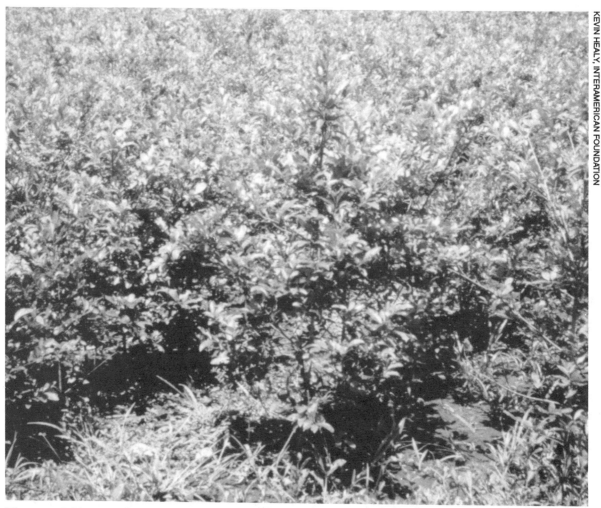

KEVIN HEALY, INTERAMERICAN FOUNDATION

The potential impact of coca control activities on nontarget species is a key concern, particularly since coca commonly is planted with or near other economic plants. Here is a coca plot with banana, papaya, and pepper on the back border.

BIOLOGICAL CONTROL

Biological control (biocontrol) uses living organisms or their byproducts to reduce a target pest population to a tolerable level. Biocontrol approaches are categorized by agent source (i.e., indigenous vs. exotic) and application criteria. The primary categories of biocontrol include:

- *Classical*—importation of exotic species and their establishment in a new habitat;
- *Augmentative*—augmentation of established species through direct manipulation of their populations or their natural products; and
- *Conservative*—conservation of established species through manipulation of the environment (20).

Some experts suggest an augmentative approach would be more likely to yield rapid short-term coca reduction, whereas classical or conservative approaches would be more likely to offer longer-lasting results. Further, the latter approaches would create a gradual target decline and allow a transition period for producers to adjust to alternative livelihoods (26).

Box 6-A—Erythroxylum Species That Are the Primary Sources of Cocaine

Cocaine is derived from certain plants of the genus *Erythroxylum* (family Erythroxylaceae). The genus name *Erythroxylum*, derived from the Greek erythros (red) and xylon (wood), denotes the reddish wood of some of the shrubs and small trees included in the genus. In all, some 250 species of *Erythroxylum* exist in tropical and subtropical habitats worldwide. Whereas most species grow in the New World, the genus is well known also in Africa and Asia. Two loosely related South American species of coca (*E. coca* and *E. novogranatense*) and varieties of these species are the primary sources of cocaine. The species differ largely in trunk, branch, and bark characteristics, whereas the varieties within species differ largely in leaf characteristics.

Although coca was scientifically described some 200 years ago, detailed studies of coca specimens were conducted only in the last century. They revealed subtle differences in leaf and stem anatomies, growth and branching habits; and characteristics of bark, stipules, flowers and fruits, breeding relationships, and geographic distributions. Coca is a perennial shrub ranging between 0.5 and 2.5 meters tall and has a short flowering and fruiting period.

Erythroxylum coca—The two varieties of this species are *E. coca* var. *ipadu* and *E. coca* var. *coca*. The former has large, elliptical leaves, whereas the latter has smaller, more pointed and broadly lanceolate to elliptic leaves with two parallel longitudinal lines on their undersides.

E. coca var. *coca*
(Bolivian or Huanuco coca)
- Source of most of the world's cocaine.
- Believed to be the ancestral taxon of all cultivated coca.
- Cultivated and found in the wild.
- Restricted arealy to narrow zone of moist tropical forest known as *montaña*.
- Little known outside South America.

E. coca var. *ipadu*
(Amazonian coca)
- Restricted to the western Amazon, and geographically isolated from other coca varieties.
- Cultivated for its leaves by a few isolated Indian tribes of Brazil, Peru, and Colombia.
- True cultivar, unknown in the wild.
- Probably a recent derivative of *E. coca* var. *coca*; the two varieties share many morphological characteristics.

(continued on next page)

By definition, biocontrol is based on a density-dependent balance—the control agent abundance is directly dependent on the availability of the target (coca). As the target numbers decrease so does the control agent population. Thus, the biocontrol methodology is an unlikely eradication technique. It could, however, provide means to reduce the amount grown in target areas, and make coca cultivation difficult (20).

Understanding the traits of the various coca species and varieties is key to selection of a biocontrol approach. Information about the life-cycle, reproduction, and metabolic pathways can be used to focus a biocontrol strategy (box 6-A). For example, the coca (*Erythroxylum*) species of interest have short flowering and fruiting periods, propagation depends on seed production, and seed viability is brief (27). These botanical features might suggest that a biocontrol agent that hinders reproduction or seed viability could reduce opportunities for expanding coca production.

Box 6-A—Continued

Erythroxylum novogranatense—The two varieties of this species are *E. novograntense* var. *novogranatense* and *E. novogranatense* var. *truxillense* and both have complex distribution patterns. *E. novogranatense* var. *truxillense* has narrowly elliptic leaves that tend to be smaller than those of the other varieties whereas the leaves of *E. novogranatense* var. *novogranatense* are larger and more oblong in shape and have a distinct bright yellow-green color. Both varieties occur only as cultivated plants and are tolerant of arid conditions, growing where the *E. coca* varieties would not survive. Neither variety of *E. novogranatense* is a major world source of cocaine.

E. novogranatense
var. *novogranatense*
(Colombian coca)

- Found today as a plantation crop only in Colombia, where it is cultivated in drier mountain areas by a few isolated Indian tribes that harvest the leaves for chewing.
- Tolerant of diverse ecological conditions.
- Figured prominently in world horticultural trade in the early 20th century, and continues to be grown in many tropical countries as an ornamental plant.

E. novogranatense
var. truxillense
(Trujillo coca)

- Grows today only in the river valleys of the north coastal Peru and in the arid upper Río Marañon valley.
- Leaves are highly prized by chewers for their excellent flavor.
- Due to difficulties of extracting and crystallizing pure cocaine, it is a minor contributor to the illicit drug market.
- Trujillo coca is used primarily in the manufacture of de-cocainized extracts for soft drink flavoring.

The ecological conditions under which coca plants are cultivated in part determine their morphological characteristics, such that a continuum of leaf sizes and shapes exists among the four primary coca varieties. Plants grown in full sun develop thicker and smaller leaves, while plants grown in partial shade develop larger, thinner and more delicate leaves. Humidity and moisture availability also can affect the size, form, and venation of coca leaves. Because of these variations it is often impossible to identify a coca variety positively from isolated leaves or leaf fragments alone. Integrated data on a number of micromorphological features of leaves and other plant parts are required, along with information on the geography and ecology of the specimen source.

Coca varieties differ in their physical properties and growth habits, as well as in the biochemical properties of their leaves. The alkaloid content of coca leaves is of particular concern. Coca leaves contain 13 different alkaloids, the most concentrated of which is cocaine, first isolated from coca leaves in the mid 19th century. Like coca, many plants contain economically important and naturally occurring alkaloids (e.g. caffeine in coffee, nicotine in tobacco, morphine in opium poppies, and piperine in black pepper).

Coca leaves on average contain about 1 percent cocaine, but typical values range between 1.02 percent for *E. novogranatense* var. *truxillense*, and 0.11 to 0.41 percent for Amazonian coca (*E. coca* var. *ipadu*). Average values for *E. coca* var. *coca* and *E. novogranatense* var. *novogranatense* are intermediary (0.23 to 0.93 percent). The potency of coca leaves with respect to cocaine content also depends on the plant's growing site. The *E. coca* var. *coca* leaves with the greatest cocaine content were found in Chinchao, in Huánuco, Peru, among the highest elevations where coca is grown. Plants grown in the *montañas* generally are thought to produce more potent leaves than plants at lower altitudes.

SOURCE: T. Plowman, "Coca Chewing and the Botanical Origins of Coca (*Erythroxylum* ssp.) in South America," D. Pacini and C. Franquemont (eds.), *Coca and Cocaine: Effects on People and Policy in Latin America*, Cultural Survival Report #23 (Peterborough, NH: Transcript Printing Company, 1986), pp. 5-33.

Agricultural Application of Biocontrol

Examining biocontrol of weeds may offer some insight into the potential of this method for coca reduction. The first practical attempt at biocontrol of weeds dates from 1863, when efforts were made to control the prickly pear cactus with an insect observed to attack the cactus in northern India. Based on these observations, the insect was introduced to southern India and later to Sri Lanka, where it was successful in controlling wild populations of prickly pear. Initially, most of the weed targets for biocontrol efforts were exotic, terrestrial species, but, increasingly, aquatic and semi-aquatic native and exotic weeds have been subjects of biocontrol research.

Biocontrol has experienced a rapid expansion in the last three decades. By 1985, 214 exotic natural enemies had been introduced into 53 countries for the control of 89 weeds. Biological agents, primarily insects and plant pathogens, have achieved substantial control for many target weeds (e.g., klamath weed, prickly pear, lantana) (17). Additional examples of successful development and marketing of weed biocontrol agents include the use of pathogens to control northern joint vetch (biocontrol agent *Collectotrichum gloeosporioides*) and stranglervine of citrus (biocontrol agent *Phytophthora*) (29). Insects have been the most common successful biocontrol agents to date, yet nematodes, fungi, and mites have also been used.

To date, 267 biocontrol projects have been undertaken worldwide and 48 percent have achieved a measurable degree of success. The majority of biocontrol projects have relied on importation of exotic organisms—classical biocontrol—and of these projects, 45 percent have been rated as successful. Whereas an introduced organism may become established, success is measured by the agents identifiable control effects on the target pest. Results of introductions tend to be mixed with only some of the introduced agents becoming established and effective (i.e., 64 percent of

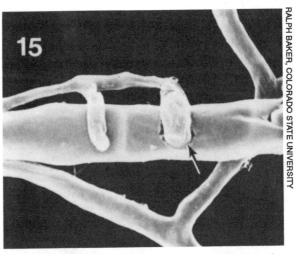

Insects are the most widely used biocontrol agents for agricultural pests, although interest in using other organisms is increasing. Shown here is a fungal parasite penetrating the hyphae of its target.

the natural enemies introduced in the biocontrol projects have become established and 26 percent of these have been rated effective). Nevertheless, nearly two-thirds of the target weed species have been brought under control using biological methods in at least one project (7).

Application of Biocontrol to Narcotic Crop Control

Agricultural biocontrol achievements have occurred under conditions where security risks and likelihood of countermeasures were not factors. The potential for achieving similar success within the framework of a narcotics control program may be less likely. Clearly, the need for international coordination and cooperation would be paramount.

Experts indicate development time for a biocontrol program for coca would be strongly influenced by the outcome of initial search for and identification of potential agents. Effective, indigenous candidates would be likely to have a shorter development period than candidates needing enhancement to meet safety and efficacy requirements. Common protocol for biocontrol research and development programs includes:

Box 6-B—Categories of Potential Biocontrol Agents

Numerous **arthropod** species feed on coca or related plants. Deliberate establishment of an arthropod pest in coca-growing regions would add to the complex of pests attacking cultivated coca. However, if heavy damage ensued, countermeasures would likely be undertaken by growers. Insects and mites generally can be controlled effectively with pesticides, particularly where there are no restrictions on the choice of materials or application rates. Stem borers and soil-dwelling root borers are more difficult to control, although there are chemical and cultural means for their control. Pesticide resistance is likely a critical requirement for these types of biocontrol agents.

Pathogenic fungi are becoming increasingly useful in classical biocontrol of weeds. However, they also can be controlled with pesticides. Alternatively, they could be used as mycoherbicides, although in this form application may become problematic.

Nematodes have been little used in weed biocontrol to date, although some gall- forming varieties have shown some promise (16). In general, nematodes are more difficult to diagnose and control than arthropods or fungi. However, little is known about nematodes attacking coca so that their use in biocontrol could require extensive research.

Viruses may offer the greatest potential because they cannot be controlled chemically, either before or after infection. Those transmitted by effective insect vectors can spread rapidly and are among the most virulent and devastating disease problems for legitimate agricultural crops. However, there is a general lack of biocontrol workers trained in virology and little has been done in this area of biocontrol. Further, currently very little is known about viral diseases of coca, or potential vectors.

SOURCE: D. Rosen, "Potential for Biological Control of Coca," contractor report prepared for the Office of Technology Assessment, November 1991.

- Search and identification of natural enemies,
- Enhancement of candidate agents (if needed),
- Screening of candidate agents,
- Production of candidate agents, and
- Application.

SEARCH AND IDENTIFICATION

The first step in a biocontrol program for coca entails international, interdisciplinary research to identify natural coca enemies (box 6-B). Existing literature reveals 44 arthropods, 24 fungi, one nematode, and one virus recorded from *Erythroxylum coca* alone (tables 6-3 and 6-4). Numerous others have been recorded from other *Erythroxylum* species, including some polyphagous (nonhost-specific) and notorious agricultural pests. However, most known natural enemies have been recorded from cultivated coca. No intensive study of the natural enemies of wild *E. coca, E. novogranatense*, and related species has been conducted (20). Approximately 250 species of

Erythroxylum occur in South America and elsewhere, 24 of them just in Peru, (14,36), and many of the organisms attacking them may prove capable of infesting or infecting coca. Other potential agents might be identified through field surveys reviewing pests and diseases associated with wild and cultivated coca.

Desired characteristics for candidate biocontrol agents include:

- *Density-dependence*—The population density of the natural enemy increases or decreases with the population density of the target species.
- *Host specificity*—Agents should be highly adapted to the target species and unable to affect nontarget species adversely.
- *Searching ability*—Mobile agents should have great capability of finding the target species.
- *Reproductive capacity*—Agents should be capable of high levels of reproduction to

Table 6-3—Insects and Mites Associated With *Erythroxylum coca*

Order	Family	Species	Activity	Known range
Acarina	Tetranychidae	*Tetranychus* sp.	Spider mites attack leaves and twigs.	Peru, Bolivia
Coleoptera	Curculionidae	*Conotrachelus* sp.	In seeds of fruits.	Cuba, Trinidad
		Mecostylus vittaticollis	Beetles feed on leaves and larvae develop as borers.	East Africa
		Pantomorus bondari	Beetles feed on leaves.	Brazil
	Scolytidae	*Stephanoderes hampei*	Beetles bore fruits for shelter.	Indonesia
		Xyleborus coffeae	Beetles and larvae tunnel in bark.	Indonesia
		Xyleborus morstatti	Twig borer.	Indonesia, Malaysia
Diptera	Trypetidae	*Trirhithrum nigerrimum*	Larvae infest fruits.	Ghana
Heteroptera	Pentatomidae	*Rhynchocoris plagiatus*	Bugs suck plant sap.	India, Sri Lanka
Homoptera	Asterolecaniidae	*Asterolecanium pustulans*	Scale insects suck from leaves and twigs. This is the pit scale—a polyphagous pest of deciduous fruit trees and ornamentals.	Brazil, Cuba
	Coccidae	*Coccus elongatus*	Polyphagous scale insect.	Taiwan
		Coccus hesperidum	Scale insects suck sap from leaves and tender tips. This is the soft brown scale—a polyphagous pest of fruit trees and ornamentals.	Brazil, Peru, Bolivia
		Lecanium sp.		Peru
		Saissetia coffeae	Scale insect feeds on twigs. This is the hemispherical scale—a pest of citrus and coffee.	Peru, Bolivia
		Tachardia gemmifera		Peru
		Tachardia lacca		Guiana
		Tachardia silvestrii		India
	Diaspididae	*Aspidiotus* sp.	Scale insect feeds on twigs. Polyphagous.	Peru, Bolivia
		Howardia biclavis		Sri Lanka
		Lepidosaphes sp.		Peru
		Quadraspidiotus sp.		Peru
		Selenaspidus articulatus	This is the rufous scale— a major pest of citrus.	Cuba
	Kermesidae	*Kermes* sp.		Peru
	Pseudococcidae	*Pseudococcus* sp.	Mealy bugs feed on growing tips, twigs, and roots.	Peru, Bolivia
Hymenoptera	Formicidae	*Acromyrmex hispidus*	Leaf-cutting ants damage young plants.	Peru
		Atta sexdens	Leaf-cutting polyphagous ants.	Peru, Venezuela
		Atta sp.	Leaf-cutting ants.	Peru
	Megachilidae	*Megachile opposita*	Leaf-cutting bees.	Indonesia, Malaysia

(continued on next page)

Table 6-3—Continued

Order	Family	Species	Activity	Known range
Lepidoptera	Arctiidae	*Rhodogastria atrivena*		Uganda
		Rhodogastria bubo		Uganda
	Cossidae	*Zuezera coffeae*	Caterpillars tunnel in twigs and stems and feed on leaves.	India, Sri Lanka, Malaysia, Indonesia
	Geometridae	*Boarmia* spp.	Caterpillars attack twigs.	Indonesia
		Hyposidra talaca	Caterpillars feed on leaves.	Indonesia
	Limacodidae	*Phobetron hipparchia*		Venezuela
	Lymantriidae	*Eloria noyesi*	Caterpillars feed on leaves, stalks, and tender tips.	Peru
		Eloria sp.	Caterpillars feed on leaves and twigs.	Bolivia
	Noctuidae	*Spodoptera litura*	Caterpillars feed on leaves. Also a pest of *Cannabis* and *Papaver*.	Malaysia, Indonesia
	Nymphalidae	*Morpho catenarius*	Caterpillars feed on leaves.	Brazil
	Sphingidae	*Protambulyx strigilis*	Caterpillars feed on leaves.	Venezuela
	Tineidae	*Eucleodora cocae*	Caterpillars feed on leaves and tender tips.	Peru
		Linoclostis gonatius	Caterpillars bore in bark.	Taiwan
		Setomorpha rutella	Caterpillars feed on leaves and tunnel in dry leaves.	Malaysia, Indonesia
Thysanoptera	Thripidae	*Neosmerinthrothrips xylebori*	Thrips found in tunnels of *Xyleborus coffeae*.	Indonesia
		Selenothrips rubrocinctus	Thrips attack leaves.	Venezuela, Brazil

SOURCE: D. Rosen, "Potential for Biological Control of Coca," contractor report prepared for the Office of Technology Assessment, 1991.

assure sufficient populations to achieve the desired goal.

- *Adaptability*—Agents should be highly adaptable to the broad range of environmental conditions in which the target species may grow (20).

A comprehensive field survey team would require at a minimum, biocontrol experts, botanists, entomologists, and plant pathologists. A smaller search team might be required to collect samples from the field and bring them back to a secure site for comprehensive examination. Field surveys for potential control agents should include observations on their role in controlling the abundance and reproduction of coca, and on their life history (e.g., reproduction, fecundity, dispersal, overwintering, epidemiology, mode of attack, target plant parts, direct and indirect damage inflicted, and existence of distinct biotypes) (4,7). Search efforts should cover at least one season's activity of the plant and as much of its distributional range as possible to note variations in predator/prey relationships and plant vulnerability at different life stages.

Throughout the search and collection of natural enemies, sound biosystematics—the identification and classification of species and the reconstruction of their evolutionary history—proves essential. When live natural enemies of a plant are being sought, or are transferred from one region to another, correct identification of the plant host and the natural enemies and recognition of infraspecific entities may be of utmost importance. Biosystematic study may show a potential biocontrol agent rejected for its seemingly broad host range, is a combination of sibling species, each with a narrow host range and one of which may be an appropriate biocontrol candidate. Many serious failures of biocontrol agents have resulted from inadequate biosystematics (7).

Table 6-4—Pathogens Recorded From *Erythroxylum coca*

Order	Species	Activity	Known range
Fungi	Armillariella mellea	Broad spectrum; causes damage to peanuts and sweet potatoes.	South America
	Aschersonia turbinata	Entomopathogenic.	Bolivia
	Aspergillus cinereus	Occurs on poorly dried leaves.	Argentina
	Bubakia erthroxylonis	Rust, causing yellowing of leaves premature defoliation, not a serious threat; also on other *Erythroxylum* spp.	Argentina, Bolivia, Colombia, Peru, Ecuador, Panama, Costa Rica; possibly Brazil, Venezuela, Cuba, Puerto Rico
	Cercosporella cocae		Argentina
	Clavulina leveillei	Occurs on roots, probably not pathogenic.	Indonesia
	Colletotrichum cocae		Argentina
	Corticium invisum	Causes black rot, also affects tea.	Sri Lanka
	Corticium pervagum	Thread-blight, kills leaves and twigs.	Sri Lanka
	Corticium salmonicolor	Causes pink disease on branches, twigs and leaves; attacks many tropical plants including rubber.	Sri Lanka, South America, Indonesia
	Fomes noxius	Ubiquitous in tropics on many hosts; causes brown root rot.	Sri Lanka, Indonesia, Taiwan
	Fusarium sp.[a]	Soil borne disease.	Peru
	Gloesporium sp.	Attacks seedlings, losses of nearly 50 percent.	South America, Indonesia
	Hypochnus erythroxyloni	Attacks basal parts of young seedlings.	Taiwan
	Hypochnus rubrocinctus	Now considered a lichen.	Venezuela
	Hypocrella palmae	Entomopathogenic.	Peru
	Mycena citricolor	Broad spectrum; particularly damages coffee in South America and West Africa.	Peru, USSR
	Mycosphaerella erythroxyloni		Argentina
	Pellicularia sasakii	Causes banded sclerotial disease on leaves.	Japan, India, Indonesia, Philippines, Taiwan
	Phyllosticta erythroxylonis		Peru, Bolivia, Colombia
	Protomyces cocae		Argentina
	Ravenelula boliviensis	Occurs on dead wood.	Bolivia
	Verticillium sp.		Peru
	Xylaria apiculata	Black root disease, infecting roots, stem bases; may cause plant death; also found on potatoes and other hosts.	Brazil, Dominican Republic, Puerto Rico, China, Sri Lanka, Indonesia, Zimbabwe
Nematoda	Pratylenchus branchyurus	Occurs in roots.	Ivory Coast
Viruses	Witches' broom	Apparently a virus transmitted by an aphid.	Bolivia

[a] *Fusarium oxysporum* has been spreading in the Huallaga Valley. Although reports vary, betweeen 10,000 and 15,000 hectares are reported to have been affected by the fungus (22).

SOURCE: D. Rosen, "Potential for Biological Control of Coca," contractor report prepared for the Office of Technology Assessment, 1991.

ENHANCEMENT OF CANDIDATE AGENTS

Enhancement of a natural enemy can improve its ability to provide the desired control safely and effectively. Conventional selection techniques can be used to develop a large, uniform population displaying a desired trait. Alternatively, genetic manipulation could be used to enhance a desired trait of a natural enemy. Currently, conventional selection and mass rearing offer the greatest possibilities for enhancing the capabilities of a natural enemy.

Arthropods are amenable to enhancement through conventional selection. Many adaptive races exist and there usually is considerable genetic variation in natural populations. Selective breeding has been used to increase tolerance for climatic extremes, alter host preferences, and increase pesticide resistance (11,12). Release and establishment of such a strain, however, could be considered equivalent to importing an exotic species (20). Pesticide resistance may be a desired trait since producers are likely to use chemicals to control pest infestations. For example, many coca producers already use insecticides to control such pests as *Eloria noyesi*.

Genetic variability is a primary concern to ensure agent vitality. Stock cultures would need to be established from abundant material collected at numerous and varied localities to maximize genetic variation. If natural variability is insufficient, it could be enhanced by irradiation or mutagenic chemicals, although mutagenesis can cause random, often deleterious, mutations and may require large numbers of organisms to be screened. Following the selection program, the improved strain should be tested to determine its ability to survive, as well as the genetic mechanism governing the selected trait (20).

An alternative to this more conventional, non-invasive method of enhancement of natural enemies would be to use genetic engineering technologies used to isolate genes from an organism, manipulate them in the laboratory, and insert them stably into another organism. In this way it may be possible to introduce a desired trait (e.g., pesticide resistance) into a natural enemy of coca. Although the technology in this area of biocontrol is not yet well-developed, significant advances have been made in recent years and possibilities for improvement exist (27).

Eventually, genetic engineering through recombinant DNA (rDNA) techniques may be more efficient than conventional selection. Someday, desirable genes may be obtained from a given species, cloned, and inserted into another species. Some work has been done in this area, particularly with fruit flies. However, developments in fruit fly research have not been duplicated with other insects. With micro-injection techniques for inserting hybrid genes into insect eggs for germ-line transformation, it is believed methodology for

genetic engineering of arthropods will be available within 5 or 10 years (35). However, conventional selection and genetic engineering are currently more feasible with plant pathogens than with arthropod biocontrol agents.

The debate over whether or not genetic engineering should be considered for a biocontrol program focuses largely on development time. Detractors suggest the complexity of genetic engineering would add to research and development time and reduce the potential for near-term production of a biocontrol agent (27).

SCREENING

Screening of candidate agents is a critical development step in a biocontrol program to determine whether a candidate can be released without the danger that it may also damage nontarget organisms. The procedure follows several steps, beginning with collection of information about the target plant and associated phytophagous and pathogenic organisms and their respective host spectra (i.e., if any of them are already known as pests of desirable plants). Information also is collected on host records of organisms closely related to the potential candidate. Only organisms likely to be host specific are selected for screening tests, beginning with those causing the greatest damage and possessing special adaptations likely to restrict host preference (20).

It is likely to be impossible to screen candidate species on all plants in coca production areas. At a minimum, potential targets chosen for the screening process would include:

- Recorded hosts of the candidate agent,
- Host plants of species closely related to the candidate agent,
- Desirable plants related to the target plant,
- Nonrelated plants having morphological or biochemical characteristics in common with the target plant, and
- Crop and ornamental plants in the target area whose pests and diseases have not been

identified and have not been exposed to the candidate biocontrol agent.

The common sequence is first to test the agent on other forms of the target species, other species of the same genus, and other members of the same subfamily, family, and order. However, laboratory tests alone are insufficient, for a broader range of plants may be accepted by the agent in the laboratory than in nature. Field tests are needed to corroborate laboratory data, preferably in the countries of origin (20).

Once an organism is screened and determined to be sufficiently host specific to be used as a biocontrol agent, it may be imported and checked for contaminants under strict quarantine. Prior to release, an agent normally is tested in the target area since climatic and ecological variations among areas make extrapolation of test results across target sites inappropriate.

Genetically engineered organisms also must go through an extensive screening process. Researchers and regulators have established five criteria for evaluating the potential environmental impact of a genetically engineered organism:

1. *Potential for negative effects*—If it is known that a recombinant organism will have no negative effects, there is no cause for concern. But predicting ecological effects, their probability, and assessing whether they are negative or positive is not straightforward.
2. *Survival*—If a genetically engineered organism does not survive, it is unlikely to have any ecological impact. It is also unlikely to fulfill the purpose for which it was engineered (unless brief survival is all that is required).
3. *Reproduction*—Some applications require not only the recombinant organism's survival but also its reproduction and maintenance. Increasing numbers could, in some settings, increase the possibility of unforeseen consequences.
4. *Transfer of genetic information*—Even if the engineered organism itself dies out, its environmental effects could continue if the crucial genetic material was favored by selection, and transferred to and functioned in a native species.
5. *Transportation or dissemination of the engineered organism*—A recombinant organism that moves into nontarget environments in sufficient numbers could interact in unforeseen ways with other populations or members of other communities (30).

PRODUCTION AND STORAGE

Stability, shelf life, and potential for mass production are key issues in developing a biocontrol agent. Agents often must be reared in a laboratory or controlled environment. Quality control is extremely important since inbreeding can have negative effects, causing future generations to lose vigor and efficacy. Cultures must be supplemented periodically with material collected from the field (19). Rearing methodologies for genetically enhanced agents would vary according to the nature of the agents. Artificial media are available for many pathogens and various arthropods, however, it may be better to rear them on the target plant to reduce the potential for undesirable adaptations.

Full exploitation of pathogenic agents is likely to require careful attention to formulation. Temperature, moisture, and growth media requirements are critical for producing and storing live agents. Formulation techniques can overcome some of the stresses associated with storage and application. For example, a well-proportioned adjuvant or surfactant may overcome certain environmental stresses, such as reduced moisture availability, to assist the activity of the agent (3).

APPLICATION

The approach (classical, augmentative, conservative) and the agent selected determine the range of suitable application technologies. Both factors will affect the timing and frequency of application. For example, under an augmentative approach application would be more frequent than under a classical or conservative approach. The biological activity of the selected agent may require that application occur during specific seasons. For example, some fungi depend on moisture availability to disperse effectively; thus, application during wet seasons could be a requirement (3). Other potential application concerns include photoperiod and dew period length, temperature, and inoculum concentration.

In general, the same application methods used for herbicides can be used to apply biocontrol agents (e.g., spray, broadcast) as well as release of mobile agents at the target. Thus, the constraints that apply to herbicide application also apply to biocontrol application (e.g., difficulty in precision using aerial application techniques). The formulation of the biocontrol agent (e.g., liquid, pellets, live insects) will determine the type of equipment suitable for application. Pathogens may lend themselves to liquid formulations and be easily applied using existing spray technology. For example, a mycoherbicide inoculum can be applied so every plant is deliberately inoculated (25). However, for a mycoherbicide to be effective, problems involving production of spores, efficacy, specificity, genetic variability, and timing of applications would have to be solved (5,24,25). Pelletized forms may be broadcast from aerial or ground-based systems.

Potential exists for developing biocontrol complexes using a number of discrete bioforms to accomplish search and attack of a target pest. For example, mobile vectors could be inoculated with a virus that would be introduced into the target as the mobile vector feeds. The mobile part of the complex would be selected for its searching ability, whereas the additional agent would be selected for its virulence. This technology is not yet well-developed but it could provide an option to simplify application. Another possibility may be combining chemical herbicides and biocontrol agents.

CONTAINMENT

Ability to contain or restrict movement of biocontrol agents once released poses a significant problem, yet would be key in addressing concerns about release of biocontrol agents. If the release of a biocontrol agent had unanticipated negative environmental, health, or economic impacts, containment could reduce the level of impact. However, only a few methods for eliminating a released agent have been identified, including applying pesticides, releasing a natural predator of the agent, and employing genetic controls (e.g., ''suicide genes,'' sterile male release). A lethal pathogen of at least 40 weeds, *Sclerotinia sclerotiorum*, has been manipulated by deletion mutagenesis to have an absolute requirement for cytosine to activate its pathogenic traits. Thus, containment can be achieved by witholding the activating compound. In another instance, a pathogen was mutated to create a lifeform incapable of overwintering or producing dispersal structures. Thus, the initial population would die off with cold weather or old age (26).

There are concerns that some containment mechanisms could compound environmental or human health problems. Applying pesticides to destroy a biocontrol agent could have adverse environmental impacts such as affecting non-target species and contaminating groundwater and surface waters. Releasing another enemy to control the coca agent also could have various unforeseen environmental consequences. Employing genetic controls would also raise concerns about the release of a genetically manipulated organism in the Andean region.

A containment mechanism, however, could be a valuable facet of a biocontrol program and could be an important research component for coca control. Identifying a natural enemy of coca could include research on ''suicide genes,'' susceptibility to pesticides, and identification of natural predators. Demonstrated ability to contain a control agent of coca could help achieve host country consent.

DEVELOPMENT NEEDS FOR BIOCONTROL OF COCA

A biocontrol program will face many obstacles, the most obvious being sociopolitical and economic constraints. The bulk of experience with biocontrol efforts has been in the realm of controlling unwanted pests. Coca is not a weed—it is a valuable crop and a source of income. Thus, coca biocontrol programs are likely to meet resistance from participants in the cocaine economy. Furthermore, biocontrol of coca hinges on cooperation and coordination with host governments. Implementing a biocontrol program for domestic marijuana production in the United States could demonstrate U.S. confidence in this technology as an eradication method (27). Such an effort might increase acceptance in potential host countries as well as highlight unforeseen pitfalls that might be associated with this technology.

Technologically, biocontrol of coca faces several constraints as well. Several key research and development priorities are identified in box 6-C. Whereas there are several possibilities for enhancing an existing enemy (box 6-D), the most sophisticated type of enhancement—genetic engineering—is not likely to be feasible for nearly 5 years. Moreover, there is no way to determine the efficacy of any given control agent until it is actually released into the target area. Levels of control can only be estimated and there are no guarantees (20).

The environmental concerns over biocontrol focus on the potential for effects on nontarget species and the likelihood of increased use of pesticides by coca producers. Additional concerns relate to the lack of knowledge of the role of coca in the Andean ecology and the potential for adverse effects resulting from its removal. Incomplete knowledge of Andean ecology further means that comprehensive screening and host-specificity testing of potential agents are likely to be difficult.

SUMMARY AND CONCLUSIONS

Eradicating coca across its current range in the Andean region is most likely an unrealistic goal given the enormity of the task and the variety of barriers. The difficult environments of the coca-growing regions compound the technological constraints to eradication. Further, the overarching sociopolitical and economic features of the producing countries suggest that even if some success is achieved through eradication efforts, production would likely shift to other areas. Nevertheless, control efforts could play a role in overall narcotics reduction by increasing incentives to adopt alternative livelihoods (27,28). Without clear risks connected to coca production, little incentive exists for farmers to adopt alternative crops or enter into other livelihoods (27). Effective production control programs, particularly biocontrol, could increase the hardships associated with coca cultivation. However, for such activities to achieve the desired effect (i.e., decrease supply) viable, acceptable alternatives should be available.

Criteria for evaluating the suitability of different coca reduction opportunities include efficacy, minimal potential environmental and human health impacts, and current and easily demonstrated technological feasibility. At the moment, no single eradication method satisfies all of these criteria. Whereas a biocontrol approach may offer the least environmentally damaging and longest-term means of coca reduction, reduction levels are difficult to determine. Experiments measuring predation levels on targets in the laboratory are insufficient to extrapolate agent behavior once released (i.e., a 40-percent efficiency in the laboratory does not necessarily translate into 40-percent efficiency in the wild). Thus, biocontrol cannot guarantee specific reduction results (27). As long as coca remains a profitable crop and conditions promoting entrance into legitimate livelihoods are lacking, it is likely that producers will increase pesticide use to protect their investment.

Box 6-C—Priorities for Biocontrol Development

Developing a biocontrol agent or complex against coca species in the Andean region would require attention to a variety of unknowns. The following list summarizes priority areas identified by a panel of experts contributing to this Office of Technology Assessment study.

1. **International, interdisciplinary search to identify natural enemies of coca**—Wide-scale search for coca predators on cultivated and wild coca that may have potential as biocontrol agents.
2. **National and international recognition of cocaine as a problem**—Campaign to increase awareness of the adverse effects of cocaine on society to increase support for efforts to control cocaine production.
3. **Host specificity screening**—Rigorous screening tests of candidate species on coca and associated plants prior to field tests to determine the specificity of the agent and reduce risk.
4. **Human and ecological health risk assessment**—Environmental assessment of the potential adverse impacts of a biocontrol program in the Andean region.
5. **Genetics, ecology, and biology of target plant and relatives**—Detailed information on coca species, related species, and plants associated with coca to augment screening and search efforts.
6. **Efficacy screening of candidate species**—Screening programs to determine the level of predation of candidate agents on coca and associated plants.
7. **Production technologies and quality control**—Techniques to produce candidate agent and ensure quality/conformity suitable to fulfill the goal of a biocontrol program.
8. **Education on biocontrol**—Education on the methodology, development regimes, and safety measures to contribute to building public support for biocontrol.
9. **Field trials**—Carefully controlled field experiments to determine the activity of potential agents in the natural environment and identify potential areas of concern.
10. **Environmental damage of coca production/processing**—Information on the level of environmental damage from coca production and processing activities to be used as a comparative for assessing the value of a biocontrol effort.
11. **Socioeconomic model**—Model to assist in determining potential socioeconomic outcome of potential policy actions and identify needs to mitigate adverse impacts.
12. **Application technology**—Technologies to apply a selected biocontrol agent in a safe and efficient manner.
13. **Identification of potential countermeasures**—Identification of actions that may be undertaken by groups/individuals against biocontrol efforts and development of mechanisms to thwart such efforts.

SOURCE: U.S. Congress, Office of Technology Assessment, "Biological Control Workshop," Washington, DC, January 23, 1992.

The United Nations International Drug Control Programme (UNDCP) investigations into potential narcotic crop control opportunities highlight host country involvement and agreement. Biocontrol was identified as an opportunity for narcotic crop control in the late 1970s by the UNDCP, but little research was conducted beyond the initial scoping phase. The UNDCP is now conducting meetings with experts to determine biocontrol's potential. Any actions that might result from these activities will be conditional on host-country agreement and cooperation in all phases (22). The U.S. Department of State notes similar agreements would be sought for U.S. bilateral eradication activities in the Andean region, but little likelihood exists for obtaining them now (27).

The potential for successful biocontrol application in the Andean countries are affected by three factors:

1. *Cooperation and coordination*—Cooperation among potential host and donor countries to develop and implement a biocontrol

---

Box 6-D—Examples of Natural Enemies of Coca

One species particularly specific to coca and indigenous to Peru, **Eloria noyesi** Schaus (Lepidoptera:Lymantriidae), could be a possibility for biocontrol research. The larva of the moth feeds on coca leaves and is a principal natural pest of coca. With a short lifecycle (30 days) and repeated breeding throughout the year, larval populations can be sustained relatively easily. **Eloria noyesi** was reported to "swarm" and destroy almost 20,000 hectares of coca in Peru, causing losses to drug traffickers estimated to be at least $37 million. Another species from Peru, **Eucleodora cocae** Busck (Lepidoptera: Tineidae), could be a possible candidate for biocontrol research as well (20). Both species meet many of the listed criteria, although further screening would be necessary.

More recently, outbreaks of **Fusarium oxysporum** in Peru have increased awareness of the potential impact fungi can have on coca production. Under normal conditions fungi and lichen infestations of healthy coca shrubs are key factors in limiting the plant's productive life (8). The **Fusarium** fungus has contributed to widespread destruction of coca plantations near Santa Rosa in the Alto Huallaga (2). Peruvian farmers in the region have complained that the fungus and the blight it produces have affected legal crops as well as coca (21).

SOURCE: Office of Technology Assessment, 1993.

---

program effectively is a key need for success. Primary needs include multilateral agreements to undertake eradication programs and broad-based public participation in the program assessment process. Experience with herbicide testing in Peru suggests greater government and public participation will be necessary (31). Incorporating public review and comment periods, broad dissemination of environmental impact reviews and methodologies, and coordinated and cooperative efforts with national groups will be critical.

2. *Information*—Information on the potential benefits and costs of a biocontrol program for the Andean countries is needed. Areas needing investigation include the effects of coca production and processing on the Andean environment and the subsequent effects on future development options, mechanisms to improve environmental assessments of potential impacts of biocontrol efforts, and the role of coca in Andean ecology.

3. *Technological feasibility*—Although biocontrol methodologies exist, technological constraints to rapid implementation are overwhelming (21). If a biocontrol program is determined to be feasible, an extensive research and development period could be required. Further, ability to conduct needed field experiments is hindered by lack of political agreements, and the technology does not afford the certainty of a specific reduction level (i.e., in many ways biocontrol may be considered "applied experimentation").

Absent the political realities hindering any coca eradication effort, the current state of biocontrol development does not seem to offer a timely mechanism for reducing coca production in the Andean nations. Although opportunities exist to develop biocontrol, existing information, cooperation, and coordination needs will continue to have a profound effect on the possibilities for success.

CHAPTER 6 REFERENCES

1. Adamczyk, T., "Chemical Eradication of Coca," Contractor report prepared for the Office of Technology Assessment, December 1991.
2. Arroyo, A., and Medrano, O., "Huallaga in Flames," CARETAS, Aug. 13, 1992, pp. 30-37, in: Joint Publication Research Service, "Peasant Army Expels Shining Path in Huallaga," JPRS-TOT-92-029-L, Aug. 28, 1992, p.10.
3. Bannon, J.S., "CASST Herbicide (Alternaria cassiae): A Case History of a Mycoherbicide,"

American Journal of Alternative Agriculture 3(2&3):73-75.

4. CAB International, *Screening Organisms for Biological Control of Weeds*, CAB International Institute of Biological Control, Silwood Park, Ascot, UK, 1986, In: Rosen, 1991.

5. Charudattan, R., "The Mycoherbicide Approach With Plant Pathogens," in *Microbial Control of Weeds*, D.O. TeBeest (ed.) 1991, In: Rosen, 1991.

6. Christensen, E., "The Environmental Impact Analysis Process and Coca Eradication Programs," Contractor report prepared for the Office of Technology Assessment, August 1991.

7. DeBach, P., and Rosen, D., *Biological Control by Natural Enemies*, 2nd Ed. (Cambridge: Cambridge University Press, 1991) In: Rosen, 1991.

8. Duke, J. A., Botanist, U.S. Department of Agriculture, Agricultural Research Service, Beltsville Agricultural Research Center, Beltsville, MD, personal communication, August 1989.

9. Executive Order 12114, "Environmental Effects Abroad of Major Federal Actions," vol. 44 Federal Register 1957, Jan. 4, 1979, In: Christenson, 1991.

10. Genter, W., U.S. Department of Agriculture, Agricultural Research Service, retired, personal communication, August 1992.

11. Hoy, M.A., "Use of Genetic Improvement in Biological Control," *Agricultural Ecosystems and Environment* 15:109-119, 1986, In: Rosen, 1991.

12. Hoy, M.A., "Genetic Improvement of Arthropod Natural Enemies: Becoming a Conventional Tactic?" in *New Directions in Biological Control: Alternatives for Suppressing Agricultural Pests and Diseases*, R.R. Baker and P.E. Dunn (eds.) (New York: Alan R. Liss, 1990), pp. 405-417, In: Rosen, 1991.

13. Krebs, C.J., *Ecology: The Experimental Analysis of Distribution and Abundance*, (New York, NY: Harper & Row, 1972).

14. Machado Gazorla, E., "El Genero Erythroxylon en el Peru. Las Cocas Silvestres y Cultivadas del Pais," *Raymondiana* 5:5-101, 1972, In: Rosen, 1991.

15. Mardon, M., "The Big Push," *Sierra*, November/December 1988, p. 75.

16. Parker, P.E., "Nematodes as Biological Control Agents of Weeds," In: *Microbial Control of Weeds*, D.O. TeBeest (ed.) (New York, NY: Chapman and Hall, 1991) pp. 58-68, In: Rosen, 1991.

17. Perkins, J.H., *Insects, Experts, and the Insecticide Crisis* (New York, NY: Plenum Press, 1982).

18. Plowman, T., "Coca Chewing and the Botanical Origins of Coca (*Erythroxylum* ssp.) in South America," D. Pacini and C. Franquemont (eds.), *Coca and Cocaine: Effects on People and Policy in Latin America*, Cultural Survival Report #23 (Peterborough, NH: Transcript Printing Company, 1986), pp. 5-33.

19. Rosen, D., Vivigani Professor of Agriculture, The Hebrew University of Jerusalem, Rehovot, Israel, personal communication, February 1992.

20. Rosen, D., "Potential for Biological Control of Coca," Contractor report prepared for the Office of Technology Assessment, November 1991.

21. Rosenquist, E., U.S. Department of Agriculture, Agricultural Research Service, Beltsville, MD, personal communication, 1991.

22. Stevenson, S., "Peru Farmers Blame U.S. for Coca-Killing Fungus," *Miami Herald*, June 2, 1992, p.A-19.

23. Szendri, K., Director, United Nations Drug Control Programme, Vienna, Austria, personal communication, September 1992.

24. TeBeest, D.O., "Conflicts and Strategies for Future Development of Mycoherbicides," in *New Directions in Biological Control: Alternatives for Suppressing Agricultural Pests and Diseases*, R.R. Baker and P.E. Dunn (eds.) (New York: Alan R. Liss, 1990), pp. 323-332, In: Rosen, 1991.

25. Templeton, G.E., and Heiny, D.K., "Mycoherbicides," in *New Directions in Biological Control: Alternatives for Suppressing Agricultural Pests and Diseases*, R.R. Baker and P.E. Dunn (eds.) (New York: Alan R. Liss, 1990), pp. 279-286, In: Rosen, 1991.

26. United Nations Commission on Narcotic Drugs, Report of the Expert Group Meeting on Environmentally Safe Methods for the Eradication of Illicit Narcotic Plants, meeting held in Vienna December 4-8, 1989, E/CN.7/1990/CRP.7, Dec. 14, 1989.

27. U.S. Congress, Office of Technology Assessment, ''Biological Control Workshop,'' held in Washington, DC, Jan. 23, 1992.

28. U.S. Congress, Office of Technology Assessment, ''Crop Substitution Workshop,'' held in Washington, DC, Sept. 30-Oct. 1, 1991.

29. U.S. Congress, Office of Technology Assessment, *Beneath the Bottom Line: Agricultural Approaches To Reduce Agrichemical Contamination of Groundwater*, OTA-F-418 (Washington, DC: U.S. Government Printing Office, November 1990).

30. U.S. Congress, Office of Technology Assessment, *New Developments in Biotechnology: Field-Testing Engineered Organisms—Genetic and Ecological Issues*, OTA-BA-350 (Washington, DC: U.S. Government Printing Office, 1988), pp. 16-17.

31. U.S. Congress, Senate, Permanent Subcommittee on Investigations, *Cocaine Production, Eradication, and the Environment: Policy, Impact, And Options*, prepared by Congressional Research Service, 101st Congress, 2d session, 1990, S. Print 101-110.

32. U.S. Department of Agriculture, Agricultural Research Service, Weed Science Laboratory, ''Coca Herbicide Screening Summary,'' Beltsville Agricultural Research Center, 1992.

33. U.S. Department of State, Department of State Foreign Affairs Manual Circular No. 807A, subpart B(2)(c), Sept. 4, 1979, reprinted Federal Register vol. 44, p. 67004 (Nov. 21, 1979) In: Christenson, 1991.

34. Weeks, J., ''Control of Coca With Herbicides in Peru'' in U.S. Congress, Senate Permanent Subcommittee on Investigations, *Cocaine Production, Eradication, and the Environment: Policy, Impact, And Options*, prepared by Congressional Research Service, 101st Congress, 2d session, 1990, S. Print 101-110.

35. Whitten, M.J., Commonwealth Science and Information Research Organization, Canberra, Australia, personal communication, 1991 In: Rosen, 1991.

36. Willis, J.C., *A Dictionary of Flowering Plants and Ferns*, 7th Ed. (Cambridge: Cambridge University Press, 1966) In: Rosen, 1991.

Appendix A: Workshop Participants

■ Crop Substitution Workshop
September 30 and October 1, 1991

Elena Alvarez
University Center for Policy
　Research
State University of New York
Albany, NY

James Anderson
Weed Science
U.S. Department of Agriculture
Agricultural Research Service
Beltsville, MD

Ray Ashton
Water & Air Research, Inc.
Gainesville, FL

Bruce Bagley
University of Miami
Graduate School of International
　Studies
Coral Gables, FL

Antonio Chavez
Independent Consultant
Lima, Peru

Howard Clark
U.S. Agency for International
　Development
Quito, Ecuador

Lee Darlington
Weed Science
U.S. Department of Agriculture
Agricultural Research Service
Beltsville, MD

James A. Duke
U.S. Department of Agriculture
Agricultural Research Service
Beltsville, MD

Victoria Greenfield
Natural Resources and Commerce
　Division
Congressional Budget Office
Washington, DC

Kevin Healy
InterAmerican Foundation
Rosslyn, VA

Ray Henkel
Department of Geography
Arizona State University
Tempe, AZ

Michael Painter
Institute for Development
　Anthropology
Binghamton, NY

Raphael Perl
Congressional Research Service
Library of Congress
Washington, DC

Douglas J. Pool
Development Alternatives, Inc.
Bethesda, MD

Eric Rosenquist
U.S. Department of Agriculture
Agricultural Research Service
Beltsville, MD

Robert Schroeder
RDA International
Placerville, CA

Sean Swezey
Agroecology Program
University of California–Santa Cruz
Santa Cruz, CA

Joseph Tosi
Centro Científico Tropical
San Jose, Costa Rica

Hugo Villachica
Independent Consultant
Lima, Peru

Ken Weiss
Chemonics, Inc.
Washington, DC

■ Biological Control of Coca Workshop
January 23, 1992

Tom Adamczyk
U.S. Environmental Protection
   Agency
Office of Pesticide Programs
Herbicide-Fungicide Branch
Washington, DC

Joseph Antognini
Weed Science
U.S. Department of Agriculture
Agricultural Research Service
Beltsville, MD

Dominic Cataldo
Battelle
Pacific Northwest Laboratories
Richland, WA

Larry Christy
Bioherbicide Research
Crop Genetics, Inc.
Columbia, MD

Lee Darlington
Weed Science
U.S. Department of Agriculture
Agricultural Research Service
Beltsville, MD

Walt Gentner (retired)
U.S. Department of Agriculture
Agricultural Research Service
Adelphi, MD

Clifford Gerwick
Biological and Biochemical
Research
DowElanco
Greenfield, IN

George Heim
Geodot Associates
Virginia Beach, VA

Dennis Linskey
U.S. Department of State
Bureau of International Narcotics
   Matters
Washington, DC

Luis Moreno
U.S. Department of State
Bureau of International Narcotics
   Matters
Washington, DC

Peggy Olwell
Center for Plant Conservation
St. Louis, MO

Paul Parker
U.S. Department of Agriculture
Mission Biological Control
Laboratory
Mission, TX

Robert Rose
U.S. Environmental Protection
   Agency
Office of Pesticide Programs
Washington, DC

David Rosen
Faculty of Agriculture
The Hebrew University of
   Jerusalem
Rehovot, Israel

Peter Van Voris
Battelle
Pacific Northwest Laboratories
Richland, WA

James L. Walker
U.S. Department of Agriculture
Washington, DC

Appendix B: List of Acronyms

ADCZP — Agricultural Development in the Coca Zones Project

AHV — Associated High Valleys, *Asociación de Valles Altos*

AID — U.S. Agency for International Development

AMS — Agricultural Marketing Service, U.S. Department of Agriculture

ANAPO — Associate of Wheat and Oil Producers (*Asociación de Productores de Oleaginosas y Trigo*)

APHIS — Animal and Plant Health Inspection Service, U.S. Department of Agriculture

ARS — Agricultural Research Service, U.S. Department of Agriculture

ATI — Andean Trade Initiative

ATPA — Andean Trade Preference Act

CIA — Central Intelligence Agency

CIAT — Tropical Agriculture Research Center (*Centro de Investigación Agrícola Tropical*)

CIFP — Pairumani Plant Genetics Research Center (*Centro de Investigaciones Fitogeneticas de Pairumani*)

CIID — International Research Center for Development (*Centro Internacional de Investigaciones para el Desarrollo*)

CIP — International Potato Center (*Centro Internacional de la Papa*)

CNE — Colombia National Council of Dangerous Drugs (*Consejo Nacional de Estupificantes*)

CNIEA — National Counsel on Agricultural Research and Extension (*Consejo Nacional de Investigación y Extensión Agropecuaria*)

CORAH — Project for the Control and Reduction of Coca Cultivation in the Alto Huallaga (*Proyecto de Control y Reducción de los Cultivos de Coca en el Alto Huallaga*)

CORDECO — Development Corporation of Cochabamba (*Corporación de Desarrollo de Cochabamba*)

CORDEP — Cochabamba Regional Development Project

COTESU — Swiss Technical Cooperation (*Cooperación Técnica Suiza*)

CRDP — Chapare Regional Development Project

DAS — Colombia Administrative Security Department (*Departamento Administrativo de Seguridad*)

DEA — Drug Enforcement Administration, U.S. Department of Justice

DIRECO — Bolivian National Agricultural Reconversion Board (*Dirección Nacional de Reconversión Agrícola*)

DOD — U.S. Department of Defense

EAI —Enterprise for the Americas Initiative

EPA —U.S. Environmental Protection Agency

FDA —Food and Drug Administration, U.S. Department of Health and Human Services

FELCN —Bolivia Special Force in the Struggle Against Drug Trafficking (*Fuerza Especial en la Lucha Contra el Narcotráfico*)

FSIS —Food Safety Inspection Service, U.S. Department of Agriculture

GATT —General Agreement on Trade and Tariffs

GSP —Generalized System of Preferences

IARC —International Agricultural Research Center

IBTA —Bolivian Institute of Agriculture and Livestock Technology (*Instituto Boliviano de Tecnología Agropecuaria*)

IBTN —Bolivian Institute of Science and Nuclear Technology (*Instituto Boliviano de Ciencia y Tecnología Nuclear*)

ICA —Colombian Agricultural Institute (*Instituto Colombiano Agropecuaria*)

IIAP —Peruvian Amazon Research Institute (*Instituto de Investigaciones de la Amazonía Peruana*)

INIAA —National Institute for Agrarian and Agroindustry Research (*Instituto Nacional de Investigación Agraria y Agroindustrial*)

INM —Bureau of International Narcotics Matters, U.S. Department of State

IVITA —Veterinary Institute for Tropical and Highland Research (*Instituto Veterinario de Investigaciones Tropicales y de Altura*)

MACA —Bolivia Ministry of Campesino Affairs and Agriculture (*Ministerio de Asuntos Campesinos y Agricultura*)

NGO —Nongovernmental organization

OAS —Organization of American States

ONDCP —U.S. Office of National Drug Control Policy

OPIC —Overseas Private Investment Corporation

PDAR —Bolivia Regional Program for Alternative Development (*Programa de Desarrollo Alternativo Regional*)

PEAH —Alto Huallaga Special Project (*Proyecto Especial Alto Huallaga*)

PRODES —Bolivia Development and Substitution Project (*Proyecto de Desarrollo y Sustitución*)

PROSEMPA —Potato Seed Project (*Proyecto de Semilla de Papa*)

PVO —Private voluntary organization

REPAP —Peruvian Amazon Research Network (*Red de Investigación de la Amazonía Peruana*)

SINTAP —National System of Technical Assistance for Small Producers (*Sistema Nacional de Transferencia de Tecnología Agropecuaria*)

SNC —Bolivia National Road Service (*Servicio Nacional de Caminos*)

SUBDESAL —Bolivia Subsecretariat for Alternative Development and Coca Substitution (*Subsecretaría de Desarrollo Alternativo y Sustitución de Cultivos de Coca*)

UMATAs —Municipal Units of Technical Assistance (*Unidad Municipal de Asistencia Técnica Agropecuaria*)

UMOPAR —Bolivia Mobile Rural Patrol Unit (*Unidad Móvil de Patrulla Rural*) or Mobile Rural Patrol Unit, Peruvian Civil Guard of Peru (*Unidad Móvil de Patrullaje Rural de la Guardia Civil del Perú*)

UNA —National Agrarian University (*Universidad Nacional Agraria*)

UNDCP —United Nations International Drug Control Programme

UNFDAC —United Nations Fund for Drug Abuse Control

UNMSM —National University of San Marcos Graduate School (*Universidad Nacional Mayor de San Marcos*)

USDA —U.S. Department of Agriculture

Appendix C: List of Contractor Reports

Overviews

The Geoecology and Agroecosystems of the Northern and Central Andes
Donald Alford
GeoResearch, Inc.
Billings, MT

Institutional Analysis of the Chapare Regional Development Project (CRDP) and the Upper Huallaga Special Project (PEAH)
Michael Painter
Eduardo Bedoya Garland
Institute for Development Anthropology
Binghamton, NY

Sociopolitical Setting

Opportunities and Constraints to Source Reduction of Coca in Colombia: The Sociopolitical Context
Bruce M. Bagley
University of Miami
Graduate School of International Studies
Coral Gables, FL

The Bolivian Sociopolitical Context for Rural Development
Kevin Healy
InterAmerican Foundation
Ballston, VA

Migration, Social Change, and the Coca/Cocaine Economy in Bolivia
Ivo Kraljevic
Chemonics, Inc.
Washington, DC

Opportunities and Constraints to Source Reduction of Coca: The Peruvian Sociopolitical Context
Cynthia McClintock
George Washington University
Washington, DC

Traditional Roles and Uses of Coca Leaf in Andean Society
Mary-Elizabeth Reeve
University of Illinois—Urbana
Huntington, MD

Economic Setting

Opportunities and Constraints to Reduce Coca Production: The Macro-Economic Context in Bolivia and Peru
Elena Alvarez
State University of New York
Albany, NY

Colombia: Opportunities and Constraints to Source Reduction of Coca and Cocaine
Francisco Thoumi
Independent Consultant
Arlington, VA

Renewable Resource-Based Alternatives to Coca

Potential Use of Neotropical Wildlife in Sustainable Development
Ray E. Ashton, Jr.
Water and Air Research, Inc.
Gainesville, FL

Diversification and Multiple Cropping as a Basis for Agricultural Alternatives to Coca Production
Stephen Gliessman
University of California
Santa Cruz, CA

Biodiversity Conservation and Forest Management as an Alternative to Coca Production in the Andean Countries
Dennis McCaffrey
Independent Consultant
Gaithersburg, MD

Fishery/Aquatic Resources in Bolivia, Colombia, and Peru: Production Systems and Potential as Alternative Livelihoods
Robert Schroeder
RDA, International
Placerville, CA

Crop Diversification in Bolivia, Colombia, and Peru: Potential to Enhance Agricultural Production
Hugo Villachica
Independent Consultant
Lima, Peru

Supporting Alternative Livelihoods

Agricultural Research, Extension, and Technology Transfer Activities: Potential Mechanisms to Enhance Crop Substitution Efforts in Bolivia, Colombia, and Peru
Antonio Chavez
Independent Consultant
Lima, Peru

Infrastructural Needs to Support Agricultural Alternatives to Coca Production
Juan DeVincenti
Architect/Planner
Bethesda, MD

Alternative Trade Organizations, Peasant Farmers, and Coca
Rink Dickinson
Equal Exchange
Stoughton, MA

Postharvest Technologies to Improve Agricultural Profitability in Bolivia and Andean Nations
Bill Stevenson
Development Alternatives, Inc.
Cochabamba, Bolivia

Primer on U.S. Agricultural and Trade Policies: Opportunities and Constraints to Crop Substitution in the Andean Nations
Elizabeth Turner

Coca Eradication and Control

Chemical Eradication of Coca
Thomas Adamczyk
U.S. Environmental Protection Agency
Washington, DC

The Environmental Impact Analysis Process and Coca Eradication Programs
Eric Christensen
Consulting Attorney
Arlington, VA

Potential for Biological Control of Coca
David Rosen
The Hebrew University of Jerusalem
Rehovot, Israel

Index

U.S. GOVERNMENT PRINTING OFFICE : 1993 - 331-054

Superintendent of Documents **Publications** Order Form

Order Processing Code:
*7082

Telephone orders (202) 783-32
To fax your orders (202) 512-22:
Charge your orde
It's Eas

☐ **YES**, please send me the following:

_____ copies of *Alternative Coca Reduction Strategies in the Andean Region (220 pages)*,
S/N 052-003-01329-1 at $12.00 each.

The total cost of my order is $_____. International customers please add 25%. Prices include regular domestic postage and handling and are subject to change.

_____
(Company or Personal Name)   (Please type or print)

_____
(Additional address/attention line)

_____
(Street address)

_____
(City, State, ZIP Code)

_____
(Daytime phone including area code)

_____
(Purchase Order No.)

Please Choose Method of Payment:

☐ Check Payable to the Superintendent of Documents

☐ GPO Deposit Account ☐☐☐☐☐☐☐ — ☐

☐ VISA or MasterCard Account

☐☐☐☐☐☐☐☐☐☐☐☐☐☐☐☐☐☐☐☐☐

☐☐☐☐ (Credit card expiration date)

Thank you fo
your orde

_____
(Authorizing Signature)   (6/9

May we make your name/address available to other mailers? ☐ ☐
YES N

Mail To: New Orders, Superintendent of Documents, P.O. Box 371954, Pittsburgh, PA 15250-7954

THIS FORM MAY BE PHOTOCOPIE

Superintendent of Documents **Publications** Order Form

Order Processing Code:
*7082

Telephone orders (202) 783-32:
To fax your orders (202) 512-22!
Charge your orde
It's Eas

☐ **YES**, please send me the following:

_____ copies of *Alternative Coca Reduction Strategies in the Andean Region (220 pages)*,
S/N 052-003-01329-1 at $12.00 each.

The total cost of my order is $_____. International customers please add 25%. Prices include regular domestic postage and handling and are subject to change.

_____
(Company or Personal Name)   (Please type or print)

_____
(Additional address/attention line)

_____
(Street address)

_____
(City, State, ZIP Code)

_____
(Daytime phone including area code)

_____
(Purchase Order No.)

Please Choose Method of Payment:

☐ Check Payable to the Superintendent of Documents

☐ GPO Deposit Account ☐☐☐☐☐☐☐ — ☐

☐ VISA or MasterCard Account

☐☐☐☐☐☐☐☐☐☐☐☐☐☐☐☐☐☐☐☐☐

☐☐☐☐ (Credit card expiration date)

Thank you fo
your orde

_____
(Authorizing Signature)   (6/9

May we make your name/address available to other mailers? ☐ ☐
YES N

Mail To: New Orders, Superintendent of Documents, P.O. Box 371954, Pittsburgh, PA 15250-7954

THIS FORM MAY BE PHOTOCOPIE